The Family *Is* the Patient

Using Family

Interviews

in Children's

Medical Care

SECOND EDITION

The Family *Is* the Patient

Using Family Interviews

in Children's Medical Care

BAYARD W. ALLMOND, Jr., MD
Associate Clinical Professor of Pediatrics
University of California School of Medicine
San Francisco, California

J. LANE TANNER, MD
Associate Clinical Professor of Pediatrics
Division of Behavioral and Developmental Pediatrics
University of California School of Medicine
San Francisco, California

with
HELEN F. GOFMAN, MD
Emeritus Associate Professor of Pediatrics
University of California School of Medicine
San Francisco, California

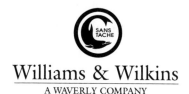

Williams & Wilkins
A WAVERLY COMPANY

BALTIMORE • PHILADELPHIA • LONDON • PARIS • BANGKOK
BUENOS AIRES • HONG KONG • MUNICH • SYDNEY • TOKYO • WROCLAW

Editor: Tim Hiscock
Managing Editor: Joyce A. Murphy
Development Editor: Alethea H. Elkins
Marketing Manager: Daniell Griffin
Project Editor: Lisa J. Franko

351 West Camden Street
Baltimore, Maryland 21201-2436 USA

Rose Tree Corporate Center
1400 North Providence Road
Building II, Suite 5025
Media, Pennsylvania 19063-2043 USA

Printed in the United States of America

Library of Congress Cataloging-in-Publication Data is available.

To purchase additional copies of this book, call our customer service department at **(800) 638-0672** or fax orders to **(800) 447-8438.** For other book services, including chapter reprints and large quantity sales, ask for the Special Sales department.

Canadian customers should call **(800) 665-1148,** or fax **(800) 665-0103.** For all other calls originating outside of the United States, please call **(410) 528-4223** or fax us at **(410) 528-8550.**

Visit *Williams & Wilkins* on the *Internet:* http://www.wwilkins.com or contact our customer service department at **custserv@wwilkins.com.** Williams & Wilkins customer service representatives are available from 8:30 am to 6:00 pm, EST, Monday through Friday, for telephone access.

98 99 00 01 02
1 2 3 4 5 6 7 8 9 10

Dedicated to

Everyone at the Child Study Unit

...especially Wilma and Donya

Wasn't that a time!

Contents

Introduction to the Revised Edition

The Family Is the Patient describes a clinical approach that has been developed over the years within the Division of Behavioral and Developmental Pediatrics at the University of California San Francisco. A brief history of that division explains the setting that has nurtured our ideas.

HISTORY OF THE DIVISION OF BEHAVIORAL AND DEVELOPMENTAL PEDIATRICS

Origin

The division, originally composed of two staff members and one trainee, was established almost 50 years ago by the late Dr. George Schade, a pediatrician at the University of California San Francisco. In the 1930s, he was one of four pediatricians selected throughout the country to receive 2 years of training with Dr. Frederick Allen and Dr. Jessie Taft at the Philadelphia Child Guidance Clinic. This training, which focused on the management of pediatric emotional and behavioral problems, was supported by the Commonwealth Foundation.

The organization hoped this project would improve the training of many more pediatricians in the management of such pediatric problems. Following training, the four pediatricians were expected to return to their respective pediatric departments and establish teaching programs devoted to this aspect of pediatrics. In 1948, Dr. Schade, with the aid of a small grant from the Commonwealth Foundation and subsequent support from the University of California and its Department of Pediatrics, fulfilled this expectation by formally opening the Pediatric Mental Health Unit within the Department of Pediatrics. The staff consisted of Dr. Schade, a psychiatric social worker, and Dr. Helen Gofman, his first pediatric fellow.

Purpose of the Division

From the beginning, the purpose of the unit was to provide opportunities for pediatricians to become better pediatricians. Pediatric house officers were taught to understand and manage behavioral problems commonly seen in pediatric practice. Particular emphasis was placed on understanding normal development and developmental differences in children. Dr. Allen had viewed a child's behavior often as a manifestation of "growth toward independence." This view, one of the early attempts to understand children using a "growth" model rather than a "pathology" model, was incorporated into teaching efforts with pediatric trainees in the unit. Influenced by Allen, the clinical approaches were concerned most often with the present rather than the past, with an emphasis on practical interventions and strategies, a format particularly appealing to pediatricians, then and now.

Mrs. Wilma Buckman (second author of the first edition of this text) joined the Pediatric Mental Health Unit in 1950 as a psychiatric social worker. In addition to her background in social work, she had served as an elementary and nursery school teacher and director and received a master's degree in child growth and development. Therefore, she underscored the unit's clinical emphasis on developmental aspects of a child's growth and behavior. She and Dr. Gofman began working together on the development of a practical teaching program for pediatric house officers in interviewing and pediatric counseling—the basic underpinning of this book and the teaching program, which continues in the division to this day.

Progress and Growth

By the 1970s, the unit (renamed the Child Study Unit in 1966) was flourishing. From two original staff members, the group had grown to 15 teaching professionals: four pediatricians, five pediatric psychologists, one psychiatrist, one neurologist, one pediatric nurse practitioner, one educational specialist, and two secretaries. Teaching programs were formalized for pediatric trainees at every level (e.g., interns, residents, postgraduate fellows, nursing students, postgraduate fellows in psychology). At that time, training focused on the evaluation of children with learning problems and on the development of family interviewing skills in pediatric settings. From this training model, the first edition of this textbook was produced in 1979.

FIRST EDITION

When we wrote the original text almost 20 years ago, comments from colleagues indicated that the book was received well and sparked the interest of behavioral pediatric teachers and students. The initial success was followed by sluggish sales and a decision by our former publisher to take the volume out of print. However, interest in the book continued, and we received countless requests for the book. Existing copies were hoarded and passed on to trainees in our own institution and to those elsewhere who were persistent or flattering enough to move us. Although requests for a revised edition continued throughout the years, there were no plans for a second edition. In 1981, the senior author began a solo clinical practice of behavioral pediatrics, which took his full energy and focus, and he steadfastly refused a rewrite. However, in 1995, continuing praise and requests for the book, originally published in 1979 and out of print since 1984, suggested even to him that a revised edition was needed.

REVISED EDITION

What's Different?

It has been interesting to review material first articulated in 1977–1979 and written as truth. We wondered how often we might experience toe-curling embarrassment at having put "that" in print. How much of what we suggested in the 1970s would stand up to 1990s theory and practice? With two exceptions, the ideas proposed in 1979 are still actively taught and used by us.

One exception is the chapter on Gestalt therapy strategies. Over the years, trainees complained that these approaches were too difficult to readily incorporate into pediatric clinical work, particularly for novice family interviewers. We also realized that Gestalt therapy strategies are not emphasized in our own current work. Thus, we dropped that chapter from this edition.

The chapter on fatal illness is also excluded, partly for the same reasons.

Reading our 1979 ideas on that subject suggested a major overhaul would be needed to improve readability and update concepts for the 1990s. Yet none of us any longer works with fatally ill children and their families, either in clinical practice or in teaching. The chapter was deleted because we wanted this edition to reflect our current teaching and clinical emphases. Other than these two areas, we still use our original material, which has weathered time, trends, fads, and our own development as clinicians.

Although our principles and guidelines for working with families may have remained relatively constant, the authors and the world of pediatrics have changed. These changes have had an impact on the production of this revision.

Authors

The writing team has undergone several changes since the first edition. Dr. Allmond withdrew from academic pediatrics in 1981 and began a full-time clinical practice of behavioral pediatrics in which he continues now. Mrs. Buckman, we are sad to say, died in 1982. The loss of her expert teaching and her companionship continues to be felt by her coauthors. Dr. Gofman retired from academic medicine and the Child Study Unit in 1983. The leadership of that unit then passed on to others with an inevitable gradual alteration in personnel and broadening of the unit's interests.

Another author has joined us for this revised edition. In the late 1970s, Dr. Lane Tanner was a pediatric fellow in the former Child Study Unit at the University of California San Francisco, when both Dr. Allmond and Dr. Gofman were still teaching. Following his training, Dr. Tanner joined the faculty and eventually assumed the major responsibility for teaching family interviewing theory and practice to pediatric trainees. He continues to perform that function and many others as Interim Director for the Division of Behavioral and Developmental Pediatrics at the University of California San Francisco.

Changes in Health Care

Not only was the unit changing dramatically, including its name (the Child Study Unit is now the Division of Behavioral and Developmental Pediatrics), so were traditional forms of health care, delivery, and funding. Managed care has now knocked at the door of almost every provider in California. Although some providers are resisting it, managed care is pervasive. Estimates predict that by the end of 1998, 60% of people living in United States cities will be covered by managed care plans (1). Although major health care reform sputtered for a time, it has not yet materialized at the federal level. These turbulent alterations in health care will affect how physicians will be able to use the principles and practices put forth in this volume. While revising this text, we have recognized that time and money will be severely constrained in the new system of health care. We believe that interested clinicians, armed with the knowledge and principles in these pages, will still be able to integrate these approaches into pediatric teaching and practice.

The practice of pediatrics also has shifted as a result of the evolving health needs of children. In a 1995 article, Dr. Robert Haggerty, author of the foreword for our original text, ventured a look at the now-and-future needs of children.

> *Forecasting the future is dangerous. Who would have predicted the epidemic of AIDS and HIV today? But the needs of children in the 21st century can be predicted fairly confidently. They will be the same as today: the need for loving adults, usually parents; a biological, social, and environmental milieu that includes access to integrated and coordinated health and human services; a supportive and safe neighborhood and community; a school system that allows each child to achieve his or her full potential; and the promise of a job as an adult that will pay a living wage and yield a sense of satisfaction. There will of course be surprises, including the reemergence of old diseases (such as drug-resistant tuberculosis) and new diseases such as AIDS, for which flexibility and willingness to change to meet these new challenges must be part of the skills of the pediatrician.*
>
> *But more central to meeting the needs of children today and tomorrow is the enormous diversity; the differences in socioeconomic status, race and ethnicity, culture, educational achievement, marital status, mobility, and disease and social problems among families. That is the reality under which pediatricians must practice. Different families have and will have different needs. For the many children lucky enough to live in two parent families with adequate means in safe communities that have good schools, the roles of their pediatricians, although not simple, will be*

different from the roles of pediatricians working with children of single parents, growing up in poverty, and surrounded by a peer culture of violence, drugs, and early sex.

For all children, it is safe to predict that in the 21st century, competence in the area of emotional health, school performance, and conflict resolution—what might be termed "prevention of the new morbidity"— will be a more prominent part of pediatric practice. (2)

One conclusion we have drawn from Dr. Haggerty's remarks is that there is definitely a place in the future for the pediatrician interested in family-focused delivery of children's health care. Instead of fading into obsolescence, the care model presented in these pages offers a learnable, relevant strategy for pediatricians to approach many of the predicted health needs for children of the twenty-first century.

Format of Second Edition

Case Studies and Dialogue

Case studies with specific dialogues are used throughout this book. This style of writing has advantages and disadvantages. One of the disadvantages is that dialogic accounts can lose some meaning when they are written. The nonverbal behavior, setting, and mood are unknown and must be imagined or ignored. This limitation is regrettable but unavoidable. Another disadvantage is that lengthy sections of dialogue may make reading cumbersome. In many of the situations, the dialogue has been "cleaned up" to facilitate the reading process. The conversations themselves are actual, and, beyond the editorial deletions, the meaning of a person's speech has not been changed. However, to ensure privacy, we have changed the names, genders, geographic locations, ages, and occupations.

Although there are disadvantages to using written dialogue, we have chosen this method of illustration for several reasons. Because this text aims to demonstrate clinical approaches that are practical and specific, we feel that our case studies must show practical skills being used during clinical interviews with specific dialogues between physicians and families.

The text is also concerned with "how" questions (e.g., how does a family member react to a comment, how does a doctor handle this situation, how does one tell a mother this particular news). Examples of clinical dialogue can effectively answer such questions more succinctly than other written devices.

Another reason for our inclusion of dialogue is to show interviewing styles. In order to be effective teachers of behavioral pediatrics, pediatricians must be willing to expose their own interviewing styles, for better or worse, through their successes and failures. Some of the cases, particularly those in the first part of the book, sound neat, easy, and almost too successful. Although we do not apologize for these successes (they did in fact occur), we have presented a few of our clinical failures to provide a balance. We hope that by exposing our failures and successes, trainees will be encouraged in their own clinical work with children and families. Taking risks ultimately separates the successful from the unsuccessful learner.

Most often an interviewer in the examples presented is referred to as "the pediatrician" or "the physician." These terms reflect several things about the authors: we are all pediatricians, we see ourselves as teachers of pediatric care givers, and we have spent our professional careers in teaching and practicing that discipline. Also, we have always felt that the audience for this volume was primarily pediatric clinicians; however, readers in other disciplines need not be offended. These terms are meant to be generic, representing any professional who may be involved in the medical and psychological care of children, using family interviewing as a tool. Thus, we invite those of all appropriate disciplines (e.g., primary care physicians, nurses, social workers, psychologists, psychiatrists, family therapists, school counselors, academicians) to be our students through this text. Any of these professionals may wish to conduct family interviews, and the substance of this book is directed to each one. These terms are used simply for consistency in writing style and as an authentic reporting of our own experiences as pediatricians in family interviews.

Parts

The text is divided into two major parts. The first part, Principles, describes the work of theorists and clinicians who have strongly influenced our clinical work and teaching approaches. To their techniques, we have added elements of our own. These combined ideas produce a clinical approach, which we present through case illustrations in Part II, Clinical Application.

Some readers may prefer to begin with the second part of the text, learning our specific clinical style first, and then turn to Part I and our discussion of many of the principles that underlie our work. Because many busy pediatricians will do this anyway, we would like to sanction such an approach to the reading of this text.

PURPOSE STATEMENT

This book is enthusiastic in its view that family therapy principles can be applied to pediatric practice for both the diagnosis and management of some pediatric problems, particularly those in the behavioral realm. Our enthusiasm stems from the development of a family systems approach that is practical, effective, exciting, congruent with our ideas about children and their families, and comfortable for us. However, do not mistake our enthusiasm for arrogance. We do not intend to discount other theoretical hypotheses or alternative clinical approaches. Instead, this text serves to introduce one method, one model, and one approach that has worked well for us.

References ˙

1. Leslie LK. Can pediatric training manage in managed care? Pediatrics 1995;96:1143.
2. Haggerty RJ. Child health 2000. New pediatrics in the changing environment of children's needs in the 21st century. Pediatrics 1995;96:811.

part I

Principles

chapter **1**

The Family as the Treatment Unit and the Pediatric Clinician as the Interviewer

THE LOCKSLEY FAMILY

Joan, age 7 years, sits quietly in her chair. She is swinging her legs back and forth as her grandmother explains the situation to Dr. Henry Abbott, the pediatrician.

Grandmother: She's not sleeping, Doctor. And neither am I—none of us has had a good night's rest in 7 weeks or so. Even if I get her in bed by 8 pm, usually about 11 she wakes up-terrified, screaming. Then I'm up all night with the poor child. And when she does settle down again, at maybe 3 or 4 am, she still thrashes and screams out—in her sleep! Why, I've had to bring her into the emergency room twice in the past 2 weeks . . . she just gets hysterical. The doctor who saw her said something about epilepsy.

Pediatrician: Well, Mrs. Locksley, I wonder if—

Grandmother: Screams bloody murder—it wakes the neighbors! We're all on pins and needles now at night. And look at the circles under her eyes . . . low blood, somebody told me.

Pediatrician: What I meant to say—

Grandmother: I've tried everything—night light, waking her up, taking her to the bathroom, stories, rocking, hot milk—my own mother used to do that. Could it be worms, Doctor?

Pediatrician: That's something to consider. Now back to—

3

Grandmother:	What could cause a child to cry out in her sleep like that? Well, I don't know if she's asleep or not. But I do know she just won't stay in bed when the whole thing starts. Oh, stomachaches—I almost forgot. She complains about that—in bed 5 minutes and then "Gramma, my tummy hurts." Then I know we're in for it for the rest of the night. Makes no difference when she goes to bed, early or late; it's the same thing.
Pediatrician:	When does she usually—
Grandmother:	I think more of this child than myself, Doctor—I want you to know that. Why, I've raised her since she was 4 years old. We're never apart, isn't that right, honey?
Joan:	(nods)
Pediatrician:	Do the two of you live alone?
Grandmother:	Well, we did, but no, my daughter, Joan's mother, lives with us now. She was separated recently. And my other daughter, divorced too, she's moved back in with me. And she has her own little girl, Cheryl, just 6 months younger than Joan. The two kids get along really well. What's that? Yes, the house is crowded, but we're making do. But Joan's business has been getting to everybody. With the last episode three nights ago, we all went to the emergency room. She certainly needs some sort of checkup, don't you think? Can growing pains ever do this?
Pediatrician:	Sometimes. The stomachaches you mentioned, just where does she complain of pain?
Grandmother:	All over, isn't that right, Joan? Show him, sweetie . . . now don't be that way. The doctor is here to help us. Speak right up and talk to the nice man; he wants to know where you hurt. There's nothing to be afraid of . . . she doesn't like doctors. Doctor, you're not going to give her any shots are you? She hates shots. Now Joan, sweetie, don't cry.

A history of sorts has been obtained; a physical examination will follow. Often in such situations, the child's sleep disorder and the grandmother's notions (being directly communicated to the patient, of course) about epilepsy, worms, growing pains, low blood, and physicians will remain.

Only the pediatrician's energy level will have experienced a decrease. This situation, although not included as an example of fancy interviewing footwork, did occur and serves to introduce a major theme in this book: look beyond the individual patient and, using the tool of a family interview, focus on the family constellation surrounding a child. Using this family perspective, the focus for diagnosis and treatment shifts from a single individual or relationship to a group of relationships called "the family."

Focusing on the family is not a new idea. It is a time-honored tradition in pediatrics to obtain a complete family history when treating a child. Indeed, pediatricians seem to be particularly family-oriented in their views of children and children's health care. No pediatrician finishes training without the realization that he or she is almost always working with at least two patients simultaneously—the child and the parent. In this sense, pediatricians and family practice physicians are already committed to the idea that working with children means working with the child's family members (often mothers). However, precious little has been written in medical literature regarding the use of family interviews or family-oriented interviewing approaches in pediatric or family practice.

We propose that because pediatric caregivers already understand that children cannot be considered or treated apart from their families, then clinicians should view the treatment unit to be the family: the family becomes **THE** patient. Further, we believe that physicians should develop a specific skill (i.e., family interviewing) for working with this "patient." This is a skill based on specific principles, as learnable as auscultation of the heart and equally as useful in clinical medicine.

THE EVOLUTION OF FAMILY INTERVIEWING

The principles of family interviewing that are discussed derive from a body of psychiatric and social work developed during the past 50 years. Family interviewing and family therapy began as an underground swell, without credentials or acceptance in the late 1940s. In 1962, Jay Haley stated the following:

> *The treatment of an entire family, interviewed together regularly as a group, is a new procedure in psychiatry. Just when family therapy originated is difficult to estimate because the movement has been largely a se-*

cret one. Until recently, therapists who treat whole families have not pub-lished on their methods, and their papers are still quite rare, although we may soon expect a deluge. The secrecy about family therapy has two sources: those using this method have been too uncertain about their tech-niques and results to commit themselves to print (therapists of individu-als have not let this dissuade them), and there has apparently been a fear of charges of heresy because the influence of family members have been considered irrelevant to the nature and cure of psychopathology in the pa-tient. As a result, since the late 1940s, one could attend psychiatric meet-ings and hear nothing about family therapy unless, in a quiet hotel room, one happened to confess that he treated whole families. Then another therapist would put down his drink and reveal that he too had attempted this type of therapy. The furtive conversations ultimately led to an un-derground movement of therapists devoted to this most challenging of all types of psychotherapy and this movement is now appearing on the sur-face. (1)

Freud himself gave a nod to the importance of family members in one of his most famous cases, "Little Hans" (2). In 1909, he undertook the treatment of that child's phobia by working exclusively with the father. Hans himself was not interviewed. However, family therapy was not born of this case. Freud preferred to work with individuals apart from their fam-ilies, and psychoanalysts eventually objected to the inclusion of families in the treatment of individuals, stating that transference between the patient and therapist could never be satisfactorily established with intrusions by other family members (3).

Harry Stack Sullivan, with his stress on the interpersonal aspects of men-tal illness, was an advocate for the importance of family members in a child's psychiatric treatment. In his work, the mother–child relationship was the focus of treatment. Sullivan's ideas helped the child guidance move-ment, which in some ways promoted family treatment but did so at the mother's expense. One negative result of Sullivan's view was the tendency to blame mothers for their children's difficulties. In the zeal to shift sights off the child and onto the mother–child dyad, the focus often became the "other one" in the relationship (i.e., the mother). The phrase, "There are no bad children, only bad mothers" was the hallmark of many child guid-ance clinics of the 1930s and 1940s.

Clinics advocating this approach treated the child as the helpless victim and the mother as the cause of the child's problems. The child would be whisked into the playroom for a weekly secret hour of play with the child psychiatrist in "the corrective emotional experience." In the meantime, the mother would spend the hour talking with a psychiatric social worker. In many clinics during the 1940s, psychiatrists and social workers did not talk together. Their work was viewed as independent of each other, and professional silence was rigorously observed to avoid contamination of individual therapeutic efforts. Fathers were almost never included in the treatment, and even when they were considered important, they were usually dismissed as "unavailable." Siblings were ignored. This form of therapy still prevails in some communities.

The 1950s produced the next surge in the growth of family treatment. At the Mental Research Institute in Palo Alto, California, four co-workers (Gregory Bateson, Don Jackson, John Weakland, and Jay Haley) were formulating a hypothesis that would become a keystone of subsequent family theory. In their now classic paper (4), they suggested that the symptoms of schizophrenia could be produced by a family's placing one family member in something called the "double bind." This "double-bind hypothesis" implicated the family directly in the development of an individual's symptoms and suggested to some a need for treatment of the entire family. The double-bind hypothesis is discussed in more detail in chapter 2.

Coincident with the publication of this hypothesis, one of the investigators, Don Jackson, introduced another term equally basic to the future development of family therapy: "family homeostasis"(5). He observed that families with a mentally ill member acted as a unit, with all members in dynamic equilibrium. Jackson perceived a balance in family relationships that was maintained by each family member in some way. Alan Leveton, for many years consulting psychiatrist to the (then) Child Study Unit, demonstrated this balance using a mobile, gently moving in the air: the whole is in balance—steady, yet moving. Some pieces are moving rapidly, others are almost stationary. Some are heavier and appear to carry more weight in the ultimate direction of the mobile's movement; others seem to go along for the ride. A breeze catching only one segment of the mobile immediately influences the movement of every piece, and the pace picks up with some pieces unbalancing themselves and moving chaotically for a time. Gradually, the whole exerts its influence on the errant parts, and balance is restored but not before a decided change in direction of the whole may have occurred. One may also notice changeability regarding closeness and distance among pieces, the impact of actual contact with another piece, and the importance of vertical hierarchy. Coalitions of movement may be observed between two pieces, or one piece may appear persistently isolated from the others; however, its isolated position is essential to balancing the entire system. Virginia Satir (whose work is discussed extensively in the following chapters) also likened a family to a mobile.

> *In a mobile all the pieces, no matter what size or shape, can be grouped together in balance by shortening or lengthening their strings, rearranging the distance between pieces, or changing their weight. So it is with a family. None of the family members is identical to any other: each is different and at a different level of growth. As in a mobile, you can't arrange one member without thinking of the others. (6)*

Jackson also acknowledged "so it is with a family"—the whole and its pieces. In his view, family members were moving constantly, maintaining a precarious balance in their individual relationships with each other. In the individual treatment of a patient in psychotherapy, he noted the following:

> *Other family members interfered with, tried to become a part of, or sabotaged the individual treatment of the "sick" member, as though the family had a stake in his sickness. The hospitalized . . . patient often got worse or regressed after a visit from family members, as though family interaction had a direct bearing on his symptoms. Other family members got worse as the patient got better, as though sickness in one of the family members were essential to the family's way of operating. (7)*

This notion of homeostasis also seemed to call for treatment to include all parts of the mobile. Following the acceptance of this term "family homeostasis," clinical work treating the entire family may have begun in earnest.

In 1958, Nathan Ackerman published the first full-length study combining theory and practice, in which he emphasized the importance of role relations within the family (8). Ackerman was already an experienced family therapy clinician by this time, having independently moved from an individual theoretical set to one that used clinical intervention with the family unit. In 1964, Satir was on the family treatment scene with her famous text titled *Conjoint Family Therapy: A Guide to Theory and Technique* (9).

By this time in the fields of psychiatry and social work, the technique of treating emotional disturbance by working with the family had been aggressively and successfully launched. In the decades since, conjoint family interviewing and therapy has continued to develop and now enjoys respect as a fundamental therapeutic tool in the mental health field.

PEDIATRICIANS AND THE FAMILY INTERVIEW

Although psychiatry has embraced family therapy, pediatrics understandably has not been so quick to use family interviewing. Pediatrics and psychiatry have a long history of mutual distrust. Psychiatric treatment is often dismissed by pediatricians as impractical, time-consuming, illogical, and not within the province of pediatrics. Traditional psychiatric treatment does not work well in a busy clinical pediatric setting. For example, few pediatricians would be eager to initiate weekly play therapy for 1, 2, or 3 years with an encopretic child. First, it would be an affront to the pediatrician's expectations of visible results over a short period of time. Second, few pediatricians would have time for such an extended course of therapy, and managed care would hardly support such a venture. Third and most important, many pediatricians would not know how to execute such therapy, nor would many want to learn.

Despite these challenges, it is not reasonable to conclude that all forms of behavioral intervention with children are beyond the pediatrician's interest, skill, and tolerance. In selected pediatric situations, family interviewing and family therapy have been practical, relatively time-efficient, effective, and definitely within the province of pediatrics. Clearly, we do not recommend that pediatricians provide the long-term care of a schizophrenic teenager via conjoint family therapy. All of the previously raised objections by pediatricians would surface within 30 minutes of the first interview. Rather, we suggest that a variety of conditions—which already appear daily in a pediatrician's office—could be successfully managed and alleviated if the pediatrician were knowledgeable of family theory and interviewing techniques.

When is family therapy appropriate in a pediatric setting? In our experience, the following cases have been successfully managed by pediatricians using a family orientation.

School phobia

Eating disorders

Enuresis

Encopresis

Sleep disorders

Behavioral aspects of psychosomatic conditions (e.g., recurrent abdominal pain, headaches)

Juvenile diabetes mellitus

Short stature

Acting-out behavior

Psychosocial complications of chronic illnesses (e.g., asthma, seizure disorders, cystic fibrosis, hemophilia)

Psychosocial aspects of fatal illness

Difficulties associated with a wide variety of neurodevelopmental disorders (e.g., specific learning disabilities, mental retardation, attention deficit hyperactivity disorder [ADHD])

Coping problems accompanying physical disabilities

Behavioral problems associated with no particular disease for which anxious parents consult physicians regularly (Note: The physician is often the first professional to be consulted in such situations.)

A review of this list reveals that we do not propose physicians expand their practices to include the treatment of serious mental illness. Rather, physicians should develop some skills to assist patients who are already sitting in their waiting rooms, whom they know well—Joan and her grandmother, for example. These two certainly would benefit from a physician trained in the techniques of family interviewing.

The physician who insists on an individual (versus a family) orientation in Joan's situation may be headed for trouble. Approaching this case from an individual focus may lead the physician to request an electroencephalogram (EEG), complete blood cell count (CBC), pinworm preparation, and possibly a barium swallow and upper gastrointestinal radiograph series. Theoretically, these tests could be followed by a chaser of antispasmodics, a tranquilizer, or both, none of which will solve the problem. Of course, we are not recommending such treatment, but such a sequence is possible in some offices.

What if the physician were to use a family approach in Joan's case? In fact, the physician did after that first meeting: all five family members were seen together. Through the initial family interview, more information was disclosed.

> ▶ Several years earlier, Joan's mother had left the child in Grandmother's care to run off and remarry. The mother had recently returned and hoped to assume a responsible mother role with Joan. By this time, Grandmother saw Joan as her own daughter and resented the return of Joan's mother. Therefore, the two quickly locked in a struggle over who would mother the child. To complicate matters, Grandmother's older daughter (with her own child) had returned to the family home to lick her wounds after a bitter separation and divorce. This mother and daughter rallied with Grandmother against Joan's mother. Joan, squarely in the middle of a battle, was handling the situation by refusing to sleep, literally jumping from bed to bed at night, staying with whomever she could entice to comfort and hold her. Her sleep disturbance and psychosomatic symptoms were automatic triggering mechanisms for beginning the contest anew each night over who would mother her.

After this information was obtained, the treatment shifted from a diagnostic evaluation of Joan's gastrointestinal tract to a family cease-fire and a clarification of specific family rules. The physician facilitated this, and after three family sessions, Joan's (and the family's) difficulties with sleep disappeared permanently. Although family counseling continued, it focused on substantially different issues.

How to gather such diagnostic family information, how to use it, and how to facilitate change in the family's behavior (all accomplished by the pediatrician in three interviews) are the focus of the remainder of this book.

FAMILY INTERVIEW TRAINING

This text is not a substitute for thorough training and experience in interviewing families. Many readers protest that such training is difficult to find, and we agree. Family interviewing training, particularly for pediatricians, is even more difficult to obtain now than when we originally wrote this text in 1979. There are several reasons for this:

1. The continued dominance of the biomedical model and limited recognition of a biopsychosocial model in medical training, academic research, and health care delivery
2. A resulting deficit of core information for medical students regarding the impact of psychosocial influences on health
3. A reimbursement system that has traditionally devalued time spent in the delivery of this model of care, along with the rapid growth of managed health care, which has enormously increased the scope and rate of this devaluation process
4. Pediatric training that tends to be centered at tertiary care sites in which the importance of the family is perhaps least apparent (and often considered least important) to trainees
5. The explosion of information that medical trainees are required to know
6. The relative scarcity of properly trained teachers and models within the ranks of teaching faculty in pediatrics

Are there too many obstacles in medical training today to prevent pediatricians from developing family interviewing skills? We hope not. That we have been asked repeatedly by trainees and graduates to publish a revised edition suggests that pediatricians want to use a family approach in clinical practice. As one of us (Lane Tanner) stated in a 1995 article:

> *the motivation and commitment by residents to work effectively with families remains high; it is often cited as a primary motivator for entering pediatrics and a special ability or interest. In addition pediatricians with experience in practice are often most vocal in expressing the need for help and training in this area. They speak of the high prevalence of family-connected problems in routine pediatric practice, of their fascination and personal involvement with the concerns of the families they treat, and of the frustrations they experience in not being as effective as they would like to be. (10)*

If the interest in family approaches to medicine is not matched by the availability of training, how is a trainee or clinician to learn the necessary skills? We believe pediatricians these days must take an active role in designing and integrating training opportunities to meet their own needs and interests. Such a role may require the trainees to develop their own "training package," using pieces from different training locations and orientations, setting realistic training goals based on anticipated needs for practice. Although creating such a training package is difficult, requiring considerable creativity, flexibility, and foresight, it is possible and worthwhile.

Five Levels of Physician Involvement

Using their experience in training family practitioners, Doherty and Baird described five levels of physician involvement with families (11). They saw these levels as a developmental sequence through which many physicians travel as they become more competent in family-oriented care. These levels can be equally useful to pediatric clinicians in designing their own training.

Level 1: Minimal Emphasis on the Family

At this level, "biomedical issues are the sole conscious focus of patient care." Families are included "only as necessary for practical and medical–legal reasons."

Level 2: Ongoing Medical Information and Advice

The focus is primarily biomedical, with regular effective communication with the family concerning medical issues. The physician is aware of the importance of the family in optimizing medical treatment, is able to identify family issues that interfere with such treatment, and is prepared to make referrals to a therapist in such cases. Physicians "develop competency in conducting family conferences to discuss the patient's medical problems and treatment."

Level 3: Feelings and Support

The physician is more active in empathically eliciting the stressors, concerns, and feelings surrounding the medical circumstances of the patient and family. Coping efforts are encouraged, and medical advice is tailored to the unique needs of the family. The physician is "comfortable in switching back and forth between medical data and family feelings and concerns."

Level 4: Systematic Assessment and Planned Intervention

With training in family systems theory and practice, the physician can assess family patterns that contribute to clinical problems, engaging families

in structured interviews to help them collaborate and cope in more constructive ways. "These skills would tend to be effective with basically well-
functioning families who are becoming disabled because of a medical or
other situational crisis." Physicians at this level can identify deeply rooted
difficulties and may facilitate appropriate referrals.

Level 5: Family Therapy

At this level, the physician has moved "beyond the primary care domain
into specialized family treatment," which requires in-depth, postgraduate
family therapy training. Family therapy allows the physician to independently engage families who have more entrenched interactional problems.

By choosing the level at which one hopes to practice, a physician can determine the type, duration, and intensity of training needed for developing the appropriate family interviewing skills. Pediatricians who place
themselves at either Level 1 or 2 will learn the basic concepts and expertise
necessary for working at these levels from most traditional medical school
curricula. To practice the care involved in Levels 3, 4, and 5, physicians will
need additional, specialized training in family interviewing and family systems medicine.

Features of Effective Pediatric Family Interview Training

In selecting or designing additional specialized training, prospective
trainees are urged to assess how well the curriculum under consideration
addresses certain basic features essential to a good training experience.
These features, we believe, are particularly relevant for the training of pediatricians in family interviewing skills.

Gain a Multilateral Family Focus

At Doherty's Levels 1, 2, and 3, the physician must learn the skill of increased awareness. The pediatrician must be conscious of the possible concerns, potential influences, and likely adaptations required of other family
members, including those not present in the examining room. For trainees
at Levels 4 and 5, the challenge is finding ways to understand the feelings
of each family member, avoiding special alliances that might preclude a
multilateral consideration. Parental conflict, adolescent rebellion, child

abuse, and medical compliance problems are examples of family issues that unfortunately encourage physicians to "take sides."

Listen to the Story and the Facts

Medical training emphasizes the separation of the "subjective" from the "objective." However, a family's understanding of a pediatric problem naturally shapes their complaint and frequently determines their reaction to the physician's diagnosis and treatment. The challenge for the clinician is to listen well, to attempt to understand the "story" of the problem as the family perceives it, and to incorporate elements of the family's story into the diagnosis and treatment plan.

Analyze Process Communication As Well As Content

Physicians become experts in gathering, organizing, and storing factual information. However, family members interact and communicate their needs often through nonverbal or "process" communication (e.g., facial expressions, body language, voice tone, expressed mood). A difficult skill for pediatric trainees to learn is the effective use of process communication during family interviewing. Reading and tracking this communication accurately while absorbing the verbal content of the interview can be challenging. In this area, direct clinical supervision (i.e., directly observed and supervised patient encounters) is necessary. Videotapes of interviews are particularly valuable because they allow the trainee and teacher to stop the action and study process and content in detail.

Tolerate Ambiguity

Families give accounts that are sometimes internally contradictory and disparate. Pediatricians, who are trained to evaluate facts, often find these inconsistencies and ambiguities frustrating. Family interview training should teach the usefulness of allowing and even highlighting such differences in developing a diagnostic formulation or intervention.

Resist the "Urge to Expertise"

Physicians, more than other professionals, often pressure themselves to solve every problem and remedy every ill. Patients reinforce this notion by encouraging such a role from their physicians. Good training in family-oriented care teaches physicians that the most effective solutions are generated from within the family. Effective clinicians are more often catalysts rather than the origins for such solutions.

Recognize and Use Subjective Experiences

Medical training teaches pediatricians little about recognizing and using personal reactions and feelings to provide a more family-oriented style of care. Appropriate specialized training actually encourages the exploration and implementation of subjective responses. Group supervision formats often help teach the "use of self" as both permissible and important in family interviewing.

Master a Core Knowledge of Family Processes and Common Family Dynamics

The type of training necessary for understanding family dynamics depends on the level of physician involvement the trainee intends to pursue. However, pediatricians of all levels require a basic understanding of complex family phenomena, such as early attachment and separation behaviors, sibling interactions, parent reactions to developmental transitions of a child, grief responses, the effects of parental illness or depression, and the underpinnings of family violence. Training programs should have a core curriculum derived from theory, research, and clinical sources in these areas.

Accept the Necessary Changes of Time and Tempo

Pediatricians are not trained in the culture of the 50-minute therapy hour. Instead, they are accustomed to brief encounters in which they take an active role. Family-oriented pediatric care requires the clinician to shift gears from doing to listening, from following a short, planned regimen to permitting a longer, more open-ended interview, with patient needs taking precedence over the traditional 15-minute segments of most office formats. This extended consultation is possible only if pediatricians are willing to bill for the time they spend and if health insurance providers are willing to reimburse. Assigning value to this work, however, begins with the family-oriented physician. An individual trained in family interviewing becomes the provider of a highly complex level of medical care. Good training should encourage this view.

We believe that any training program, formal or informal, devoted to teaching a family-oriented approach to pediatricians should, at the very least, encompass and address each of these fundamental physician issues.

References

1. Haley J. Whither family therapy. Family Process 1962;1:69.
2. Freud S. Analysis of phobia in a five year old boy. In: Strachey F, ed. The Complete Works of Sigmund Freud. London: The Hogarth Press, 1964;10:5–148.
3. Foley V. An Introduction to Family Therapy. New York: Grune and Stratton, 1974.
4. Bateson G, Jackson DD, Haley J, et al. Toward a theory of schizophrenia. Behav Sci 1956;1:251.
5. Jackson D. The question of family homeostasis. Psychiatr Q Suppl 1957;31:79.
6. Satir V. The New Peoplemaking. Mountain View, CA: Science and Behavior Books, 1988;137.
7. Satir V. Conjoint Family Therapy. 3rd ed. Palo Alto, CA: Science and Behavior Books, 1983;3.
8. Ackerman N. Psychodynamics of Family Life. New York: Basic Books, 1958.
9. Satir, Conjoint family therapy, 3.
10. Tanner L. Training for family-oriented pediatric care. Pediatr Clin North Am 1995;42:193.
11. Doherty WJ, Baird MA. Developmental levels in family-centered medical care. Fam Med 1986;18:153,155.

Communication and the Family

CONJOINT DRAWING

Two residents in pediatrics, Dr. Karen L. and Dr. Fred A., arrive at the Division of Behavioral and Developmental Pediatrics for the beginning of their training period. It is their first day and their first teaching session. At the moment, both are silent, engaged in an assigned nonverbal task. A 2-feet by 3-feet sheet of butcher paper is spread on a table, and a box of crayons is provided. With minimum explanation, they have been asked to "do something with the paper and crayons for 30 minutes, without talking to one another or to me." Their requests for clarification are answered mostly by shoulder shrugs. Their uncertainty, discomfort, and anxiety are met by a reassuring tone of voice from the instructor. Otherwise, the two trainees are left to struggle with the task on their own. Within 3 minutes, they begin working in earnest, oblivious to the clock and the presence of the instructor, and they are not concerned with the silliness of the task. In fact, they appear to be enjoying themselves. She is busy drawing a country scene with mountains and trees, and he is occupied with a tall fence around a structure.

The conjoint drawing technique is often used with families in the course of family work (see chapter 5); however, we also use it as a teaching device with our trainees in family interviewing. This method has proved effective for focusing trainees on communication. We begin our study of communication by insisting on silence, so our residents can experience that even "nontalk" is communication. Because many of our residents arrive for their training after an exhausting, intense rotation in the pediatric intensive care nursery, they are weary and still immersed in the life-and-death issues of caring for critically ill infants. This nursery rotation is a hard act to follow.

How can we introduce residents to a very different facet of training so that they will find it stimulating enough to include in their practice of pediatrics? An experiential task helps residents shift their orientation from blood gases and intubation to the study of family communication. The conjoint drawing facilitates this shift in focus by arousing curiosity and anxiety. In most cases, curiosity prevails and trainees complete the task, usually with enthusiasm and even playfulness. In fact, no one has ever refused to participate.

Not just a device to attract interest, conjoint drawing more importantly focuses on two elementary aspects of communication: content and process. It is with these terms and the drawing that we introduce trainees to a study of family communication.

CONTENT AND PROCESS

The content of communication refers to the literal, denotative aspect of that verbal message. Process describes the way in which the content is expressed, including all aspects of a communication outside the words and the specific subject matter. Process encompasses the tone of voice, body language, facial expression, hidden meaning, and general feeling tone. In short, process is all that is implicit in a message. If content relates to "words," process is the "music" of a communication; if content is the "figure," process is the "background." Content includes the "what" or verbal part of the message whereas process contains the "how" or nonverbal signals.

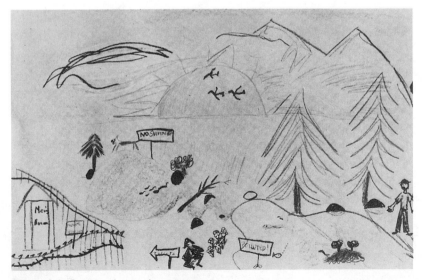

Figure 2.1. Conjoint drawing by trainees.

Using the conjoint drawing illustration, the picture is easily recognized as the content of that particular communication, and the process comprises the ways in which that particular picture was developed and drawn. We return to the two residents, now energetically engaged in their mutual project. Their completed drawing is shown in Figure 2.1. The content consists of a landscape with mountains, sun, clouds, trees, a stream, a pond, animals, and a fence-enclosed men's room. The description of "how" that drawing arrived on the paper (i.e., the process) is more interesting and says much more about how these two individuals were relating to one another during the nonverbal communication task.

▶ Initially, the trainees were not pleasantly engaged. There was a strained silence, particularly after both participants realized they were being asked to perform the task on their own without assistance from the instructor. They both fiddled with the crayons for a few seconds. Within 1 minute, however, Dr. Karen L. stood up, leaned over the paper, and drew the horizon line of mountains that extended across the entire paper. She rapidly added the large sun in the middle of the drawing, then sat back and glanced at her coworker. Dr. Fred A. sat nervously removing the wrapper from his black crayon. He had yet to put a mark on the paper. Karen turned to her work and energetically began to fill in her landscape with trees and other objects. Periodically she would sense her partner's inactivity and draw the beginning of an object on the paper close to him. Fred was quickly losing available space by default; Karen's drawing was taking up more and more territory. Reluctantly, he began drawing, careful not to complete or adorn any of the items that Joan was offering as mutual projects. Instead, he began to draw slowly and deliberately something of his own . . . a pond. This seemed to stimulate Joan's cooperative urge, and she offered him even more figures to which he might add his own touches. He did not. Undaunted, she began to add to what he was drawing. When his pond was invaded by her trees and rocks, he promptly put up a "NO SWIMMING" sign and moved on to draw a house deep in his territory. Karen returned to her side for a while but eventually returned to work on Fred's house. At this, he labeled his structure "MEN'S ROOM." This time, when Karen moved back to her mountains and trees, Fred started constructing a fence to surround his men's room, and he worked diligently on the fence until the end of the task. Karen's final touch was adding finials to his fence posts, completing the construction of a barrier obviously intended for her.

When discussing their experience, both residents were able to see parallels between their drawing behavior and some aspects of their more general styles of communication in life. Joan saw herself as a helper who reached out to draw others closer, realizing in the process that her impulsiveness, aggressiveness, and persistence sometimes pushed people away. Fred acknowledged that he often lost out in relationships by withholding, waiting to be invited, and being a loner. Both had unwittingly acted out these styles of communication and behavior in the process of their nonverbal content interchange on the paper.

Recognizing Content

Physicians are beautifully schooled in the ways of content; as content gatherers they are without peer. The discipline of medical education emphasizes the importance of obtaining a thorough history. Third-year students beginning their clinical rotations have been well primed. In their first experiences with "a new patient workup," students can overwhelm patients, preceptors, and classmates with elaborate medical histories that read like the rough draft of a master's thesis.

The pursuit of medical data is reinforced by the structure of medical teaching itself. Case presentations, rounds, and clinical pathological presentations are often competitive exercises in content. The competence of student physicians is judged by such things as the quantity and thoroughness of one's presentation, the completeness of material placed on the board for discussion, and the demonstration of exceptional familiarity with the literature. The more data and the more stunningly presented, the more favorably physicians-in-training are viewed by peers and teachers. The ability to accumulate and organize content is a priority in medical training. Content is a physician's friend.

Recognizing Process

Not so with process. Of course, there is a place in the traditional medical write-up for such items as general behavior of patient, mental status, and reliability of informant. However, these observations are not weighted equally with history of presenting illness or past medical history, both of which are primarily concerned with content. The patient's communication process is rarely noted in a formal medical history write-up.

During a first conjoint family interview, many physicians will focus on the content of that interview. Afterward, these physicians admit to feeling hopelessly lost in family conversations that apparently discuss who takes out the garbage on weeknights or defines family rules for watching television. Ensnared in the "problems" that the family brings into the interview situation, novice interviewers are diverted from a focus on the process of the interview being played out. Yet the process is there and should be considered before and during the family office visit.

Process to Note Before the Office Visit

Who initiates the referral? Who takes responsibility for seeking assistance from the physician? How does that person sound on the telephone (e.g., desperate, angry, obsequious, suspicious)?

Who attends the first interview? Who is missing in spite of a specific request from the physician that all members attend? Who seems to speak for the missing member?

Who determines when the interview will take place? Is the time based strictly on the physician's or the family's schedule (e.g., "Sorry, Jane has a clarinet lesson that afternoon, Doctor. No. Thursday isn't good either.")?

Process to Note in the Office

How does the family enter the interview room? Who leads the way? Who holds back? Do the parents seem to be in charge, or are the children controlling the situation by disruptive behavior or some other tactic?

What is their seating arrangement? Does one family member sit apart from the others? Do the parents sit together, or is the identified patient sandwiched between them? Is one child sitting close to one parent and far from the other? Do the children appear physically close to or alienated from one another?

Who begins the interview? Again, who seems to be in charge of the family? Do family members listen to one another? How are disruptions handled and by whom?

As the family's story is told, what are their feelings? Are they allowed to give their version and, if so, by whom? Are changes in facial expression and feeling tone noticed, acknowledged, and accepted? How do family members react when strong feelings are displayed (e.g., tears, anger)?

What is the family's general tone (e.g., somber, angry, chaotic, anxious)? What is the family's general appearance and dress? Is that appearance consistent among all family members? What individual and collective body language is displayed? Do closeness and touching occur? How do family members handle themselves spatially in the interview room?

All of these observations are seen simultaneously while hearing that Alfred, age 6 years, has been throwing up at school for the past 3 weeks. To focus on that fact alone without regard to process is to miss important information regarding that family's particular structure—the family's mobile or shifting balance of relationships, the pattern of family homeostasis. A clear understanding of these characteristics forms the basis for subsequent therapeutic interventions by the physician.

THE COMMUNICATION MODEL OF VIRGINIA SATIR

Although understanding the difference between content and process is an important start in family interviewing, it is not enough to determine a family's structure of relationships or communication pattern. The physician needs other concepts to guide observations of family function. The ideas presented in the work of Virginia Satir are useful. This author contributed significantly to the emergence of family therapy with the publication of the 1964 textbook *Conjoint Family Therapy* (1). As a result of this book and her subsequent writings and workshops, Satir was recognized as a major force in family therapy and is still considered a founder and guiding light in the field.

Satir's book begins: "Family therapists deal with family pain. When one person in a family (the patient) has pain which shows up in symptoms, all family members are feeling this pain in some way" (2). In agreement with the basic notion of family homeostasis proposed by other communication theorists, she feels that the marital relationship is one of the major influences in a family's homeostatic balance, referring to the marital pair as the "architects" of a family. If there is pain in a marital relationship, then dysfunctional parenting occurs, often resulting in a child with overt symptoms. Because Satir concerned herself almost exclusively with these interactional issues in the appearance of behavioral symptoms, there are no references in her work to the role of traditionally recognized intrapsychic factors in symptom development. From her 1964 writing alone, it may be concluded that she believed this pattern of dysfunction was the exclusive route for the development of behavioral symptoms in children.

In *Peoplemaking,* published in 1972, Satir expanded her view on the origins of behavior: "Any piece of behavior at a moment in time is the outcome of the four-way interplay of the person's self-worth, and his place in time and space and situation" (3). Today, even this expanded view seems restrictive, omitting much of what is now known about attachment theory and the importance of biological determinants of behavior. Satir did not emphasize these deep forces, which influence communication patterns; forces such as the nature of the attachment relationship between parent and child along with the powerful, transgenerational pattern of attachment, care, and communication that travels down through every family through the years. And what about specific characteristics presented to the family by the child in terms of the child's individual temperament, behavioral individuality, and developmental pattern? These factors are innate and represent the child's contribution to family relationships. Children are not passive recipients of parenting. Their temperament and developmental pattern (with or without developmental deviation) affect the parenting they receive, influencing for better or worse the parent–child relationship. Extensive work on the individual behavioral style and temperament can be found in the work of Chess, Thomas, and Birch (4,5). We believe that a child's temperament must be included as a variable in any hypothesis regarding the origin of behavioral difficulties and symptoms. The important role of temperament in understanding children's behavior and in conducting family interviews is discussed further in chapter 6, Common Behavior Problems.

However, even with these omissions, Satir's work has held up surprisingly well as a foundation upon which to design some of our clinical approaches to working with children and families. We continue to use her ideas daily in family interviews. Returning to her original 1964 model (which assumes that dysfunctional parenting is present in a given situation), we agree with the next step in Satir's hypothesis: one member of the family, often a child, may be so significantly affected by the dysfunctional parenting that he or she develops symptoms. That child then becomes the "identified patient," and the symptoms are an "SOS" by the child about parental pain and family imbalance. The symptoms indicate a child who is distorting his or her own emotional growth in an effort to alleviate and absorb the parents' pain.

Maturation: Functional and Dysfunctional Communication

Satir described individuals as either functional or dysfunctional, depending on their degree of maturation, "the most important concept in therapy" (6). She defined maturation as the state in which a human being is fully in charge of himself or herself. A mature and, therefore, functional person is one who is able to make choices and decisions based on accurate perceptions of the self, others, and context, acknowledging these choices and decisions as one's own.

Functional Communication

A functional person communicates clearly with others, is in touch with and able to express what he or she feels, and can accept responsibility for what he or she feels, rather than denying or attributing it to others. A functional individual views the presence of "differentness" between oneself and others as an opportunity for learning, rather than a threat. This person can negotiate, successfully clarifying communication. A person who communicates in a functional manner can:

- Firmly state the case
- At the same time clarify and qualify what he or she says
- Ask for feedback
- Be receptive to feedback when given

Dysfunctional Communication

A dysfunctional person, on the other hand, is one who has not learned to communicate properly. The dysfunctional individual may:

- Deliver unclear and perhaps conflicting messages
- Be unable to clarify meanings
- Be unable to listen to feedback

• View differentness as a threat

A dysfunctional communicator tends to overgeneralize and make false assumptions. Satir described several false assumptions:

False assumption 1: One instance is an example of all instances.
"Why don't you ever . . ."
"I always have to . . ."
"Nobody wears that!"
False assumption 2: Other people should share my feelings, thoughts, and perceptions.
"I don't see how you can stand . . ."
"You should know how I feel about that."
False assumption 3: My perceptions are complete.
"Makes no difference what you tell me. I won't believe it."
False assumption 4: My perceptions will not change.
"That's the way he is. Period."
"Oh well, that's life."
False assumption 5: There are only two possible alternatives; things are or are not.
"If you cared for me, you wouldn't do that."
"You're either for me or against me."
False assumption 6: Characteristics of behavior define the person himself.
"She's a greedy person."
"He is an extremely hostile individual."
False assumption 7: I can get inside the skin of others.
"What she means to say is . . ."
"You don't really want that; what you want is . . ."
"I know what you're thinking."

A functional individual on the receiving end of any of these dysfunctional openers would ask for clarification and qualification, rather than responding in kind. However, the dysfunctional sender would react with an open rebuff, restatement of his or her original case, an attack on the questioner, or simple evasion of the question. From that point, the interchange would deteriorate, no matter how functional one member of the communication pair might be. Satir said, "if verbal communication is to be reasonably clear, then both the sender of a message and the receiver have the responsibility to make it so" (7).

Satir conceded that we all generalize when we communicate and that anyone who perpetually clarifies and qualifies is just as dysfunctional as the person who rarely does so. A sender who too rigorously asks a receiver for feedback may end up in the position of being inundated by feedback. Similarly, a receiver who continually asks for a sender to clarify would seem testy, uncooperative, and irritating. It is perhaps a matter of degree, as expressed by Satir. "Absolutely clear communication is impossible to achieve because communication is, by its very nature, incomplete. But there are degrees of incompleteness. The dysfunctional communicator leaves the receiver groping and guessing about what he has inside his head or heart" (8).

Self-esteem and Parental Validation

Observe the following interchange at a breakfast table:

Alice:	I don't suppose you want another cup of coffee, George.
George:	This stuff tastes like hot water!
Alice:	You never have two cups.
George:	Pass the sugar, Alice.
Alice:	Anybody who likes sugar in coffee must be sick.

George and Alice, according to many of the characteristics cited, are having a dysfunctional interchange. Sidney, their 4-year-old son seated at the table, agrees. According to Satir's idea that the development of dysfunctional communication is connected to the family behavior that surrounds a child, Sidney may be on the way to dysfunctional interchanges of his own. One reason for this is that modeling behavior by parents is very influential. If their messages to each other and to their children are unclear and contradictory, then children in such a position (e.g., Sidney) learn to communicate in an unclear, contradictory way. However, modeling dysfunctional behavior is not the only thing that determines the development of faulty communication. Satir postulated that communication difficulties are closely linked to problems in the development of one's self-esteem during childhood.

Self-esteem, as with maturation, was one of Satir's essential concepts. In fact, she acknowledged a fundamental difference in her views from those of psychoanalytic thought when she stated:

> *I do not postulate sex as the basic drive of man. From what I have ob-*
> *served, the sex drive is continually subordinated to and used for the pur-*
> *pose of enhancing self-esteem. . . . The need to feel esteem about the self*
> *is so important that adult mates will do without sexual satisfaction or*
> *fail to demand it in a vital relationship if sexual behavior, or demands*
> *for it, lead to threatened self-esteem. One sees this over and over again*
> *when counseling marital pairs. (9)*

Self-esteem and Mastery

Satir divided self-esteem into two areas: esteem for the self as a masterful person (i.e., able to do for oneself) and esteem for the self as a sexual person. Our discussion is limited to self-esteem regarding mastery, in which Satir offered an excellent summary of the formative role of a parent in the emergence of a child's self-esteem. She saw parents, or at least one parent, as essential to validate a child's developmental growth. Validation occurs when a parent notes the existence of growth, communicates verbally or nonverbally that he or she has noticed, and gives the child increased opportunity for using the abilities emerging from that growth. A child learns not only to feed himself or herself, tie shoes, and go to the store alone, but in a larger sense, he or she becomes increasingly able to make decisions, reason, create, form and maintain relationships, plan ahead, and tolerate frustration and disappointment. In other words, the sense of self-mastery expands. Parents must time their validation carefully, Satir warned. To ring true and enhance self-esteem, validation must fit the needs, abilities, and readiness of the child.

The development of self-esteem in mastery can go awry when a parent does not validate developmental growth or offers validation inappropriately. In such cases, this invalidated part of a child's growth remains an unintegrated fragment, often labeled by the child as that part of himself or herself that is unimportant, incomplete, inadequate, or bad. The lack of parental validation can occur in a variety of ways: a parent may fail to see the emerging ability, allow no opportunity for its emergence, or fail to comment on its emergence when manifest. Validation may also fail when a parent perceives growth prematurely, anxiously urging its expression before the youngster is actually capable. Validation can be seriously jeopardized if one parent contradicts the validating messages of the other.

Constructive parental validation fits the needs, abilities, and readiness of the child. Validation should be clear, direct, and specific and is given in a relatively matter-of-fact way. One parent does not contradict or depreciate the validation of another. With such constructive parental validation, a child's self-esteem flourishes. Satir felt strongly that adequate self-esteem is essential if children are to grow toward independence, realize their potential and uniqueness, and develop a functional style of communicating with others.

Without feelings of competence and mastery, individuals experience considerable anxiety and uncertainty. Unfortunately, self-esteem for these people is based on what others think; thus, a sense of autonomy and individuality is seriously compromised. Yet a person so crippled often works hard at disguising feelings of low self-esteem from others, particularly from those deemed important to impress, such as a parent, spouse, or future spouse. The individual with low self-esteem is uncomfortable in any situation that calls for compromise and commitment to a joint outcome (i.e., marriage) because any additional sacrifice of self seems an intolerable diminution of something already in short supply—the self. This individual appears poised to receive any evidence of differentness in someone close as a personal insult or a sign of being unloved. Thus, differing opinions, feelings, and thoughts have a way of becoming larger than life and so problematic that they may be constantly argued over or treated as though they do not exist.

Unfortunately, as Satir pointed out in a chapter titled "Low Self-Esteem and Mate Selection," two individuals with mutually low self-esteem usually seek out one another in relationships, with the predictably unhappy outcome of dysfunctional communication for themselves and for their children.

The Induction Process

Satir believed that dysfunctional communication between spouses results from mutual feelings of low self-esteem caused by a failure of parental validation during childhood; however, the connection must be made between the dysfunctional communication of such parents and the subsequent symptom development in their child. To explain the connection, Satir postulated an induction process that is unwittingly used by the parents, the keystone of which is "the double-level message."

Double-level Messages and Double Bind

Double-level messages are statements that say one thing and mean another.

"I can't stand watching this TV program." (while continuing to watch)
"You little devil!" (with a smile and a hug)
"Oh, I really shouldn't." (holding out a plate for seconds)

Often quite harmless and entertaining, double-level messages are used by everyone and do not necessarily lead to difficulty, particularly in situations where clarification is possible. "Thus, by itself, double-level communication need not lead to symptomatic behavior. But under certain conditions, especially where children are involved, it can produce a vicelike situation, which has been termed the 'double bind'" (10).

As mentioned in chapter 1, "double bind" was introduced in a classic paper (11). Stated in its briefest form, a double bind is a paradoxical injunction. The terms "double-level message" and "double bind" must not be confused because they are not the same. The former is nothing more than a message, whereas double bind is a situation or an environment. A double-level message is based on simple contradiction; one may choose either element of the discrepant message. A logical choice is possible. With a double-bind, no choice is logically possible. Foley elegantly captures the essence of a double bind in his illustration borrowed from Greenberg: "Give your son, Marvin, two sport shirts as a present. The first time he wears one of them, look at him sadly and say in your Basic Tone of Voice: 'The other one you didn't like?'" (12). For Marvin, there is no possible choice.

For such no-win situations to have symptom-producing effects on a child, several conditions are necessary:

a. *First, the child must be exposed to double level messages repeatedly and over a long period of time.*
b. *Second, these must come from persons who have survival significance for him.*
   Parents are automatically survival figures because the child liter-

ally depends on them for physical life; later, his need for love and approval from them becomes invested with like meaning.

In addition, the way the parents structure their messages to the child will determine his techniques for mastering his environment. It is not only his present, but his future survival which is in their hands.

As a result, he cannot afford to ignore messages from them, no matter how confused.

c. *Third, perhaps most important of all, he must be conditioned from an early age not to ask, "Did you mean that or that?" but must accept his parents' conflicting messages in all their impossibility. He must be faced with the hopeless task of translating them into a single way of behaving. (13)*

In such a family, the parents often fail to recognize the child's feelings, emerging abilities, needs for nurture, and validation as a worthy individual. Satir felt these parents miss this because they themselves are not receiving appreciation of their own feelings, abilities, and need for support from one another in the marital relationship, and they did not receive such validation in their own childhoods.

When these conditions are present over an extended period, they do not all need to be present to ensure a double-binding situation. Even the presence of one is apparently sufficient to put the child in a bind.

There are three options to a child in a double-bind situation. None are appealing:

First one concludes the "victim" is overlooking something in the situation. He searches and searches but the more he tries to understand, the more confused he becomes. A second possibility is to become absolutely literal and follow each and every injunction to the letter. The basic premise underlying this approach is that things do not make sense anyhow, so why worry. Anyone familiar with institutional living, for example, the army, will recognize this response. A third option is to withdraw from human involvement so that all incoming material is blocked out. The "victim" is caught because he cannot discuss the messages with an outside party. He cannot . . . talk about his communication and thus escape his field. The "victim" therefore remains trapped and unable to escape. (14)

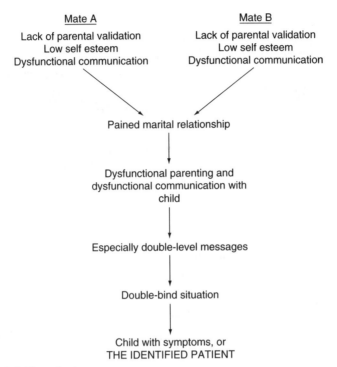

Figure 2.2. The induction process.

When an individual in response to feeling double-bound adopts a style of relating that is predominantly confused, literal, or withdrawn, others eventually notice (e.g., "Frank sure is acting funny"). Such behavior is labeled "sick," "crazy," or "bad." The induction route has been traveled completely when a patient is identified, first in the family and eventually in the doctor's office (see Figure 2.2).

The Interviewer's Approach

According to Figure 2.2, symptoms in a child are directly related to faulty styles of family communication. Satir considered family therapy to be the study and subsequent alteration of maladaptive family communication methods:

> *If illness is seen to derive from inadequate methods of communication (by which we mean all interactional behavior) it follows that therapy will be seen as an attempt to improve these methods. . . . The emphasis will be*

on correcting discrepancies in communication and teaching ways to achieve more fitting joint outcomes. This approach to therapy depends on three primary beliefs about human nature:

First, that every individual is geared to survival, growth, and getting close to others and that all behavior expresses these aims, no matter how distorted it may look. Even an extremely disturbed person will be fundamentally on the side of the therapist.

Second, that what society calls sick, crazy, stupid, or bad behavior is really an attempt on the part of the afflicted person to signal the presence of trouble and call for help. In that sense, it may not be so sick, crazy, stupid, or bad after all.

Third, that humans beings are limited only by the extent of their knowledge, their ways of understanding themselves and their ability to "check out" with others. Thought and feeling are inextricably bound together; the individual need not be a prisoner of his feelings but can use the cognitive component of his feeling to free himself. This is the basis for assuming that a human being can learn what he doesn't know and can change the ways of commenting and understanding that don't fit. (15)

This optimistic view conveys Satir's strong belief in the capacity for growth in every individual and her reluctance to view symptoms within a disease or psychopathology framework. According to Satir, people were not sick or bad; rather, communication and interactional rules were bad, producing family pain. Medical and psychiatric labels had no usefulness in her work.

Avoiding Labels

We agree that avoiding such labels has certain advantages, as summarized by Foley:

To take the label off a person and to put it on a way of interacting is to defuse a potentially volatile situation. Instead of saying that John is the cause of the family's problem, saying that some rules in the family are causing a problem has a twofold effect. First, it takes the label of scapegoat off John and makes him part of the family system and not the cause of its pain. This gives him some breathing room and opens up the possibility of his changing. Second, the parents do not have to feel that they have been failures in their parental role. They have been guilty, perhaps, of over-looking certain procedures in the family, but they no longer have to feel guilty of failing as human beings . . . they can retain their feeling of self-worth as persons and as parents. The distinction is important because instead of locking the system into itself by reinforcing the labels of identified patient and failing parents, it opens up the possibility of change in the system. (16)

This represents the heart of Satir's work: revealing to families their own possibilities for change and facilitating that change.

Directing Communication

Using Satir's approach, a physician functions as a resource person, an impartial observer who can report to the family what he or she sees and hears. This same person serves as a model of clear communication, using functional communication with family members and explicitly teaching individuals the rules for functional interchange. How this is accomplished partly depends on an individual's interviewing style, but regardless of style, certain things are essential.

1. Unclear communications must be clarified.
   "I don't understand what you mean."
   "Would you boil all of that down into one sentence, and then say it directly to your son."
2. Feedback is both demonstrated and encouraged.
   "I like the strength in your voice as you discuss this."
   "I see confusion in your face. Am I reading you right?"
3. Double-level messages are explicitly labeled.
   "You just said to Frances that you didn't mind, and then you turned away with your body."
   "The tears in your eyes don't match your words."
   "If you are angry at Deb, why has your voice gotten so soft?"
4. All the false assumptions of communication are challenged.
   "What do you mean he should know how you feel? He's not a mind reader."
   "Ever, never, always—those words have a way of putting folks on the defensive. Try telling Marge again, leaving those words out."

5. Each individual is encouraged to take responsibility for their actions, thoughts, and feelings.

"Neil, start over again and begin your sentence with the pronoun 'I.'"

These guidelines allow an interviewer to repeatedly examine, alter, and redirect communication. And by commenting on what one hears, sees, and feels in the family's midst, the interviewer also models new ways of communication for the family.

Establishing Authority

Satir considered it extremely important to quickly establish her authority in the interview. When children were involved, she preferred that parents set limits for their children in the interview. Satir developed specific rules that she explained to the family.

> *I do make it my responsibility, however, to communicate clearly the rules of behavior that apply in my own bailiwick, the therapy room*
>> *No one may hit or play with the microphone or the recording equipment.*
>> *No one may destroy any chairs, window blinds, etc.*
>> *No one (including parents) may speak for others.*
>> *Everyone must speak so he can be heard.*
>> *Everyone must make it possible for others to be heard. "You are hurting my eardrums" I will say, or "You will have to take turns talking or I can't do my work."*
>> *The parents will often ask me to set a rule about leaving the therapy room. Mother will ask, "Is it all right if he leaves?" I will say, "Yes," and then instruct the child on how to find the water fountain or toilet.*
>> *I also set rules on how often a child may leave the therapy room. Usually one trip to the toilet, and one trip to the water fountain will give Johnny or Patty all the chance they need to explore.*
>> *I also shorten the length of the therapy session to conform to the ages of the children. (17)*

The Interviews

The Initial Phase: Introduction and History

For Satir, therapy with a family had a reliable developmental pattern. Initial contact was usually with one family member on the telephone. She gathered enough information to understand the concerns and set up the first appointment, usually with the parents alone. Satir wrote in her original text that the first two appointments were most often with parents, which underscored her notion that the parents were the "authorized leaders" of the family.

During the first session, she would ask questions to establish the parents' expectations of treatment. Each spouse was asked, "What would you like to accomplish here?" She then explained the importance of a family view with comments such as, "No one person can see the whole picture because he is limited to his own perspective. By having everyone together, we can get the whole picture more clearly. Every person has a unique contribution to make that cannot be duplicated by anyone else." She explored with the spouses' complaints, usually about their child (i.e., "the problem"), and concluded by acknowledging the parents' confusion and good intentions regarding the child and their efforts.

In the second interview (sometimes at the conclusion of the first interview), Satir proceeded to what she termed a family chronology, an extensive exploration with the family of their history as individuals and as a group. The chronology would begin with each parent's relationship as children with their parents. Satir felt this was an invaluable device for helping families relax and become less frightened. Recollection of the past, particularly of those pleasant times before the family's present trouble started, often reassured the patients, at times rekindling hope that things might get better.

We have not implemented this part of Satir's approach routinely, preferring to begin with families and their problems in the present. We return to historical events only as the situation warrants. In the previous edition of this book, we stated that we did not conduct any initial interviews without the children—another departure from the technique proposed by Virginia Satir. However, we have returned to the Satir format of conducting an initial meeting with parents and without children to assess the appropriateness of a conjoint family interviewing approach. If family work seems indicated, all or selected children are included in subsequent meetings.

Returning to Satir's model, she noted that when children were included, there were specific issues that she hoped to confront immediately. She wanted family members to recognize each other as individuals and make them aware that there would be disagreements. Satir was careful to integrate the children into the interview process, respecting children by greeting them separately, honoring all questions from them, and asking each child specific questions about the reasons for their coming to the family interview. Often, the first family interview ended on a positive note, having family members acknowledge good feelings when pleased by what another has done or said. For many families, Satir found this was a departure from their usual style of blaming and criticism. Such groups had forgotten how to offer positive feedback.

The Middle Phase: Accountability and Responsibility

After the initial phase, family therapy according to Satir would settle into a middle period, during which the therapist has important work to do. He or she must create a setting in which people can, often for the first time, risk looking clearly at themselves and their behavior. This is done in several ways. The interviewer demonstrates that whereas the family is fearful, the interviewer is not, particularly when it comes to asking questions and taking responsibility for what is not being discussed. By doing so, the interviewer models clear communication, provides direction, and at the same time shows patients how they look to others. When asking for and giving information, the interviewer does so in a matter-of-fact, nonjudgmental way. One endeavors to build self-esteem in family members through validation of their appropriate behavior. One lessens any sense of threat that family members feel toward the interview by setting clear rules for interaction in the session. In making the interview a relatively safe place, one discourages the need for defenses among family members. At the same time one is very cautious and conservative with material that is obviously charged, proceeding slowly at such times.

While establishing the therapy room as a safe and honest place for the family, the interviewer is also encouraging members to assume personal responsibility and accountability in order to handle communication and behavior in a more functional manner. The interviewer does this by reminding individuals of their ability to be in charge of themselves. Blaming others is discouraged, and each family member's use of "I" is encouraged, emphasizing the responsibility for the self as essential for the formation and maintenance of functional relationships.

The Completion of Treatment

The concept of using and behaving as an "I" was so important to Satir that she considered it a determinant for when family treatment would end.

Treatment is completed:
  When family members can complete transactions, check, ask.
  When they can interpret hostility.
  When they can see how others see them.
  When they can see how they see themselves.
  When one member can tell another how he manifests himself.
  When one member can tell another what he hopes, fears, and expects from him.
  When they can disagree.
  When they can make choices.
  When they can learn through practice.
  When they can free themselves from harmful effects of past models.
  When they can give a clear message, that is, be congruent in their behavior, with a minimum of difference between feelings and communication, and with a minimum of hidden messages.

. . . In short, treatment is completed when everyone in the therapy setting can use the first person "I" followed by an active verb and ending with a direct object. (18)

References

1. Satir V. Conjoint family therapy: a guide to theory and technique. Palo Alto, CA: Science and Behavior Books, 1964.
2. Satir V. Conjoint family therapy. 3rd ed. Palo Alto, CA: Science and Behavior Books, 1983:1.
3. Satir V. Peoplemaking. Palo Alto, CA: Science and Behavior Books, 1972:xi.
4. Chess S, Thomas A, Birch HG, et al. Behavioral individuality in early childhood. New York: New York University Press, 1963.
5. Carey J, McDevitt S. Coping with children's temperament. New York: Basic Books, 1995.
6. Satir, Conjoint family therapy, 3rd ed, 117.
7. Satir, Conjoint family therapy, 3rd ed, 88.
8. Satir, Conjoint family therapy, 3rd ed, 92.
9. Satir, Conjoint family therapy, 3rd ed, 69–70.

10. Satir, Conjoint family therapy, 3rd ed, 46.

11. Bateson G, Jackson D, Haley J, et al. Toward a theory of schizophrenia. Behavioral Science 1956;1:251.

12. Foley V. An introduction to family therapy. New York: Grune & Stratton, 1974.

13. Satir, Conjoint family therapy, 3rd ed, 46.

14. Foley, 15.

15. Satir, Conjoint family therapy, 3rd ed, 124–125.

16. Foley, 101.

17. Satir, Conjoint family therapy, 3rd ed, 184–185.

18. Satir, Conjoint family therapy, 3rd ed, 227–228.

chapter 3

Structural Views of the Family

THE MALONEY FAMILY

As she sat with her parents, Jennifer Maloney, age 9 years, reminded the pediatrician of illustrations long ago in *A Child's Garden of Verses*—pretty, nicely dressed, dainty, innocent. The pediatrician's impression of Jennifer was vastly different from the way in which her parents were to describe her. This was the sixth physician or therapist whom they had consulted regarding their only child and her difficulties, which had lasted for the past 7 years. Mrs. Maloney was close to tears as she told the story. Mr. Maloney was silent and seemed indifferent or frightened.

Jennifer had developed "a sleeping problem" even before she was one year old, often drawing up her legs in sleep and seeming fretful. The parents were told by their first pediatrician that she had colic, so they adjusted the feeding formula several times. The behavior continued, and by the time she was 2 years old, Jennifer's parents were convinced that she was having "nightmares" when she would scream out in her sleep during the night. Mrs. Maloney would go immediately to the bedside and try to comfort her child, but Jennifer was "very hostile" during these episodes, and comforting did not work.

By the time she was 5 years old, these nocturnal episodes occurred as often as three times a week. By this time, several physicians, including a family doctor, a pediatrician, and a child psychiatrist, had advised that these spells were most probably night terrors and that Jennifer would eventually "grow out of it." She did not, and the episodes seemed to occur more frequently. Enuresis began to accompany these outbursts when Jennifer was 6 years old. A neurologist (the second) described in his report: "The usual sequence of events is that the girl goes to bed at 7:30. Somewhere around 11:30 to 12:30, the girl begins to 'holler—thrash in her bed—looks frightened—speaks but no one can understand her.' Mother usually goes to her side but is unable to comfort her. This episode may last from 1 minute to, on one occasion, 15 minutes. She then resumes sleeping."

Additional problems began when Jennifer began school. She became anxious about the smallest details (e.g., what clothes she would wear, how she would perform that day in reading, whether her paper was neat enough, what would happen on the playground, how she would get along with friends, whether the teacher would like her). In fact, she was an excellent student and did well with both peers and teachers, but she became so anxious regarding all aspects of her school career that she refused to go—and school was directly across the street from the Maloney's house. The school counselor was contacted, and some mornings Jennifer would literally be dragged by Mrs. Maloney to the street and transferred to the school counselor, who would continue the coercion into the school building. Many mornings Jennifer just did not attend at all because she was "too upset." Night terrors, enuresis, school phobia—the list was growing.

Mrs. Maloney was desperate, as were the physicians. The inevitable result was that medication (e.g., imipramine for the bed wetting, tranquilizers for the anxiety) was prescribed. Psychotherapy was also suggested, and for the past 6 months, Jennifer had been in twice-weekly individual play therapy with a child psychologist.

According to the parents, progress had been minimal. The mother told each doctor that she felt as though she were on a treadmill in which no one really understood what the family was going through, and the only course of action was a referral from one specialist to another. Until now, no one had met with the family together.

TREATMENT

The Initial Interview

Several things surfaced during the initial family meeting with a pediatrician trained in working with families. He observed that Jennifer enjoyed talking about her "anxieties and worries" and her "therapist." She was willing to discuss her experiences of the past several years and viewed herself as "the patient." Her parents agreed, with Mrs. Maloney adding to the patient image with a lurid, hand-wringing description of Jennifer's difficulties. The sleep situation became the focus, until Jennifer's illness seemed one more family member to be handled.

Mr. Maloney, as mentioned, remained silent. When the doctor directly asked his opinion, Jennifer would roll her eyes, and Mrs. Maloney would follow with an interruption, restatement, or correction. The pediatrician noted that the father was the last of the three to enter his office, and he seemed to be holding back. When in the office, Mr. Maloney seated himself some distance from his family. The mother and daughter, on the other hand, were entwined with frequent touching and eye contact. Mrs. Maloney's field of vision was completely occupied by Jennifer. The father's position in the interview and in the family was remote, discounted, and peripheral.

Mrs. Maloney and Jennifer were close even though the connection between them would turn out to be a bond of frustration and conflict. Seating arrangement, body posture, eye contact, and the content of the interview itself displayed their mutual dependence. Jennifer had a way of visually checking with her mother before she spoke, which was a triggering mechanism for Mrs. Maloney to enter the conversation and finish Jennifer's sentence. At other times, the mother would speak for Jennifer (e.g., "Now, Doctor, I know Jennifer won't tell you this, but she's not at all sure about this meeting with the whole family. She would rather see you alone. She really prefers to have her own doctor to talk to."). Because this statement was repeated three times by Mrs. Maloney during the first interview, it was clear that someone, not necessarily Jennifer, was uncomfortable with a family meeting.

When asked directly, the family discussed their versions of the nighttime scene. In many respects, their story was similar to that reported by their pediatric neurologist. At approximately 11:30 PM, Jennifer would begin screaming in her room. Mrs. Maloney would rush in, find herself unable to soothe her daughter, and become worn down by the experience. However, the pediatrician heard additional important information.

Mother:	Well, you see, Doctor, my husband and I don't always agree on what should be done. Do you realize, Lester, what could happen to that child? She could injure herself. She gets so physically violent, Doctor, that she actually throws herself out of bed. She did hurt herself that one time. I can't let that happen.
Father:	I know, that's right. But I still think you go in there too soon. We've never tried just leaving her alone.
Doctor:	Tell me a little more about what you have done and what you're doing now when these episodes occur.
Mother:	When she screams out like that, I do go, I admit; I can't let her scream like that. She's not even awake. When I try to quiet her, then she gets angry with *me*, really violent sometimes, slapping and kicking. I bring her a glass of water,

and she throws it at me. Then, of course, the commotion gets really loud. And he hears it and thinks, "Oh, geez, they're at it again." And so he comes in like Godzilla and terrifies her. You just can't do that with children, Doctor. Then she ends up being scared of her own father. No patience—he has no patience. Then I have even worse problems getting her settled down after her father comes in. He's shouting at me and at her . . . I'm shouting . . . Jennifer's screaming. Sometimes we're up for hours like that.

The pediatrician concluded the hour by telling the Maloneys that they had a complex family problem that would require considerable work to change. When he offered his help and suggested beginning by seeing the parents alone in 1 week, another dialogue took place.

Mother:	But Doctor, what will *we* do in 2 days when Jennifer goes back to school? That's our next crisis. How will *we* get ourselves to school?
Jennifer:	(in a small voice) Maybe I'll just have to go alone.
Father:	Right.
Mother:	Are you sure you're really ready?
Doctor:	Mrs. Maloney, I would like you instead to tell Jennifer, "I am confident that you are ready."
Mother:	Oh, I do want to have confidence in her.
Doctor:	Tell her that, *now*.
Mother:	(to Jennifer) I do have confidence about your going to school?
Doctor:	Could you say it once again and remove the question mark from your voice?

She did, but the doctor was unconvinced and the hour ended.

The next day, the doctor received a telephone call from Mrs. Maloney. She was frantic and said that things had deteriorated badly after their visit. Jennifer had a terrible sleep disturbance that night, and the two of them had been up from 3 AM to 6 AM. The child was furious, saying to her mother, "How dare that man say this is a family problem! It's a mother–daughter problem!" Mrs. Maloney asked for an appointment alone.

Mother:	There are just so many things I wanted to say that I couldn't say in front of my husband.
Doctor:	Mrs. Maloney, I certainly agree that the family is in a serious crisis at the moment. I don't believe things can wait for a week. I would like to see you and your husband tomorrow.
Mother:	Absolutely, Doctor. And if my husband can't come, could I come alone?
Doctor:	No, Mrs. Maloney. I will need you both here.
Mother:	All right. But now what will we do about our sleeping problem? I don't think we can go through another night like last night.

The pediatrician assured her that he realized it was a trying time. Although immediate solutions would be welcome, he had none, except to suggest that spending more than 15 minutes in Jennifer's bedroom at night was too long.

The next day Mrs. Maloney arrived on time for the appointment alone. She relayed her husband's unwillingness to come, making sure the doctor understood it was a basketball game on television that took priority. The physician held his ground at the door, politely refusing to see her or begin working with the family without Mr. Maloney. She accepted his refusal with grace and a glance that said, "At least now you know what I have to put up with at home."

The Second Interview

Both parents arrived for their next scheduled appointment. The interview began with a discussion of trust; neither trusted the other's management of Jennifer. Mr. Maloney saw his wife as oversolicitous and ineffectual, and Mrs. Maloney viewed her husband as an angry, overreacting ogre with children.

Therapeutic Strategies

After listening, the physician unfolded his therapeutic strategy:

1. He acknowledged Mrs. Maloney's frustration and obvious exhaustion in dealing with the problem almost singlehandedly for years. In his medical opinion, he did not feel that she could continue much longer. It was not humanly possible.
2. He further felt that Mr. Maloney was crucial to the survival of his wife and family and that only he could help solve this family problem. It could be done by no one else.

3. However, Mr. Maloney could help his family only with the assistance of his wife. In this sense, Mrs. Maloney was also crucial to the solution. She was in an important position that could enable her husband to teach Jennifer one of the most important lessons fathers teach daughters: respect for men. Only the father could impart this to the child. And only the mother could provide the opportunity. Did she want her daughter to learn this lesson? (Mrs. Maloney readily agreed.)

4. Mrs. Maloney was to allow her husband to manage Jennifer's sleep disturbance. This would accomplish two important goals: it would allow Jennifer to see her father's competence and nurturing abilities, thus enhancing the child's respect for him, and it would provide Mrs. Maloney a rest for her exhaustion.

When asked to adhere to these strategies, both parents agreed tentatively. The discussion then turned to specific ways in which Mr. Maloney would deal with Jennifer at night. First, he would determine that Jennifer was not suffering physically, then he would leave her bedroom, assuring her that all was well and that he trusted her own ability to calm down. He was willing to do this several times a night if necessary and assured his wife that he would not be physically or verbally abusive. He was realizing for the first time that his past lack of control stemmed from his impatience with his wife's efforts and a disappointment in himself for playing such a peripheral role in parenting. The pediatrician validated Mr. Maloney's feelings and his new realizations.

Mrs. Maloney, although willing to relinquish the manager role to her husband, admitted honestly that she was not sure she could handle Jennifer's crying without checking on her. She said she might have to leave the house. The pediatrician applauded this suggestion, telling Mrs. Maloney that he wished he had thought of it and asked if she would be willing to go for a short ride in the car at such times. "I would have to," she acknowledged. The second hour ended with a return interview scheduled.

The Third Interview

In 2 weeks, the parents returned. Mrs. Maloney looked rested, less frantic, and Mr. Maloney seemed pleased. They reported that the plan was presented to Jennifer primarily by her father, with her mother in attendance. There had been no sleep disturbance since that time. They vaguely remembered two or three nights of transient whimpering, which Mr. Maloney treated by staying in his own bed.

Mrs. Maloney recalled an interesting episode a few days before this third appointment. For years, the family sat in the same seats when riding in the car, with Jennifer always placed between her parents on the front seat. She now considered that "my place." On this particular day, she came to the car to find her mother and father sitting next to one another for the first time. When Jennifer was offered a window seat, she was outraged, responding "I know what that doctor's trying to do; he's trying to get you two together!" Clearly, Jennifer was having mixed feelings: anger (at losing first place) and relief (as her nighttime behavior indicated).

During this third interview, therapeutic strategies for Jennifer's return to regular school attendance were discussed. Flushed with their nocturnal victory, the parents agreed to follow the same basic plan: decentralize the mother, enhance the father, and increase Jennifer's feelings of adequacy. These next stages of the plan were discussed in these terms:

1. Jennifer would be required to attend school daily.
2. Between waking and 9:25 AM would be her own time at home. She could use it to dress herself in her own choice of clothes. (Her mother had been picking out her clothes the night before and dressing Jennifer in the morning.) She could also use the morning time to eat breakfast and do anything else she wished.
3. At 9:25, she would be expected to go out the door for school, period (i.e., with or without the proper clothes, with or without breakfast). This would be Jennifer's choice. Mrs. Maloney would see that Jennifer left on time.
4. If difficulty developed, Mr. Maloney would be called at work to come home and assist. Mrs. Maloney would not be required to handle the problem alone any longer.

The Fourth Interview

At the fourth interview, Mr. and Mrs. Maloney reported that Jennifer was hysterical with the presentation of this plan. Nonetheless, they held their ground and were obviously pleased that school attendance had been regular and without incident ever since. Mr. Maloney had not been called and was relieved, and Mrs. Maloney felt successful.

The Fifth Interview

By the fifth interview, everyone was feeling better. The father was freely discussing his pleasure at taking a decisive stand in the work of his own family. The mother was pleased beyond words that she was finding a man, husband, and father in the family's midst, and, consequently, she had less need for her nagging, critical attitude. Their daughter appeared relaxed and was sleeping well and attending school. Her parents were able to let her go and turn their energies toward helping her enhance relationships with peers in such things as staying over at a friend's house, which Jennifer previously refused because of her "problem at night." Sessions were mutually terminated after ten visits. There was no recurrence of symptoms.

The therapeutic work and a successful outcome with Jennifer and her parents did not rest only on the use of a communication model as presented in chapter 2. The physician also relied heavily on ideas concerned with the structure of the family. Salvador Minuchin and Jay Haley were particularly prominent in the development of so-called structural family therapy in the 1970s when both were working at the Philadelphia Child Guidance Clinic. Their writings during that period have significantly influenced our approach to interviewing. A summary of the views of each man during that time illustrates their similarities and differences. The relationship of each to the interviewing model based on the communication theory of Satir should become apparent. It is the blending of approaches developed by these individuals (i.e., Satir, Minuchin, Haley) that continues to define our basic clinical direction with families today.

SALVADOR MINUCHIN AND STRUCTURAL FAMILY THERAPY

We first became interested in Minuchin's work when we learned of his effective treatment of primary anorexia nervosa through short-term family therapy. This illness has often struck panic in the hearts of clinicians when faced with a determined, starving adolescent and her desperately anxious parents. Therefore, it was refreshing to read in some of Minuchin's reports that short-term family therapy (the median course of treatment was 6 months) was successful in more than 80% of cases referred to him for treatment (1).

In 1974, a summary of his work with families, anorectic or otherwise, appeared in *Families and Family Therapy* (2). This book was followed in 1981 by another text, *Family Therapy Techniques* (3). These two books describe Minuchin's basic structural approach to families. The usefulness of family approaches in specific psychosomatic disorders was the focus of a third book, *Psychosomatic Families: Anorexia Nervosa in Context* (4), which will be discussed in chapter 9.

Minuchin states that therapy based on a structural framework is directed toward changing the organization of a family. He also describes structural therapy as a therapy of action: "the tool of this therapy is to modify the present, not to explore and interpret the past" (5). The target of treatment is the family system or structure (i.e., the invisible set of functional demands that organizes the way in which family members interact). The therapist joins this system and uses himself to transform it, changing the position of the system's members and altering the family structure. According to Minuchin, a family is a system that operates through repeated transactional patterns, which establish how, when, and with whom family members relate. These ideas are shared by other family theorists, including those primarily interested in communication. Minuchin would be comfortable with our metaphor of the family as a mobile (see chapter 1).

Three Axioms of Family Therapy

When the structure of the family is transformed, the positions of family members change accordingly. Consequently, each individual changes. While agreeing with other family therapists that man is not an isolate, Minuchin further states that family therapy rests on three axioms.

1. An individual's psychic life is not entirely an internal process.
2. Changes in a family structure contribute to changes in the behavioral and the inner psychic processes of the members of that system.
3. When a therapist works with a patient or a patient's family, his behavior becomes part of the context. Therapist and family join to form a new therapeutic system, which then governs the behavior of its members.

These three assumptions provide the foundation of Minuchin's approach. To illustrate the structural therapist's view, Minuchin cites the example of Alice in Wonderland:

> *In Wonderland, Alice suddenly grew to a gigantic size. Her experience was that she got bigger while the room got smaller. If Alice had grown in a room that was also growing at the same rate, she might have experienced everything as staying the same. Only if Alice or the room changes separately does her experience change. It is simplistic, but not inaccurate, to say that intrapsychic therapy concentrates on changing Alice. A structural family therapist concentrates on changing Alice within her room. (6)*

Subsystems and Boundaries

In Minuchin's view, every family system is characterized by subsystems of the family. A subsystem may consist of one individual, two persons (e.g., husband and wife, mother and child), or more (e.g., three children, two children with one parent). The specific subsystems are separated by boundaries, a term fundamental to structural theorists. Minuchin defines the boundary of a subsystem as that collection of rules that defines who participates and how. For example, a boundary simultaneously defining a spouse subsystem and a parental subsystem is declared when a father tells his son, "Albert, I will be with you in 15 minutes. Until then, I would like you to leave us alone. This is a time when your mother and I need some privacy to talk."

This example illustrates a clear boundary. However, boundaries may also be diffuse (i.e., unclear) or rigid (i.e., too clear and unyielding), leading to relationships characterized by overinvolvement, conflict, or coalition. Minuchin feels that the boundaries of subsystems must be clear for proper family functioning. He postulates that all families fall somewhere on a continuum, the extremes being inappropriately diffuse boundaries or overly rigid subsystem boundaries. Most families fall in between these extremes, in what he terms the "normal range of clear boundaries." Other families, operating at either extreme, are "enmeshed" (i.e., overly diffuse boundaries) or "disengaged" (i.e., overly rigid boundaries).

Almost all families at some point exhibit qualities of enmeshment, disengagement, or both. For example, as children grow and begin to separate from the family, disengagement is appropriate, following a time when enmeshment had been preeminent and satisfactory. This development is normal in Minuchin's view.

However, an unshifting stand at either extreme produces family symptomatology. Minuchin summarizes the problem in this way:

> A highly enmeshed subsystem of mother and children, for example, can exclude father, who becomes disengaged in the extreme. The resulting undermining of the children's independence might be an important factor in the development of symptoms.
>
> Members of enmeshed subsystems or families may be handicapped in that the heightened sense of belonging requires a major yielding of autonomy. The lack of subsystem differentiation discourages autonomous exploration and mastery of problems. In a child particularly, cognitive-affective skills are thereby inhibited. Members of disengaged subsystems or families may function autonomously but have a skewed sense of independence and lack of feelings of loyalty and belonging and the capacity for interdependence and for requesting support when needed.
>
> In other words, a system toward the extreme disengaged end of the continuum tolerates a wide range of individual variations in its members.

But stresses in one family member do not cross over its inappropriately rigid boundaries. Only a high level of individual stress can reverberate strongly enough to activate the family's supportive systems. At the enmeshed end of the continuum, the opposite is true. The behavior of one member immediately affects others, and stress in an individual member reverberates strongly across the boundaries and is swiftly echoed in other subsystems.

Both types of relating cause family problems when adaptive mechanisms are evoked. The enmeshed family responds to any variation from the accustomed with excessive speed and intensity. The disengaged family tends not to respond when a response is necessary. The parents in an enmeshed family may become tremendously upset because a child does not eat his dessert. The parents in a disengaged family may feel unconcerned about a child's hatred of school. (7)

The clarity of boundaries within a family becomes a useful parameter for the evaluation of family functioning. Some families turn in on themselves, developing their own "safe" world, with increased communication and concern among family members. As a result, distance decreases and boundaries are blurred. Such a system may become overloaded and lack the resources necessary to adapt and change under stressful circumstances. Another family may develop overly rigid boundaries, which causes difficult communication across this family's subsystems and handicaps the protective functions of the family.

Three Subsystems of Boundaries

Minuchin describes three subsystems in families that should have clearly defined boundaries.

1. The spouse subsystem. This system must achieve a boundary that protects it from interference by the demands and needs of other systems. This is particularly true when a family has children. The adults must have a psychological territory of their own—a haven in which they can give each other emotional support.
2. The parental subsystem. A boundary must be drawn that allows a child access to both parents, while excluding the child from spouse functions. Some of the most intense family conflicts occur over this boundary. Parents cannot protect and guide without at the same time controlling and

restricting. Children cannot grow and become individuals without re-
jecting and attacking. The process of socializing a child is inherently
conflictual. Conflict or not, a family with clear parental subsystem
boundaries never loses correct sight of who is the parent and who is the
child.

3. The sibling subsystem. Within this system, children experiment with
   peer relationships. Children learn how to negotiate, cooperate, and
   compete in this setting, preparing them for similar experiences outside
   the family. Therefore, Minuchin describes the sibling subsystem as the
   child's "first social laboratory."

By assessing family subsystems and boundaries, the structural family
therapist develops a rapid diagnostic picture of the family. This understanding orients therapeutic interventions, which are designed to unbalance the existing system, breaking up repetitive patterns, changing align-
ments, and allowing for constructive problem solving. In the case of the
Maloneys, the therapist had specific goals: to engage the father in parenting and to diminish the spousal conflict, enhancing the relationship between husband and wife. He also hoped to clarify the boundary between
mother and daughter and to decrease their coalition against the father. The
therapist achieved these goals by using himself to unbalance the system.
First, he affiliated with the father, then blocked the mother–child transactions by conducting sessions without the child and suggesting the mother's
withdrawal from Jennifer at night. The physician also encouraged the
mother and father in a coalition against the child.

Joining and Accommodation

At this point, it may seem that structural therapy is little more than a rude
chess game, with the therapist moving people around randomly. Although
Minuchin and Haley are explicitly concerned with strategies, manipulations, moves, and operations, their approaches are not random. Haley addresses this theme in *Problem-Solving Therapy* (8).

> *If successful therapy is defined as solving the problems of a client, the ther-
> apist must know how to formulate a problem and how to solve it. And if
> he or she is to solve a variety of problems, the therapist must not take a rigid
> and stereotyped approach to therapy. Any standardized method of therapy,
> no matter how effective with certain problems, cannot deal successfully with*

the wide range that is typically offered to a therapist. Flexibility and spontaneity are necessary. Yet any therapist must also learn from experience and repeat what was successful before. A combination of familiar procedures and innovative techniques increases the probability of success. (9)

Both authors believe that successful therapy depends partly on specific and learnable principles.

According to Minuchin, the therapist's job is to facilitate the transformation of the family system. The process involves three major steps:

1. The therapist joins the family in a position of leadership.
2. The therapist unearths and evaluates the underlying family structure.
3. The therapist creates circumstances that allow transformation of the structure.

Timid trainees should note Minuchin's view of the therapist's responsibility:

When the therapist joins the family he assumes the leadership of the therapeutic system. This leadership involves responsibility for what happens. . . . The family will be the matrix of the healing and growth of its members. The responsibility for reaching this state, or for failing to do so, belongs to the therapist. (10)

In our experience, therapists have too often dismissed their therapeutic failures by saying, "Well, what could I expect; the family wasn't really motivated, wasn't ready for help . . . too resistant." Yet when patients do well in counseling, the therapist usually takes credit. Why then, when a family does not do well, is that failure generally ascribed to the patient and not to the therapist? We agree with Minuchin and Haley, who deplore such summations as irresponsible therapy.

Sensitivity, balance, and timing are important in helping a family alter their structure:

The concept of transformation deals with large movements in therapy, which take place over time. The therapist must know how to map his goals. But he must also know how to facilitate the small movements that carry the family toward those goals. He must help them in such a way that they are not threatened by major dislocations. A person's ability to move from one circumstance to another depends on the support he receives; he will not move toward the unknown in a situation of danger.

Therefore it is vital to provide systems of support within the family to fa-
cilitate the movement from one position to another. (11)

With the Maloney family, the goal was to eliminate Jennifer's sleep disorder and fear of school. These goals represented the "large movement," set
in motion by many small movements (e.g., the mother was supported and
given a rest, the father was requested to enter the scene more actively, Jennifer was excluded from sessions, the mother and father were encouraged
in a cooperative effort).

Minuchin defines certain processes that are essential for successful work
with families, regardless of therapeutic styles. Methods that create a therapeutic system and establish the therapist in a position of leadership are
known as "joining and accommodation operations." Minuchin considers
these operations essential, without which restructuring cannot occur.

"Joining and accommodation are two ways of describing the same
process" (12). Joining is the process of engaging with the family, touching
them and being touched, requiring the therapist to follow their path of
communication, discovering what is open and closed. The therapist must
attend to individual dilemmas and pain, experiencing the pressures of the
family system; yet, he or she must be able to disengage from the system,
maintaining enough freedom to develop effective therapeutic goals. Thus,
joining a family requires a therapist to adapt, which Minuchin terms "accommodation." Specific accommodation techniques vary, but Minuchin
cites three: maintenance, tracking, and mimesis.

Maintenance

Maintenance refers to providing planned support for the family structure
as seen by the therapist. The physician's validation of Mrs. Maloney's good
intentions, hard work, and exhaustion is an example of this technique because the physician is validating the existing family patterns. Also, when a
therapist openly enjoys a family's humor or expresses affection for them, he
is using maintenance operations. Maintenance has to do with confirming
individuals, subsystems, or the entire family.

Tracking

Tracking occurs when a therapist follows the content of a family's communications and behavior, encouraging the members to continue. "In its sim-

plest form, tracking means to ask clarifying questions, to make approving comments, or to elicit amplification of a point. The therapist does not challenge what is being said" (13). Tracking confirms the family members by eliciting more information. The therapist does not initiate an action; he leads by following. This technique is presented as a joining procedure because used alone, it is not enough to promote family change. A family session in which only tracking is used will likely bore the interviewer and frustrate the family, which is often the case with our beginning interviewers. Tracking is often a safe retreat for these beginners, particularly with "content-oriented" physicians who track information excessively. In such cases, joining has occurred to the exclusion of any restructuring within the session.

Mimesis

Mimesis (i.e., imitation) is used to accommodate a family's style and affective range. The interviewer adopts the family's tempo of communication, slowing or quickening the pace depending on how the family operates. The therapist may use personal references to blend with the family: "I can't stand carrots either," or, "My own mother was like you in that respect." Such statements from the interviewer "increase the sense of kinship, indicating that both therapist and family members are . . . more human than otherwise" (14).

Restructuring Techniques

Restructuring is the process of using therapeutic interventions to confront and challenge a family to change. It differs from joining: joining diminishes distance between the therapist and family and is soothing; restructuring confronts issues and is often upsetting. In joining operations, the therapist is an actor in the family play. In restructuring, while still an actor, the therapist also is the director, creating, suggesting, confronting, and changing. These procedures are the highlights of therapy, and their success depends on a prior satisfactory joining between the therapist and family. There are at least seven restructuring techniques, according to Minuchin.

Actualizing Family Transactional Patterns

By assuming a leadership role in the family sessions, the therapist risks becoming the recipient of all communication. The family tends to view the therapist as the expert through whom all transactions must pass for judgment, correction, and approval. The results can be stultifying.

Doctor:	Georgie, did you know that your mother has strong objections to your wetting the bed?
Georgie:	I don't give a damn.
Doctor:	Mrs. Ayres, did you know that Georgie doesn't give a damn?
Mother:	(sob)
Doctor:	Georgie, did you realize that statements like that make your mother sad?

We agree with Minuchin that describing in this way should be avoided because it constricts the therapist. The physician will be too busy to observe and formulate goals or execute strategies. Also, families tend to become repetitive in their well-rehearsed descriptions of "the problem." An effective therapist moves beyond such verbal descriptions, giving directives and enabling actual transactions to occur between family members in the interview.

There is considerable value in making the family enact instead of describe. The therapist can gather only limited data from the family's descriptions. To amplify the data, a therapist must help them transact, in the interview, some of the ways in which they usually resolve conflicts, support each other, enter into alliances and coalitions, or diffuse stress. (15)

Minuchin refers to this method as "enacting transactional patterns." To facilitate this enactment, the therapist can direct certain family members to interact with each another around a given issue by saying, "That's an issue that involves you and Susan. I would like you to talk with one another." In some cases, families cooperate when directed to discuss issues directly with each another, but often they are not cooperative because they may fear a confrontation, or that they will not be listened to, or believe they must speak to the therapist in order to be heard. Therefore, the therapist must be persistent and have several methods available for encouraging direct communication. This dialogue is an example of a family that is hesitant to pursue direct communication:

Doctor:	That's an issue that involves you and Susan. I would like the two of you to talk to each other about that now.
Mother:	Oh, Doctor, Susan and I have discussed this thing many times at home, haven't we dear?
Susan:	(mumble, shuffle)
Doctor:	I'm sure that you have. In fact, it's one of the reasons that you've asked for my help. Will you discuss it once more, this time in front of me, so that I can hear you and help you figure out a solution?
Mother:	I feel so silly. It's so. . . . artificial.
Doctor:	I agree (silence).
Mother:	(after a pause) Oh . . . you still want me to say something?
Doctor:	(Now pushing his chair back and choosing not to look at any family member, he stares at his shoe.) Yes, even though it's silly, talk to your daughter now about this most important aspect of her growth, stealing from your purse.
Father:	Doctor, I was wondering . . .
Doctor:	Mr. Thompkins, it's probably very hard to sit silently. At the moment, your wife and Susan need to discuss this. Can you allow them to do this?
Father:	Of course.
Mother:	(long silence, then tears as she begins) Oh, Sue . . .

This procedure with variations may have to be repeated gently and firmly many times until the family learns that direct communication is required in the session.

As mentioned, a family's seating arrangement in the office offers important information about their relationships, structure, alliances, and coalitions. The manipulation of their chosen family space is another technique for helping the family to enact, rather than describe. In the above case, if Susan and her mother are seated on either side of Mr. Thompkins, the therapist may remove him from the middle to a chair next to the therapist so that "Susan and her mother can more easily talk directly to one another." This enables the therapist to place a quieting hand on Mr. Thompkins when he interrupts their transaction for the second time.

> *Positioning can be an effective way of working with boundaries. If the therapist wants to create or strengthen a boundary, he can bring members of a subsystem to the center of the room and have other family members move their chairs back so that they can observe but cannot interrupt. If he wants to block contact between two members, he can separate them or, he can position himself between them and act as go-between. Spatial manipulation has the power of simplicity. (16)*

Marking Boundaries

The therapist may have to protect not only subsystem boundaries but individual boundaries as well. Minuchin and Satir clearly agree that the following should be established early in the course of an interview:

The therapist and family should listen to what a family member says and acknowledge his or her communication.

Family members should talk to each other, not about each other.

Family members should not answer a question directed to another or talk about other family members.

Family members should not require one member to act as the memory bank for all the family.

Subsystem boundaries can be marked in several ways. In the case of Jennifer Maloney, the therapist marked the spouse boundary by excluding the child from the sessions while encouraging a more appropriate boundary between father and daughter by placing Mr. Maloney in charge of the nighttime episodes. He strengthened a parent boundary between Jennifer and her mother when he applauded the mother's suggestion that she withdraw by taking a ride in the car at night.

Escalating Stress

The purpose of increasing stress in an already stressed family is to give the therapist "and sometimes the family members themselves, an inkling of the family's capability to restructure when circumstances change. His input and his expert prodding produce new contexts, or changed circumstances, to which the family must adapt under his eye" (17). Minuchin suggests four methods

The simplest maneuver is to dam the flow of accustomed communication. When Mr. Thompkins is silenced so his wife and daughter can discuss stealing without interruption, something different may come of that conversation. This is called "blocking transactional patterns."

A second technique has the therapist increase stress by "emphasizing differences and disagreements." The therapist may say, "Whew! You two obviously don't agree on that issue! Will you discuss it now?"

A family often minimizes or avoids open conflict in subtle, yet predictable ways. A therapist may want to avoid this automatic "derailing" by the family and increase their stress through what Minuchin terms "developing implicit conflict." A child who persistently interrupts when his parents approach conflict with one another may need to be silenced. A spouse may need to be encouraged to stand his or her ground and not give up so quickly.

Minuchin terms the fourth method for escalating stress "joining in alliance or coalition." In the example immediately preceding, the therapist and the spouse being encouraged to stand his ground are temporarily joined in coalition. This method requires careful planning and an ability to disengage, so that the therapist is not sucked into the family war and alliances. There is also risk with this technique because coalition with one family member may alienate other family members. The whole family may not return. Alliances with individual family members should always be transitional and temporary.

Assigning Tasks

A therapist may use tasks within the session and may also assign homework. When the therapist requests that two individuals "talk about it now," he is assigning a task. Nonverbal tasks may require family member to participate on a project such as the conjoint drawing mentioned in chapter 2. When the family accomplishes assigned tasks at home, "they are in effect taking the therapist home with them. The interviewer becomes the maker of rules beyond the structure of the session" (18). Tasks must be carefully developed to fit the family and further the therapeutic goals. In the Maloney family, the task was to practice a new method for handling nighttime sleep disturbance. The assignment required a careful appraisal of the family's structure and a goal for restructuring. The use of tasks in family counseling is discussed in more detail later in this chapter.

Using Symptoms

Symptoms can be handled several ways by the therapist. Focusing on the symptom is a familiar role for physicians, and the family is comfortable with this method because often everyone is convinced that "things in our family would be perfect if Jennifer would sleep through the night and go to school." Although focusing on the symptom is clearly essential in some situations (e.g., fire-setting, school phobia, starvation, refusal to take lifesaving insulin), careful attention to family structure must be maintained. A careful blending of the two is illustrated elegantly in a famous case from Minuchin's former group at the Philadelphia Child Guidance Clinic. Haley was the therapist's supervisor in this case, which is summarized in the writings of both men and is also available as a film. As Minuchin tells it, a school age child:

> comes into therapy with a dog phobia that is so severe he is almost confined to the house. The therapist's diagnosis is that the symptom is supported by an implicit unresolved conflict between spouses, manifested in an affiliation between mother and son that excludes the father. His strategy is to increase the affiliation between the father and son before tackling the spouse subsystem problems. Therefore he encourages the father, who is a mailman "and therefore an expert in dealing with dogs," to teach his son how to deal with strange dogs. The child, who is adopted, in turn adopts a dog, and the father and son join in transactions around the dog. This activity strengthens their relationship and promotes a separation between mother and son. As the symptom disappears, the therapist praises both parents for their successful handling of the child. He then moves to work with the husband-wife conflicts. (19)

We agree with Minuchin's view that a focus on symptoms as an entry into the family system of interactions produces more than superficial changes.

A therapist may even want to exaggerate a symptom in some cases. In an interview by one of our staff with the family of a child hospitalized for psychosomatic nausea and vomiting, each time parental conflict was approached, the child retched, disrupting the interview and producing a chaotic scene. The therapist encouraged the child's vomiting, handed him a wastebasket, and even asked him to vomit more, deliberately requesting the family to wait while John threw up. The vomiting stopped and did not return for the remainder of the interview.

De-emphasizing the symptom is also useful, according to Minuchin. Implementation of this strategy is found in his work with anorexia nervosa: "At times it is possible to use the symptom as an avenue away from the identified patient. The technique of having lunch with an anorectic patient and her family, for example, facilitates the creation, within the field of eating, of a strong interpersonal conflict, which then takes precedence over the symptom" (20). With most anorectic patients, Minuchin conducts a family luncheon interview in the early stages of therapy. He and the family eat together, usually before the child's discharge from the hospital. In the course of this interview, many noneating issues are addressed. In the process of what is often a heated interview, the anorectic patient frequently begins to pick at her food and eventually puts some in her mouth. This action is not usually directly commented on by the interviewer. The effectiveness of this successful intervention from the 1970s is more striking when recognizing the evolving complex layers surrounding both the pathogenesis and treatment of anorexia that are available now but were not at the time of Minuchin's work.

Symptoms can be used in other ways as well. A therapist may move to a new symptom. For example, when discussing a child's avoidance of school, the mother revealed her own reluctance to be home alone during the day. The interviewer then moved to this issue. A therapist may occasionally relabel a symptom. A child who has run away from home may benefit (and so may the parents) from having her action described by the therapist as a desperate maneuver to get close to her parents through the reunion that has just occurred with her return.

Manipulating Mood or Encouraging the Problem Interaction

Delineating a family's predominant mood is part of determining its structure. A therapist can use this knowledge for restructuring. For example, the therapist can exaggerate a family mood to illogical extremes. In our own work, two overprotective parents were encouraged to such an extent by the therapist that even they wanted to back off after a time:

Mother:	I want her home 20 minutes after school is out. Children should not be unsupervised. They get into trouble.
Doctor:	Maybe 20 minutes is too long unsupervised, Mrs. Jarvis.
Mother:	Well, she has to have some time to get from school to the house. It's several blocks.
Doctor:	But 20 minutes . . . I don't know. I agree with you; kids can get into a lot of trouble and in less than 20 minutes. Have you considered picking her up in the car at school?
Father:	Excuse me for interrupting, Doctor, but I think you're wrong there. First of all, Madelyn works and couldn't possibly pick up Ellen. And second, Ellen has to learn that we trust her by herself. Twenty minutes! That's such a little while. If you can't trust your own child for 20 minutes . . . ?
Mother:	Exactly.
Doctor:	I see. Since you brought that up, what are some of the other ways in which you are letting Ellen know that you trust her own abilities?

Support, Education, and Guidance

Support, education, and guidance are self-evident. Minuchin includes them last in his list of restructuring techniques and gives them less than a page. Yet these maneuvers are among those most familiar to physicians and should not be minimized. However, because they can be frustratingly ineffective with a dysfunctional family, neither should they be used to the exclusion of other techniques. Support is essential in work with families, but it is not enough by itself to do the trick.

JAY HALEY AND PROBLEM-SOLVING THERAPY

Haley is another individual who has strongly influenced the development of our clinical approaches. As a family therapist, he became interested in power struggles among family members, but more particularly those between a therapist and the patient (i.e., the family). In *Strategies of Psychotherapy*, he suggested that any relationship is by definition a power struggle because those involved are constantly struggling to define or redefine their relationship (21). The relationship between a therapist and a patient is also a power struggle, where the therapist must win or control if change is to occur. His tactics (the word is his) for producing change are rooted in paradox and hypnosis. Haley acknowledges his debt to Dr. Milton Erickson's innovative development of indirect hypnotic methods in psychiatric treatment (22,23).

It is not this portion of Haley's work, but rather his later views that we wish to review. In his book *Problem-Solving Therapy* (24), he elaborates a therapy approach that:

> *focuses on solving a client's presenting problems within the framework of the family. . . . The therapist's task is to formulate a presenting symptom clearly and to design an intervention in the client's social situation to change that presenting symptom. . . . The approach here differs from other symptom-oriented therapies in that it emphasizes the social context of human problems. (25)*

"Solving problems" is important to Haley, and he does not beat around the bush: "The first obligation of a therapist is to change the presenting problem offered. If that is not accomplished, the therapy is a failure" (26).

Giving Directives

A cornerstone of Haley's therapeutic approach is developing the ability to give directives successfully. Giving directives or tasks serves several purposes. First, because the main goal of therapy is to get people to behave differently, directives are a way of creating such changes. Second, directives may be used to intensify a relationship between a family and their therapist. "By telling people what to do, a therapist becomes involved in the action. He becomes important because the person must either do or not do what the therapist says" (27). Third, directives are used to gather information. A family reveals itself according to how it responds to directives given.

A directive includes anything done in therapy by the therapist to the family, ranging from a simple nod to an elaborate homework assignment.

Some therapists are uncomfortable about giving directives because they feel perhaps they should not take the responsibility for telling someone what to do. It is important to emphasize that directives can be given directly or they can be given in a conversation implicitly by vocal intonation, body movement, and well-timed silence. Everything done in therapy can be seen as a directive. If an individual or a family in an interview is talking about something and the therapist says, "tell me more about that," he is giving a directive. If the therapist only nods his head and smiles, encouraging them to continue, that is also a directive. If someone says something the therapist does not like, he can tell the person not to say that any more—and that is telling him what to do. If the therapist turns his body away from the person and frowns, he is also telling the person that he should not say that sort of thing. (28)

According to Haley, there are several types of directives, which are outlined in the following categories:

A. Telling people what to do when the therapist wants them to do it
    1. Telling someone to stop doing something
    2. Telling someone to do something different
        a. Giving good advice
        b. Giving directives to change the sequence in a family.
B. Telling people what to do when the therapist does not want them to do it—because the therapist wants them to change by rebelling.

Telling someone to stop doing something is one of the most difficult directives to enforce, Haley states.

If the therapist tells someone to stop usual behavior, he must usually go to an extreme or get other family members to cooperate and change their behavior to support him in this task. Often it is like trying to stop a river from flowing; one can try to block it, but the river will go over and around the block and the therapist will drown. (29)

He is even more pessimistic about giving good advice. "Giving good advice means the therapist assumes that people have rational control of what they are doing. To be successful in the therapy business it may be better to drop that idea" (30). In our experience, good advice is often useless in helping families change.

Thus, if the objective is to have a family do the task, the therapist should use a directive that will change the sequence in a family and motivate the members to do it because there is something to gain. Previously, we have introduced several terms that, although different, relate to each other. Jackson refers to "family homeostasis," Satir uses the term "family system," Minuchin discusses "family structure," and now Haley introduces "family sequence." These terms reflect how each of these clinicians has conceptualized the family unit. Homeostasis suggests a balancing process. System involves balancing through communication patterns. Structure suggests an emphasis on configuration and organization. Sequence reflects Haley's view that family members operate with one another in predictable, repetitive sequences, which are based on each family's specific organizational pattern. A therapist, hoping to effect change in a family, must determine the family's sequence and change it.

Haley offers some advice for designing tasks. Although designing tasks may seem difficult at first, the process gets easier with practice and experience. Whatever the task, it should be simple enough that the family can do it. The best task is one that uses the presenting problem to make a structural change in the family. Using this approach, the focus is on respecting and using what the family considers important (i.e., the problem) and what the therapist thinks is important (i.e., an organizational change). The steps in designing a task include thinking about the presenting problem in terms of the sequence in the family and finding a directive that changes both.

For instance, a common problem is when a child (e.g., Jennifer Maloney) refuses to go to school. Haley suggests that the necessary first step is to determine that the problem does not stem from a school situation.

Second, the therapist must motivate the parents to work together by having them agree that the child must go to school. At this point, it is made clear that a decision to attend school is made by the parents, not the child. The therapist needs to pull the parents together in relation to the child.

The therapist then gives a directive that takes the family's usual sequence around the problem into account. The Maloney's sequence is an example:

1. The father insisted that the child go to school; he then left for work.
2. Jennifer manifested anxiety.
3. The mother, alone with Jennifer, felt overwhelmed and gave in.
4. The father subsequently criticized his wife for her helplessness.

5. The mother protested that father was insensitive.
6. The father continued to insist that the child go to school and again left for work.

Various directives are possible in such a sequence. The responsibility for taking the child to school might be given to the father or mother. The therapist might say that the mother must see that the father take the child to school. It may be appropriate that both parents escort the child to class. In the Maloney case, responsibility was given to the mother for getting Jennifer to school, with the father available to help.

In this straightforward task, Haley states that a crucial issue is anticipating what will happen. The therapist can review with each parent how he or she will take the child to school. The parents are then asked to discuss how the child will probably behave (e.g., temper, tears, upset stomach). The mother is asked what she will do when the child becomes upset; likewise, the father is asked to consider his reactions. The contingencies are all discussed beforehand in a "dry run" in the office. The family may even be asked to practice the task in front of the therapist.

Motivation

Haley offers specific suggestions for motivating a family to follow a directive. He may urge them directly to follow through in order to find a solution to their dilemma. However, even families in profound pain are not always cooperative. In these situations, more indirect methods may be necessary. For example, the therapist may encourage family members to "talk about how desperate their situation is. Rather than reassure them it is not so bad, the therapist can agree with them that it is quite bad. If the situation is made to appear desperate enough, they will listen to the therapist and do the task he offers" (31). The therapist must also fit the task to the family. Some families with a flair for the dramatic will warm to a task if it is described as huge and overwhelming. A resistant family, on the other hand, may find a small task easier to accomplish. Attention to a family's general style (e.g., informal, organized, cautious) suggests direction for presenting a task successfully. A family that is hopelessly pessimistic may be pushed into success if the therapist agrees with their pessimism: "I don't think this family will be able to carry this off. I am suggesting it, but I want you to know that I have grave doubts that you can do it at this time."

Specific Directions

The therapist should be precise and specific when giving directions. Directions should be clearly defined rather than suggested: "I would like you to . . . " brings more success than, "You might like to think about. . . ." Minuchin says specificity is important for two reasons: it helps to get the task done, and it if is not done, the therapist needs to be sure that it has not gone unfinished simply because the instructions were confusing.

Family Participation

The best directives involve all family members. For Jennifer's school difficulties, everyone was assigned some job: Jennifer was responsible for her own time before school, Mrs. Maloney was responsible for getting her out the door at 9:25, and Mr. Maloney was assigned the task of being available by telephone to assist as needed.

> *A good task has something for everyone. Even if the therapist specifically asks someone to stay out of the task, this request is still giving the person something to do. The task should be structured like any other piece of work. Someone is needed to do the job, someone to help, someone to supervise, someone to plan, someone to check to see that it gets done, and so on. (32)*

Haley also recommends that family members review their part in front of the therapist as further assurance that the task is understood. The therapist should anticipate noncompliance on the family's part and handle it in advance by reviewing the many ways in which each member might defeat successful completion of the task. Following the family's agreement to the plan, a therapist may do this by asking each person, "How could you contribute to the failure of the project? What are some ways?" If none are forthcoming, the therapist may make his own suggestions regarding sabotage efforts. When these efforts are explicitly discussed before the event, they are seldom used to defeat the task.

Reporting the Results

The therapist should always ask for a report at the next interview. Haley suggests that if the family has done the task, congratulations are in order and the interview should continue from there. If the family has only partially done their job, an exploration of this partial failure is necessary. Haley feels strongly that failure to do what a therapist asks should never be treated lightly. To allow a family to do so suggests that what the therapist has requested is not important. This then makes the therapist less important and makes it less likely that they will do the next assigned task.

Paradoxical Directives

Paradoxical tasks involve telling people what to do when the therapist does not want them to do it because the therapist wants them to change by rebelling. This approach is based on the idea that some families who come for help are resistant to that help. With all families, some resistance to change is met in treatment. The members are good at getting a therapist to try and fail. The therapist is then pulling at the family members to improve while they are resisting and provoking him to go on pulling. This situation is frustrating for both the therapist and the family (33).

A paradoxical task always has two levels: *change* and *do not change*. A brief example from our own work illustrates this technique. A family arrived asking for help with their two boys, ages 7 and 9 years. The boys fought constantly, and nowhere was it more troublesome than at the dinner table. Usually within 10 minutes, the entire family was engaged in a dispute, with resulting alienation and indigestion among all four. The therapist suggested that this family needed to fight for some reason, and because their fights were so exhausting, they should never fight on an empty stomach. Therefore he was asking them to fight even more, particularly at the dinner table. He designed a task in which the family was to have a serious fight at the dinner table every night for 14 consecutive nights. Specific roles were assigned to every family member. The family failed magnificently at the task. Two meager altercations were all they could produce, and they noticed that they were no longer involved in arguments with one another at other times. The therapist subsequently moved to other issues, and fighting did not return as a family issue.

Haley believes that families such as this achieve the goal of therapy to prove to the therapist that they are as good as other people. He believes that the therapist must accept the change when it happens and let the family put the therapist down by proving him or her wrong.

If he wants to ensure that the change continue, he might say to the members that probably the change is only temporary and they will relapse again. Then the family will continue the change to prove to him that it is not temporary. . . . He can do the same by encouraging a relapse. He can say to the family, I can see you've changed and are over the problem, but I think this has happened too fast. I would like you to have a relapse and this week go back to the way you were before. . . . To make this directive reasonable to family members, the therapist might say that too fast a change is upsetting. (34)

Eight Steps to Successful Paradoxical Intervention

Haley cautions that considerable skill is necessary in using a paradoxical approach. Although issues are serious and distressing, the therapist must be able to conceptualize them in playful and fanciful ways. Haley lists eight stages of a successful paradoxical intervention:

1. As in all directive therapy, the therapist works toward establishing a relationship defined as one to bring about change.
2. The therapist helps the family clearly define the problem to be treated.
3. The therapist sets clear goals of treatment.
4. The therapist offers a plan that makes the directive reasonable in the family's view.
5. The therapist gracefully disqualifies the current authority (i.e., a family member) on the problem. Usually someone is trying to help the patient solve the problem. That person must be defined as not doing the right thing.
6. The therapist gives the paradoxical directive.
7. The therapist observes the family's response and continues to encourage the usual behavior. If the family improves and is less symptomatic, the therapist labels that as not cooperating.
8. As changes continue, the therapist avoids credit for the change. Otherwise, relapses will occur.

In our work, we find the use of directives very effective. The majority of directives we employ are those in which we intend the family to do what we ask. Our use of paradoxical tasks with families is considerably less frequent. For further understanding of paradox and its use in family interviews, we suggest the work of Maria Selvini Palazzoli and her coworkers. That group, in Milan, Italy, raised paradoxical strategy to the level of an art form with the publication of *Paradox and Counterparadox* and subsequent writings (35). Their approach requires considerable training and is probably more complex to implement than is desired by most trainees.

Family Organization and Hierarchy

Haley notes that the people in a family, with their common history and future, follow organized ways of behaving with one another. Family members followed patterned, redundant ways of behaving, forming a hierarchy. A family hierarchy at its simplest level consists of a generation of parents who nurture and discipline a second generation (i.e., the children), who then become parents and nurture and discipline a third generation. The family must deal with the issue of hierarchy, and rules should be developed regarding who is primary and secondary in status and power. Haley believes that when an individual displays symptoms, the family organization has a hierarchical arrangement that has become unclear and confused.

> *If there is a fundamental rule of social organization, it is that an organization is in trouble when coalitions occur across levels of a hierarchy, particularly when these coalitions are secret. When an employer plays favorites among his employees, he is forming coalitions across power lines and joining one employee against another. (36)*

In this illustration by Haley, the hierarchy has become unclear. When family members cross hierarchical, generational boundaries to form coalitions, the family is in trouble, resulting in symptomatology in one or more family members. For example, Mrs. Maloney and her daughter had certainly, with their coalition, toppled the generational organization and hierarchy of the Maloney family. How do coalitions across generational lines produce symptoms? To answer this question, one must understand what Haley has to say about family sequences.

Family Sequences

We have referred to Haley's use of the term "sequence" in describing a family's behavior. He feels that family members organize themselves around repetitive sequences of behavior and that these sequences ultimately develop into repeating cycles. These sequences can reflect dysfunction when the following conditions are present (in a family of at least three individuals) and interfere with the usual clear hierarchy of a family's organization:

1. The three people responding to one another are not peers but of different generations.
2. The member of one generation forms a coalition across generations with another family member and against a generation peer.
3. The coalition across generations is denied or concealed.

Certain problem sequences are common in Haley's experience. One example involves three generations:

The classic situation is made up of grandmother, mother, and problem child. That is the typical one-parent family situation among the poor and middle-class when a mother has divorced and returned to her mother. In the classic example the grandmother tends to be defined as dominating, the mother as irresponsible, and the child as a behavior problem. The typical sequence is as follows:

1. Grandmother takes care of grandchild while protesting that mother is irresponsible and does not take care of the child properly. In this way grandmother is siding with the child against the mother in a coalition across generation lines.
2. Mother withdraws, letting grandmother care for the child.
3. The child misbehaves or expresses symptomatic behavior.
4. Grandmother protests that she should not have to take care of the child and discipline him. She has raised her children, and mother should take care of her own child.
5. Mother begins to take care of her own child.
6. Grandmother protests that mother does not know how to take care of the child properly and is being irresponsible. She takes over the care of the grandchild to save the child from the mother.
7. Mother withdraws, letting grandmother care for the child.
8. The child misbehaves or expresses symptomatic behavior. (37)

This sequence was deftly executed by Joan Locksley, her mother, and her grandmother in chapter 1.

Haley feels that this same sequence can present itself in a family without a grandparent—one in which there is a single parent and many children. In such families, often one child (usually the oldest) is designated a "parent-child" (i.e., a parent figure to the younger children). This child, like the mother in the previous example, often ends up temporarily in charge of others, only to be labeled as irresponsible and incompetent. The previous sequence then asserts itself and repeats.

Two-generation conflicts also produce recognizable, symptomatic sequences, the most common of which involves one parent in coalition with a child against the other parent.

1. One parent, usually the mother, is in an intense relationship with the child. By intense is meant a relationship that is both positive and negative and where the responses of each person are exaggeratedly important. The mother attempts to deal with the child with a mixture of affection and exasperation.
2. The child's symptomatic behavior becomes more extreme.
3. The mother, or the child, calls on the father for assistance in resolving their difficulty.
4. The father steps in to take charge and deal with the child.
5. Mother reacts against father, insisting that he is not dealing with the situation properly. Mother can react with an attack or a threat to break off the relationship with father. The threat to leave may be as indirect as "I want a vacation by myself," or as direct as "I want a divorce."
6. Father withdraws, giving up the attempt to disengage mother and child.
7. Mother and child deal with each other in a mixture of affection and exasperation until they reach a point where they are at an impasse. (38)

For Haley, family therapy in any of these situations involves the ability to change the identified sequences. This type of therapy is best accomplished in stages, he maintains. The therapist combines his observations of the family's hierarchy and repetitive sequences, then develops strategies for change. The goal is to change a sequence by preventing coalitions across generational lines. When these coalitions are prevented, the family is required to function differently.

A RETURN TO THE MALONEY FAMILY

The treatment of the Maloney family represents a blend of the approaches suggested by both Minuchin and Haley. Minuchin's influence in this case was discussed earlier. According to Haley's view, the Maloneys are a proto-type of the family he describes as having a "two-generation conflict" or an overintense parent–child dyad that alternately includes and excludes the other parent. In these cases, Haley suggests that a therapist may initiate changes in the family sequence by using the peripheral person (entering through the father–child relationship), breaking up the dyad with a task (entering through the mother–child relationship), or entering directly through the parents with a focus on their relationship. Jennifer's pediatrician chose the first technique of using the peripheral person (i.e., Mr. Maloney). The pediatrician suggested that Mr. Maloney enter the nighttime scene, handling Jennifer's "night terrors," providing his wife with a rest. Mr. Maloney had tried to deal with Jennifer previously and met with opposition from his wife. He had then criticized Mrs. Maloney for being over-protective, reinforcing in her eyes the belief that he could not possibly have the sensitivity to understand the situation. Activating the father again by the therapist required careful thought so that the mother would not be an-tagonized. She could not be made to feel, for example, that Mr. Maloney was being brought in because she had failed. For Mrs. Maloney to accept her husband's participation, the pediatrician did several things:

1. He validated her efforts to date.
2. He sympathized with her exhaustion.
3. He supported her key position in the suggested task; only her husband could teach her daughter respect for men, but only she could provide the opportunity for that to take place.
4. He appealed to her sense of good mothering by asking her cooperation in having her daughter learn one of life's essential lessons, respect for men.

The pediatrician, the task, and the family were successful in producing a decided change in this family's sequence. Jennifer and her parents ulti-mately passed through three stages with the therapist before sessions were terminated.

1. Stage one: coalition among therapist, peripheral person, and child
2. Stage two: involvement between therapist and adults, without child
3. Stage three: disengagement of the therapist from the adults and from the family

Haley notes that these stages are required in most instances of problem-solving therapy. The process of change cannot be made in one leap.

Regarding the Maloney family, stage one was discussed in the summary of their treatment. Jennifer, Mr. Maloney, and the pediatrician became involved in an activity, while Mrs. Maloney was gently shifted to the periphery. The second stage involved the mother, father, and pediatrician, while Jennifer dropped out of the adult struggle and was free to pursue life with her peers. Jennifer being excluded from sessions after the initial interview was one indication of stage two. But stage two also included four or five sessions devoted to husband–wife discussions of their marital relationship and how each could derive more satisfaction in that relationship. Their increasing satisfaction with one another led logically to stage three, when the pediatrician could disengage from the couple, leaving them involved with each other and feeling that they no longer needed the pediatrician's help. Jennifer continued to develop good relationships with friends.

References

1. Minuchin S, Rosman B, Baker L. Psychosomatic families: anorexia nervosa in context. Cambridge, MA: Harvard University Press, 1976.
2. Minuchin S. Families and family therapy. Cambridge, MA: Harvard University Press, 1974.
3. Minuchin S, Fishman HC. Family therapy techniques. Cambridge, MA: Harvard University Press, 1981.
4. Minuchin S, Rosman B, Baker L. Psychosomatic families: anorexia nervosa in context. Cambridge, MA: Harvard University Press, 1976.
5. Minuchin, 14.
6. Minuchin, 11.
7. Minuchin, 55.
8. Haley J. Problem-solving therapy. 2nd ed. San Francisco: Jossey-Bass, 1987.
9. Haley, 8.
10. Minuchin, 111.
11. Minuchin, 119.
12. Minuchin, 123.
13. Minuchin, 127.
14. Minuchin, 128.
15. Minuchin, 141.
16. Minuchin, 143.
17. Minuchin, 147.

18. Minuchin, 151.
19. Minuchin, 153.
20. Minuchin, 154.
21. Haley J. Strategies of psychotherapy. New York: Grune & Stratton, 1963.
22. Haley J. Advanced techniques of hypnosis and therapy: selected papers of Milton H. Erickson, MD. New York: Grune & Stratton, 1967.
23. Haley J. Uncommon therapy: the psychiatric techniques of Milton H Erickson, MD. New York: WW Norton & Company, 1973.
24. Haley, Problem-solving therapy.
25. Haley, Problem-solving therapy, 1.
26. Haley J. Problem-solving therapy. 2nd ed. San Francisco: Jossey-Bass, 1987:35.
27. Haley, Problem-solving therapy, 2nd ed, 56.
28. Haley, Problem-solving therapy, 57.
29. Haley, Problem-solving therapy, 60.
30. Haley, Problem-solving therapy, 61.
31. Haley, Problem-solving therapy, 63.
32. Haley, Problem-solving therapy, 66.
33. Haley, Problem-solving therapy, 77.
34. Haley, Problem-solving therapy, 78.
35. Palazzoli MS. Paradox and counterparadox. Northvale, NJ: Jason Aronson, 1990.
36. Haley, Problem-solving therapy, 111.
37. Haley, Problem-solving therapy, 117.
38. Haley, Problem-solving therapy, 121–122.

part **II**

Clinical Application

chapter 4

Designing the Clinical Setting for Family Interviewing

WHEN TO CALL A FAMILY INTERVIEW

Before determining who will attend the session, one must settle the question of exactly when a family interview is needed. Our trainees, undertaking their first experience as interviewers, almost universally ask that question, partly because of performance anxiety and partly because of the need to learn when family interviewing is appropriate. We suggest to the trainees that they examine their degree of involvement with a family to answer that question. Three clinical situations usually dictate their degree of involvement.

Clinical Situation 1

In this situation, concerns are brought up in the course of well-child or episodic medical visits. The practitioner, usually with one parent and the child, focuses on the problem as stated and offers guidance, conventional wisdom, advice, and counsel, all within the confines of the office schedule and usual practice demands. This level of care requires perceptive listening and effective history-taking skills. The practitioner must also have a sound knowledge of predictable child behavior and development and a familiarity with parent management techniques. Family interviews are not usually needed in these cases.

Clinical Situation 2

Situation 2 occurs when the clinician suspects that the advice offered is not sufficient. This may be noticed when the advice is ignored, stated problems recur or intensify, problems begin to center on relational issues, or the clinician is confused about the problem and its cause. At this point, we encourage our trainees to broaden their inquiry toward a family focus. A family interview is often useful in these cases.

Clinical Situation 3

The pediatrician realizes, in this situation, that after conducting one or several family interviews, the child and family will require further professional assistance. At this point, the pediatrician may decide to continue treatment with more elaborate therapy efforts or to refer the family to someone else with more specific training and skills to continue the work.

The concept of degrees of involvement with a family has some advantages, offering different domains of knowledge and comfort zones for clinicians to embrace or avoid while developing their clinical approaches to children. The concept also provides a predictable sequence by which to gauge patient needs and clinician effectiveness. At any point, a clinician may review whether the care being provided is appropriate to the clinical concern brought by the family. Finally, because success in each situation is usually helped by work in the preceding situation, the concept can also serve as a triage device for determining those families in need of family interviewing.

ATTENDANCE ISSUES

Parents

Having determined that a family interview is indicated, the physician must then decide who should attend, within and even outside the immediate family. Until the mid-1980s, fathers of children with behavioral issues generally were thought to be unavailable, uninterested, unaware, and uncooperative. Stereotypes of fathers from that time included the hard worker who was too busy to participate in his children's medical care and the insensitive man who bristled at the mention of behavioral difficulties in his children. These behaviors were reinforced by mothers who made their own stereotypic excuses for their husband's uninvolvement (e.g., "He's working 12 hours a day, 7 days a week," "He and I don't see eye to eye on this," "He's out of town," "He doesn't trust doctors," and "He doesn't know I'm coming in."). In spite of these prevailing attitudes, when we began family work in the 1960s, we discovered that fathers were not nearly as hopeless as we had been led to believe. It became clear that attendance at family interviews was a direct function of the interviewer's expectations. We insisted that both parents attend, and by and large, they did.

Today, of course, the roles and rules of parenting have shifted, with responsibilities no longer clearly divided along gender lines. When attendance problems arise based on work commitments and scheduling conflicts, it is just as often the mother who is the problematic nonattendee. Whether it is the mother or father who is protesting participation in a family interview, clear interviewer expectations regarding attendance is an effective mobilizer. We, our trainees, and our entire staff expect that both the mother and father will attend the family interview, and they do.

Clearly stated expectations by the physician are not used as threats with parents. Instead, expectations communicate the importance of a parent's role in the family and the essential contribution of that individual's perspective. Satir stated, "Once the therapist convinces the husband that he is essential to the therapy process, and that no one else can speak for him or take his place . . . in family life, he readily enters in" (1). This statement, although reflecting gender roles of the past, is accurate and applies to wives and husbands.

We are considerably cautious in accepting either parent's vigorous stand (usually on the telephone before the first interview) that the other parent will not attend. This parent's claim may indicate his or her need to control the interview, the family, and the interviewer. We usually request to speak to the other parent directly, offering to call at work or in the evening. This gentle insistence on the need for input from that parent for help with a solution often succeeds, motivating both parents to attend the initial interview, which is the most difficult single step. Subsequent participation depends on the problem and the therapist's ingenuity at accommodating and using that parent in a solution of the family's difficulty. We have found that concessions (e.g., late afternoon and evening appointments) usually solve the conflicts with work responsibilities.

Divorced Parents

With a divorced couple, we often encourage both parents to attend the initial session if they have a relationship that allows such a meeting and if both individuals are actively involved in the parenting of their children. The interviewer must use discretion as to the continuing participation of both divorced parents in subsequent interviews. Having divorced individuals bring their new partners to the interview can be useful or dicey and should be discussed in advance. Such sessions can become volatile.

Children

There is some controversy over which children, if any, should be included in family interviews. Satir began treatment by seeing parents alone for one or two sessions, establishing their expectations of therapy and shifting the focus from the identified patient to the family as a whole. She subsequently included the children, often determining by age who would become regular participants in ongoing meetings. Other therapists, believing that children's behavioral difficulties reflect a marital neurosis, exclude children from the beginning and work exclusively with the parents. Still others prefer to work with only the identified patient and the parents, bringing in other children as the situation warrants.

In 1979, we always requested that both parents and all children attend at least the first interview in order to observe the family system with all of its members. Now, our stance is more flexible. We usually meet with parents alone for an introductory session. If family work seems indicated, we arrange the first conjoint family interview to include at least both parents and the identified patient. Siblings are invited to attend from the outset as the situation warrants. Harry Aponte has said that "those who are asked to attend are those necessary to get the job done" (2). We agree with this statement, despite its apparent opposition to the theoretical view that *all* family members influence a family system. Aponte's method acknowledges the realities of scheduling in a busy clinical practice. When the rule is that everyone must attend every meeting, family interviews can be delayed repeatedly. Cancellations and rescheduling often halts the family's progress.

Although working with only part of the family may be more efficient, there are some pitfalls. For example, the Bensons originally asked for help with their 8-year-old daughter, Brenda, who refused to attend school. No mention was made of James, aside from the fact that he was Brenda's twin brother. Following our former dictum that everyone in the family must attend the initial interview, James came along. His withdrawal and depression were obvious. Such information would have been missing from the family's story without James' attendance.

Others

If grandparents or other relatives are living at home and appear to be a part of the family system, they are encouraged to participate in family interviews. Some family therapists, particularly the late Carl Whitaker and the late Murray Bowen, emphasized the three-generational aspect of most families. Each wrote extensively on this subject (3,4).

An individual's "family" is not necessarily limited by bloodlines. It is a logical idea that therapy with an individual should include everyone who is important to that person's basic structure of relationships. This approach, called network therapy, was developed by Ross Speck and Carolyn Attneave (5). Network therapy may include conjoint interviewing of 10 to 20 individuals, those within the family and outside it who are strongly involved in the patient's life. Network therapy is not a concept we have used. Our need for order has steered us away from interviewing crowds.

TIME AND MONEY ISSUES

We understand that the ideas and approaches suggested in this text cannot be compressed into a typical office follow-up visit, which may already include an interval history, reexamination of a 3-year-old with bilateral otitis media, and her refusal to provide a urine specimen. One of our first rules for trainees entering a family interview is that they must provide for their own comfort during work with the family. We call this "making room for oneself." Unless interviewers attend to their own needs quickly, a family session disintegrates into at least, boredom, and at most, chaos. This rule applies equally to physicians in a clinical practice setting. Their attention to time is essential for both their comfort and success in the interview. Redesigning certain office procedures may be necessary.

Billing Time

Our family interviews generally last for 1 hour, although some families (e.g., those with young children) may be seen for 30 minutes. There are some clinical situations when a 2-hour appointment has worked well. Each interview seems to require some settling-in time for the family as they get down to business. One hour usually allows for this settling-in process. Whatever time period is chosen, it must be protected by the physician and office staff. We do not accept calls or interruptions, except for emergencies, during a family interview.

We also recognize that time is a precious commodity for the pediatrician, who may be able to make considerable "room for oneself" regarding office time but experiences great discomfort if the office rent is not being paid. Therefore, we are not proposing that a doctor see families for 60 minutes, charging only for the customary 15-minute follow-up visit. The physician has a responsibility to himself and his staff to charge for his time, which may mean the billing equivalent of four 15-minute appointments. Some may question whether families will use services charged in this way. The answer is an overwhelming yes, according to our experience and that of our graduates who have entered clinical practices. Specific settings in which pediatricians have successfully used family interviews with a fee-for-service billing system have included university medical center outpatient clinics, private solo pediatric practices, small group pediatric practices, large prepaid health care facilities, state-supported health care clinics, and consultative pediatric practices limited to family counseling for behavioral and developmental disorders.

Health Care Reimbursement

If families have shown themselves willing to pay for the pediatrician's time and talent, what about third-party payers, particularly those prominent in the 1990s? It remains to be seen just how managed care and capitation as reimbursement mechanisms will affect a physician's ability to incorporate family interviews into the economics of a clinical pediatric practice. Managed care and capitation are seen by many, including us, as antithetical to the delivery of good quality, comprehensive medical care. However, Laurel Leslie has suggested that the treatment of some mental health problems by primary care physicians, including pediatricians, may become an economically desired component of managed care, one even encouraged by some health maintenance organizations.

A fundamental premise of managed care is that generalists provide less costly health care than subspecialists. Primary care physicians who have

*training in preventive care and are able to treat minor surgical, derma-
tologic, and mental health problems are in demand. Training in these areas already has been identified by physicians as desirable. . . . Generalists
are also perceived as providing more cost-effective care than specialists because of their focus on common causes of patients' complaints and their
reduced use of tests and procedures. . . . Several of the managed care groups
in California have expressed interest in hiring generalists with expertise
in particular subspecialties who might spend a percentage of their time
following the patients in their subspecialties. (6)*

Were such a role for primary care providers encouraged, pediatricians
might well find themselves in the cat-bird seat for practicing with a family
orientation, using family interviews and being adequately reimbursed for
the services provided.

A project in Oregon illustrates a successful managed care pilot program
for children with emotional and behavioral disabilities. This project re-
portedly delivered comprehensive, family-centered services (including
family therapy) to children with emotional difficulties at a cost of less than
half the average monthly cost of equivalent outpatient Medicaid services.
Although the report does not specify what sort of health care provider performed the family interviews, we are encouraged by two implications. The
first implication is that managed care has considered the discipline of family therapy worthy of inclusion in a health care package. The second is that
the cost effectiveness of such an approach has been documented. *Families
at the Center of the Development of a System of Care* by Naomi Tanner is also
encouraging, describing the development of a family-designed system of
care for children with emotional or behavioral disabilities in Essex County,
New York, presenting the practical steps taken to build a system based on
what families say they need and want (7,8). Managed care and family interviews may have a future together after all.

Value of Service

Regardless of the external economic forces that determine an approach to
clinical problems, the concept of expectations, an internal force, remains
very important. If pediatricians have been trained in the principles of a
family orientation and have effectively conducted family interviews, then
those physicians will expect and view family interviewing to be a valuable,

even essential part of quality pediatric care. This expectation will lead them
to be more effective advocates and teachers with the decision makers in
managed health care administration, most of whom are unfamiliar with the
notion of the pediatrician as the family interviewer. It is possible that these
decision makers will turn out to be no more hopeless than we found fathers
to be, when presented with clear expectations from physicians regarding
the value of a family model in the delivery of children's health care. Physicians must respect that the service they provide through family interviewing may be of substantial value to the family and to the provider. Those
physicians who refuse appropriate reimbursement for such a skill may be
afraid they are incompetent, are aware of their incompetence, have low self-
esteem, or are independently wealthy. The first type of physician should get
some training, the second should get out of the business, the third needs
his own therapist, and the fourth should spread it around. A physician who
is charging appropriately for time and services provided will have fewer
worries about "taking time away from the practice."

Scheduling Considerations

The decision as to when in the day to schedule interviews depends on several variables. Working parents, as mentioned previously, are generally
available in the late afternoons or evenings. Physicians also may want to
consider at what time of day they are best able to focus the energy required
to wrestle with a family. Group pediatric practices, in which individuals often enjoy some flexibility in determining specific time commitments, lend
themselves well to the institution of one-night-a-week evening clinics.
Nursing and other office staff are not required, and the individual physician can see two or three families in an evening without interruptions.

OFFICE EQUIPMENT

Space

Family interviewing does not require heavy expenditures for the interested
clinician. Office space, a few toys, comfortable chairs, and tissues comprise
the necessary equipment. Space can be a problem, particularly in an office
designed for efficiency with several small pediatric examining rooms, which
are usually long, narrow, and inhospitable. Those rooms can handle a fam-

ily of two parents and three children only if the interviewer is willing to work in single file. It is preferable to have a space in which the family can spread out comfortably. The area should be large enough for the therapist to manipulate space as needed. In some offices, the waiting area can be used for this purpose, particularly if interviews are held after regular office hours.

Toys

A simple assortment of toys work well as enticements for reluctant children to enter the interview room. Also, anxious or fidgety children are often able to handle an interview if they can fiddle with toys through the hour. In addition, the use of toys and play by the children and their parents can provide diagnostic information. Some useful questions regarding children's play include the following:

Are the children allowed to play?
Do they know how to play?
Is their play appropriate for their age?
How do siblings handle the competitive and conflicting aspects of play?
Do the parents have a capacity for playfulness?
How are limits set on the children's play and by whom?
What are children communicating to the interviewer about the family
    through their play?

All of these questions can be answered through careful observation of a family's manipulation of toys. Examples of inexpensive play materials include hand puppets, puzzles, blocks, toy soldiers, cars, board games, and drawing materials.

Some therapists prefer to conduct family interviews around a large table, with drawing materials available at each session for the children. Even when children appear to be uninterested in the discussion, their drawings are often dramatic illustrations of their nonverbal participation in the topic being discussed. For example, during an interview with a family of two parents and their two boys, ages 6 and 8 years, the younger child worked diligently and silently on his drawing. His parents were discussing their recent marital separation and the inability of each partner to control anger with each other and the boys. Within minutes, the younger son, encouraged by the therapist, described his picture to the group. He said it was a picture of the hospital clinic building with a huge fire on the second floor (i.e., the interview location) "burning everybody up." Four individuals were shown to have perished in the flames. A little boy had leaped out of the window to save himself, but he too was dead on the sidewalk. In cases such as this, we do not consider a child's play irrelevant in the session. We urge trainees to set aside time in which children, seemingly occupied in their own play, may discuss their particular drawings or play products, incorporating into the interview what has been communicated through play.

Recording Equipment

The only item that may be expensive in family interviewing is the recording equipment, which may range from the simplest cassette audiotape recorder to an elaborate video system. We use both video and audio recordings in our training work with pediatricians. For clinical practices, we also recommend that interviews be recorded (with the family's permission) at least on audiotape. The use of videotape, although desirable, may be logistically cumbersome. Recording is useful with families because interview segments can be played back to illustrate specific therapeutic points. Feedback for individual family members regarding communication processes can be effectively provided through tape playback. Also, audio recording helps a family return to an important topic after straying from the subject.

We strongly urge recording interviews for the interviewer's continuing growth and supervision. Family interviewing is intellectually and emotionally difficult, and conducting interviews in isolation can lead to stagnation and bad interviewing habits. Whitaker recommended that a family therapist find a group of colleagues with whom he or she can review experiences and receive feedback (9). This suggestion is echoed by David Waters and Edith Lawrence. A cornerstone of their clinical work with family therapy is to promote a partnership between the interviewer and family members. They also stress,

> *our belief in partnership extends beyond therapy to other relationships. As therapists, we believe strongly in the need for therapists to support, challenge, and encourage one another. Developing a network (formal or informal) of professionals who work to bring out the best in themselves and each other seems natural and necessary to us. As therapists, we need to expand our experience of openness, creativity and partnership. The therapist with no access to a trusted forum (individual or group) for releasing*

some of the pressures and issues that therapy raises is in the same position as an isolated client. (10)

An interviewer can play back tapes for his or her own review, but it is better to find someone (e.g., spouse, coworker) to share in the process. Ideally, a group of family interviewers should gather and provide feedback, enhancing the individual growth of its members. Such a group was successfully developed by some pediatricians in Rochester, New York, as an antidote to the "dissatisfied pediatrician" syndrome. In an effort to enrich their clinical experiences and escape the potential tedium in clinical pediatrics, these physicians incorporated abbreviated counseling for behavioral problems into their individual practices and met one evening per month to review tapes and techniques. The group grew steadily over a 5-year period to include as many as 25 pediatricians (including one of our authors, Bayard Allmond). A written description of this project appeared in 1968 (11).

Collaborative Office Rounds (COR)

Many features of that successful Rochester experience now are offered in the Collaborative Office Rounds (COR) groups initiated in 16 cities nationally by the federal office of the Maternal and Child Health Bureau. COR, usually composed of eight to twelve practitioners who meet at least monthly for 1 year or more, are led by a behavioral and developmental pediatrician and a child psychiatrist. The clinical experiences and dilemmas of the practitioners usually serve as the central focus of discussion. One of our authors, Lane Tanner, a leader of the COR group for pediatric practitioners at the University of California San Francisco, has found that interviewing dilemmas and complex family issues are among the most common concerns brought to the group. It is impressive how, within this group, professional growth emerges from the mutual sharing, problem solving, and support through the discussion of difficult cases. COR represents a model that is replicable in most communities. Although leaders with interviewing and therapy expertise are helpful to such an enterprise, we believe that much could also be accomplished by general pediatric clinicians meeting on their own in a similar format.

Additional information about these COR programs may be obtained from: Michael Fishman, MD, Maternal and Child Health Bureau, 5600 Fishers Lane, Room 18A-55, Parklawn Building, Rockville, MD, 29857.

References

1. Satir V. Conjoint family therapy. 3rd ed. Palo Alto, CA: Science & Behavior Books, 1983:6.
2. Aponte H. Personal communication: June 1977.
3. Whitaker C. A family is a four-dimensional relationship. In: Guerin P, ed. Family therapy: theory and practice. New York: Gardner Press, 1976.
4. Bowen M. Family therapy in clinical practice. Northvale, NJ: Jason Aronson, 1978.
5. Speck R, Attneave C. Family network: retribalization and healing. New York: Pantheon Books, 1973.
6. Leslie L. Can pediatric training manage in managed care? Pediatrics 1995;96:1144.
7. Tanner N. Families at the center of the development of a system of care, 1996. Available from: National Technical Assistance Center for Children's Health and Mental Health Policy, Georgetown University Child Development Center, 3307 M. Street, NW, Suite 401, Washington, DC 20007.
8. Author not cited. Children's mental health. Oregon managed care demonstration reduces costs, improves services. Advances in Family-Centered Care, 3:3, 1996.
9. Whitaker C. The hindrance of theory on clinical work. In: Guerin P, ed. Family therapy: theory and practice. New York: Gardner Press, 1976.
10. Waters D, Lawrence E. Competence, courage, and change: an approach to family therapy. New York: WW Norton, 1993:122.
11. Sumpter E, Friedman S. Workshop dealing with emotional problems: one method of preventing the "dissatisfied pediatrician syndrome." Clin Pediatr 1968;7:149.

chapter 5

The Initial Interview with a Family

PRE-INTERVIEW ISSUES

The Telephone

Mrs. Ruggles is on the telephone with her pediatrician.

Mother:	It's Harry this time, Dr. King. . . . This is really embarrassing, but I find he's been stealing from my purse, and not just nickels and dimes. Last Friday for the second time, I found $20 gone. Can I bring him in so you can talk to him, please? You're so good with all the kids—Harry adores you. Remember when you had to sew up his thumb last summer? Well he swears to everybody that you're the only doctor who can do that without hurting.
Pediatrician:	How old is he, Mrs. Ruggles?
Mother:	Eight; he's just starting the second grade.
Pediatrician:	What's your husband's reaction?
Mother:	I don't dare tell my husband about this. You know Milt. He gets so tense with the kids, and he's just had that surgery in the last year for his colitis. We don't like to get him upset. . . . That would just kill him. He doesn't know about the other times.
Pediatrician:	There have been other times?
Mother:	To be honest, this has been going on for 6 months or more I think. I didn't call you—you're so busy, and it wasn't a big thing—I thought I could take care of it. The first time was

> right after Christmas. Harry took $15 that his brother,
> Greg, had gotten for a Christmas present. He promised that
> if I didn't tell his father, it wouldn't happen again. We had to
> swear Greg to secrecy, too. Then there was a second time,
> but that was only $1.50 . . . Now recently this business with
> the $20 from my purse. I just can't get through to him. But
> now if you could just have a little talk with Harry—the two
> of you alone—I'm sure he would listen to you."

If Dr. King agrees to a "little talk with Harry," he is in trouble. There are
so many family issues at stake beyond Harry's stealing: Mrs. Ruggles' collaboration with her son and "protection" of her husband, her attempts to
manipulate the physician into an approach that will continue this collaboration, her communications that suggest that she is openly or unwittingly
encouraging her son's behavior, her direct messages to her son regarding his
behavior. How is it that she "can't get through to him?" How will the physician help her or Harry by succeeding where she has failed? What messages
has brother Greg been receiving throughout this situation? What about the
father and his apparent position of weakness and vulnerability in the family? None of these issues could be handled by a "little talk with Harry alone."
The family's participation is essential for a resolution of their dilemmas.

The Ruggles family illustrates our view that the initial interview begins
before the family enters the office. For many physicians, the first contact is
a telephone conversation with one parent, during which considerable mischief can occur if the physician is not prepared. The caller is often intent
on giving the physician the "real" story, sharing secret agendas or confidences, and enlisting the physician to take sides. These maneuvers, if successful for the caller, will alter the interviewer's perspective of the family and
may seriously compromise his or her effectiveness in the family interview.
For example, it would be duplicitous to work with a family regarding a
child's dishonesty if the interviewer has come to some private agreement
with one spouse not to reveal to the other that the child has been stealing.

To minimize the possibility of pre-interview alliances with one family
member, we discourage lengthy discussions of a parent's version on the telephone. After obtaining a brief description of the situation and supportively
acknowledging the feelings of the caller, the physician may tactfully dis-

courage further discussion of "the problem." The remainder of the call can be used to explain which family members will be required for the first interview, to arrange a time, and to discuss the length of appointments, fees, and insurance. We prefer to make these arrangements ourselves rather than through a nurse-receptionist because this dialogue with the calling family member often yields valuable information regarding that individual's willingness to consider a family approach and his or her ability to communicate to other family members the interviewer's interest in working with the family as a group.

Failure to Appear for the First Family Interview

A family's failure to attend the first interview has a direct bearing on case understanding and should be carefully included in the interviewer's data. A missed appointment should not be ignored and reestablishing contact should not be left to the family. The following questions can be pursued in a follow-up telephone call by the interviewer.

How well does the family know the physician? Do they trust him?

Does a missed initial family interview indicate that the family collectively is frightened of a joint encounter? Or is just one member refusing to attend?

What combination of influences has led to the family's nonappearance?

The physician should handle these telephone interactions directly because the family's behavior becomes important diagnostic information as the interviewer develops a formulation of the family system and its relationship to the voiced concerns.

Occasionally, even after careful preparation by the interviewer and apparent agreement from the caller, only a portion of the family attends the scheduled interview. The arriving family members usually indicate their intention to proceed without the missing members. In these cases, the family may be demonstrating its particular collection of alliances and alienations and its desire to maintain such a system. Interviewers need to use discretion in deciding whether or not to proceed under such circumstances. In our experience, if the missing person is either a spouse or the identified patient, proceeding with the interview is risky, and the subsequent inclusion of the missing members is often impossible. The interviewer should not hesitate to cancel such an interview before starting, rescheduling it at a time when the absent member will attend. However, if the missing member is a child other than the identified patient (e.g., a sibling with another commitment for the same time), we are not averse to beginning family work without that individual. However, even in this situation, the interviewer may express displeasure at meeting with the incomplete family and request that subsequent sessions include the absent member.

Depending on the circumstances, a physician may charge a family for a missed initial (or subsequent) appointment or an appointment canceled because only a portion of the family arrives at the office. This is acceptable, provided that the family was informed of this policy.

Anxiety: Family and Interviewer

The pre-interview issues are important, but they do not occur with all families. Usually the initial telephone contact with a concerned parent goes smoothly. The parent is forthright in requesting help from the physician, and the suggestion of an initial family meeting is accepted usually without question. In these cases, which for us constitute the majority, family members also manage to get themselves to the office on time for the visit.

For many of our beginning trainees, the major concern is that the family *will* arrive. For the novice interviewer, even after observation and preparation, conducting a family interview can be a harrowing experience. In the novice's mind, there are so many "what if's."

What if the family fails to arrive?
What if there are 10 of them?
What if they will not be quiet?
What if they will not talk?
What if I cannot control the situation?
What if the family starts to fight?
What if I cannot figure out what's going on?
What if I do not know what to say?
What if the family falls apart during the interview?
What if the session becomes chitchat that seems to lead nowhere?

Such doubts about competence and performance are common in any learning situation. We urge the physician interested in developing family interviewing skills to choose an uncomplicated first case. A family with whom the physician already feels somewhat comfortable and one that presents an apparently "simple" child-rearing issue would be a good beginning experience. Venturing into more serious, heavily conflict-laden family problems (e.g., delinquency, anorexia nervosa) should wait until the physician has more experience and comfort. Some physicians may choose never to work with such complex cases, even after extensive experience in family interviewing.

Physician anxiety may stem from more than mere case complexity. Although a physician in training has already developed excellent interview fact-finding (or content) skills, now he or she must learn to deal with process as well. Learning this new skill means experiencing the anxiety that comes with mastering any new task. A firm grasp of the principles underlying effective family interviewing and the practice of using them will gradually lessen the clinician's level of tension.

Until experiential knowledge accumulates, the interviewer will most likely be anxious in anticipation of a family interview. However, we encourage those interviewers to persevere, knowing that they and the family will survive the experience. We suggest that physicians continue to practice family interviews long enough not only to feel the anxiety of a first interview but also to enjoy the flush of accomplishment. After a particularly good session, one of our trainees likened his reaction to his experience of successfully intubating a premature infant for the first time: "pure exhilaration."

Beginning interviewers may find it helpful to know that usually their own anxiety is surpassed by that of the family. The family's "what if's" cover an even broader range than those of the physician:

What if the doctor says it is all my fault?
What if she thinks I am overanxious or stupid?
What if she does not like me and the way I treat my child?
What if she will not agree with me?
What if our family secret is revealed?
What if I do not maintain control of myself? What if I do not maintain control of my family?

Families are usually frightened and defensive at the beginning of an interview. They are risking exposure and scrutiny from "the outside." Yet, they want help with some sort of difficulty that has prompted their visit. Consequently, families often feel two ways about family therapy: eager for help and fearful of the process. When interviewers acknowledge a family's apprehension and grasp its ambivalence, they may be successful in reducing that family's anxiety, allowing the family to feel safe and begin working toward a solution.

OPENING STAGE OF AN INITIAL INTERVIEW: GREETING AND INTRODUCTION

The process of making a family comfortable is the social stage of an interview, and it begins when the family is ushered into the interview room. Each family member is greeted separately by name with both eye contact and physical contact (e.g., a handshake) initiated by the interviewer. The family is allowed to choose its own seating arrangement. A brief period of small talk may ensue. Minuchin refers to this as "living room behavior, conforming to cultural rules of politeness" (1).

At this point, the interviewer may discuss any recording equipment to be used. Because we routinely use audiotape or videotape in our interviews, we generally have the equipment running by the time the family enters the office. This obviates the awkward need to flip switches and adjust microphones when the family is seated. Recording can be presented to the family by saying, "You will note that I am using a tape recorder today. I am taping this session for two reasons: I may want to play back a certain section for us to review together, and I will use the recording for my own review after the session is over. I do not keep the tapes on record; they are erased after I review them." Objections to the use of tape devices are rare. However, if even one family member expresses a reluctance to be taped, the machine is turned off.

During this greeting stage, the interviewer also makes observations.

What is the general mood of the family?
How do the parents seem to be doing with the children? Are they severe and demanding, or are they ignoring and permissive to the point that the children are out of control?
How does the family appear to be organizing itself as the preliminaries of the interview unfold? Who speaks? Who speaks for others?
How do they seat themselves?

Such observations are important. However, we believe that diagnosis is an ongoing process and agree with Haley's statement:

*It is important to gather information but it is also important to keep con-
clusions tentative. The therapist may be misled and therefore ideas should
not be too firm. Observation gives information that can be tested as the
session continues. A therapist who gets too set in one idea is not free to
consider other ideas. (2)*

THE SECOND STAGE: DISCUSSION OF CONCERNS

As quickly as the therapist senses that the family can tolerate it, the social
stage of the interview should progress to a discussion of the presenting concerns. Generally, the interviewer initiates this discussion, thereby establishing the physician's authority. By asking a general question (e.g., "What
brings the family here today?" or "What help would this family like from
me?"), the physician may learn useful information, such as who in the family takes charge, who is most concerned, or who is the spokesperson for the
group? We try to avoid the word "problem" when initiating a discussion
(e.g., "What's the problem?") because it tends to invite blame. When accusations are exchanged, the therapist may well lose the good will of the
accused.

Even with carefully worded questions, the identified patient may still
be blamed by other family members. Blaming is one of the most common
defense mechanisms that a therapist encounters as an interview begins. After all, usually the family has asked for counsel because of the behavior of
one individual, so their inclination to blame that person is understandable. Unfortunately, such blame can be extremely damaging to the therapist's work. Children have repeatedly been made to feel bad and deserving
of punishment at home for the symptomatic behavior that has prompted
the visit. If the interview continues this process and parents and siblings
are allowed to blame the child in front of the physician, the child will withdraw from the interview process, becoming sullen, silent, and uncooperative.

The simplest way to change a family's blaming stance is to comment on
its first appearance in the session. For example, "You know, Mrs. Gilroy, I
am uncomfortable that Alice must be feeling pretty bad about this whole
situation. I am beginning to understand your exasperation as well. Could
you rephrase your worry in a way that does not blame her?" This intervention may require repetition with other family members as well.

A physician may wish to open with a less general inquiry, informing the family of the interviewer's intention to focus on the family unit rather than the individual. For example, "I am glad the entire family was able to come in today. I spoke briefly on the phone with you, Mrs. Watson, but I wanted to delay further discussion until we had this opportunity to meet. I know that each of you has feelings and opinions that are important if things are to get better in this family. I would like to ask each of you, and I will start on this side and go around the room, what brings you here today and what changes would you like to see take place in this family."

Interviewers may also choose a specific family member to receive the opening question. Haley, for instance, often directs his beginning question to that adult who seems less involved with the problem. He further states:

> Generally it is not a good idea to start with the problem child and ask him why the family is there. He will feel that he is too much on the spot and it may look as if the therapist is blaming him for everyone being there. It is better to deal with him later. (3)

This has not been our experience, and we often begin this second stage of an interview with a question directed toward the identified patient, such as: "Frankie, tell me what you understand about today's visit. Why is the family here today?" This child is usually particularly worried, having learned at home that "he" is the reason for this session. Although the question may increase the child's anxiety, the therapist then may demonstrate through careful listening his or her interest in the child's viewpoint.

When asked this opening question, a child often will look at one or both parents and shrug his shoulders, indicating that he does not know why the family is there. This reaction provides an opening for a discussion of how the child and other family members were prepared for the initial visit. Were they simply dragged along or was an attempt made to explain the nature of the visit? The interviewer may explore these questions directly by saying, "All right, Frankie, I would like you to pick either your mother or father and ask one of them to explain to you what brings the family here today." This request serves several purposes. First, the child is not chastised by the doctor for "pretending not to know when in fact he does." The child may be genuinely confused as to why the appointment has been made, having been told nothing more than "you will go." Second, the child indicates which parent he is willing to approach with the question. Third, the dialogue between these two family members can be observed, without the interviewer participating directly. Fourth, the interviewer is able to see some of the communication process between the chosen parent and the child. Some observations may include:

Do they communicate functionally or is it a dysfunctional interchange, laced with double-level messages, assumptions, or generalizations?

Does the parent talk in a manner appropriate for the child's understanding?

Is the explanation congruent with what the interviewer has learned on the phone, or are there alternate versions?

In this way, the family's actual communication style is demonstrated in front of the therapist.

THE THIRD STAGE: INTERACTION

This interactional stage has now been set in motion and directed by the interviewer. While the family talks together, its system and structure are revealed. Rather than "talking about" their problem with the therapist, they enact it, and the physician is able to observe firsthand how family members behave with one another.

Some families begin this process on their own. Without any specific help from the interviewer, they begin discussing among themselves feelings, thoughts, and opinions. However, most families do not initiate such discussion, and the interviewer must directly help family members interact with one another, discouraging questions that force the therapist to take sides (e.g., "Don't you think I'm right, Doctor?"). Families tend to use the interviewer as a central receptor of messages and moralistic judge, which is a difficult position to avoid. Physicians and patients are accustomed to the physician occupying the "director's chair" clinically. Although the physician should remain in control of the interview, he or she must learn to direct in a more subtle way, facilitating the family's own interaction by allowing the family story to unfold. This role may feel awkward to new family interviewers, and the family may be less than delighted with such a stance, but we feel it is essential for understanding the family structure, relationships, and communication style.

Direct Communication

How does a physician adjust to this new subtle role? The simplest technique involves redirecting comments from family members with a firm suggestion. For example, "That sounds like a message for George. Tell him that now, Gloria." Gloria may do it without hesitation, but more commonly she will protest this direct communication by doing the following:

1. Continuing to talk as though she did not hear
2. Stating that she does not understand what the doctor means
3. Saying that she and George have discussed it a thousand times previously
4. Making assumptions either about herself or about George (e.g., "He knows what I mean"; "He wouldn't understand"; "I can't talk to him about this")
5. Politely putting the doctor and his suggestion in their place (e.g., "That seems so artificial")
6. Impolitely putting the doctor and his suggestion in its place (e.g., "No, I won't. I don't like your telling me what to do")

The interviewer should be ready for such protest and should insist on direct communication. By this time in the interview, the family is beginning to reveal its communication difficulties, providing both diagnostic information and material that the interviewer may use in therapeutic work with the family. For example, if Gloria protests against speaking directly to George by making assumptions, the interviewer's job is to help Gloria drop assumption-making from her communication style.

This method of direct communication between family members must be repeated and encouraged several times, often with each family member. With time, family members become accustomed to it as an important rule of the interview. A mistake we see beginning trainees make with this strategy is that they give up too quickly, successfully redirecting an individual at the start and then later allowing that individual to resume a style of directing comments to the interviewer. When the mistake is recognized and the trainee attempts a maneuver to redirect, resistance may have increased. Direct communication is more effective if taught persistently from the beginning.

As mentioned earlier, one advantage of direct communication is that the interviewer is freed from an active role in any conversation. This detachment enables the interviewer, outside the family system, to observe the family's interaction and begin developing strategies. Another advantage is that direct communication can help them overcome their difficulties in expressing feelings to each other. The family is forced to communicate feelings directly to each other instead of funneling their emotions through the physician, thus learning skills for direct expression and the reception of feelings.

Other Communication Techniques

Along with the oral directive, an interviewer may need to use other means to underscore an emphasis on direct communication. The physician may ask two family members to move their chairs so that they are facing one another as they speak, requesting that any family members seated between the two participants move back so nothing interferes with direct communication between these individuals. An interviewer may request that the two people hold hands or touch as they talk so that contact between them is maximized, and each clearly has the other's attention. The interviewer and the family will discover that communication in such a position becomes less threatening. If a family is particularly resistant to direct communication, the interviewer may want to move his or her own chair out of the family circle, demonstrating that they, not the interviewer, are expected to participate in the interchange.

Communication Style

When family members have begun to talk directly to one another, the interviewer may begin to reshape their communication style. For example, the interviewer may request that each individual concentrate on using the pronoun "I" when talking with others (e.g., beginning sentences with "I need," "I see"), underscoring each individual's responsibility to communicate their own thoughts and feelings. The interviewer may also ask family members to concentrate on present thoughts, actions, feelings, rather than resorting to repeated reports and complaints about the past.

With all of these communication techniques, the physician must discern how fast the family seems able to tolerate interventions. With a particularly frightened family, the sessions may proceed slowly. However, even with the most tentative family group, we generally continue to encourage their direct talk to one another. This is often the first lesson for the family, and it may take several sessions to learn.

Conjoint Family Drawing

Aside from its use in resident training (see chapter 2), we also use conjoint drawing when working with families in order to assist their interaction during the interview. This technique encourages participation in a task by all family members; the less talkative members are not edged out. Because the task is nonverbal, for excessively talkative families the task eliminates unproductive chat to reveal often important nonverbal behavior. This format usually appeals to children; they participate enthusiastically. This method often reveals elements of the family's ability or inability to be playful with one another while performing such a "childish" task. Conjoint drawing provides an additional chance for the interviewer to pull back and observe, organizing and planning strategies as the drawing emerges.

This procedure has been used in several clinical situations, including marital therapy (4), the treatment of schizophrenia (5), and various other family problems (6). Although specific instructions to the family may vary, one source suggests the following:

> *Each family member is to select a felt pen of a different color and is not to exchange for any other color pen. I would like for you as a family to draw a picture as you see yourselves now as a family. You can draw the picture any way you want to, but I'd like to encourage you to be as creative and original as you can in representing yourselves as a unique family. You can draw the persons any size and place them in any position on the paper. They may be drawn touching each other, or separate. You can draw yourselves or each other, whichever you think best describes your family. (7)*

In these instructions, the interviewer specifically tells the family what to do. Our own directions to families are considerably more general. A large sheet of drawing paper is taped on top of a flat table around which a family is seated. A box of crayons is provided, and each family member is asked to choose a separate color and not to change colors. Then, the therapist instructs the family: "I would like the family to do something with the paper and crayons for the next 20 (25 or 30) minutes. What you draw is up to you. However, there is to be no talking, either with me or with one another throughout this time. We will talk when the time is up. Okay, you may begin."

Some individuals are embarrassed at having to expose their allegedly poor artistic skills. The interviewer (after making a mental note of the self-deprecator) may state that the task is not a test of anyone's artistic ability, but other comments, explanations, and suggestions should not be offered. The interviewer should then be quiet, and in a short time the family will do likewise.

With families, just as with trainees, the interviewer's observations and subsequent discussion with the family should focus on the process more than the content of the drawing. Interviewers should note:

Who initiates the drawing and who seems responsible for organizing the task and the group?

How are responsibilities shared for developing a theme and carrying it through?

Does each individual have sufficient drawing space? How are issues of spatial territory handled on the paper?

Do subsystems of the family appear, two or three individuals working jointly on a project that does not include others?

Do the children seem to have a say in the development of the drawing? Do they have such a say that the process seems largely under their control, with the parents remaining inactive or passive? Or is it the other way round?

Does one family member shift from one subsystem to another, seemingly unable to find a place to enter in?

How are reluctant participants handled and by whom?

The answers to these and other questions are added to the interviewer's growing collection of data regarding the family and its particular structure.

When the drawing is completed, the family is usually eager to discuss their experience, which should take approximately 30 minutes, particularly if the family includes several children and two parents. The interviewer may request that each family member offer a summary of his or her own feelings during and as a result of the task. To get them started, the physician can ask each person to list three adjectives that describe the experience (e.g., silly, frightening, boring). The interviewer may also ask each person to walk around the drawing, comment on the contribution of each family member, and listen to that member's response. The commentator thus initiates a dialogue with each family member regarding the drawing and the process. Because everyone is given a turn to comment, the interviewer is able to observe the specific communication style for every possible dyad in the family.

Specific content issues of the drawing can be discouraged by emphasizing the use of the word "how" in each family member's description of the experience. This focuses on the "how's" or the process rather than the "what's" of the picture itself. Even during this discussion, family members should be directed to speak to each other, not to the interviewer. If the interviewer successfully directs the discussion to sharing of how the drawing occurred, the trap of "explaining" the symbolic significance of specific items in the drawing can be avoided. Such explanations can resemble conversations in a gypsy tearoom. We recommend that they be saved for that environment and that interviewers limit their scope in this task to an understanding and discussion of the family's process during the drawing.

A family may also be encouraged to view the family drawing task as a learning experience about itself. The interviewer may ask each person to describe something learned about the self during the process and something learned about how the family works together.

The conjoint family drawing can be repeated at intervals throughout work with a family. This technique usually will reflect alterations in a family's basic set of relationships. The clinical usefulness of this drawing task is illustrated by the following case study:

THE HARRIS FAMILY

The Harris family entered family therapy because one child, 8-year-old Kelly, "has no initiative, just won't do anything on her own, is dependent and whiny," particularly with her mother. The whole family agreed to participate in sessions, including both parents and two other children, Steve, age 11 years, and Rona, age 9 years. These two children were described as cooperative, resourceful, and independent, in contrast to their "balky, immature" sister. Mrs. Harris openly complained that Kelly's clinging, whining, and demanding were driving her "crazy." She felt guilty and ashamed that, because of Kelly's behavior, she often appeared to reject her daughter, which only made matters worse. The whole family agreed that a veritable battleground had developed between the mother and Kelly. It was unclear what role the rest of the family played in the situation.

During the first family interview, the family completed a family drawing (Figure 5.1). They were asked to "work together on this piece of paper without talking for the next 20 minutes." Each family member chose one color, and their positions around the table are illustrated in the drawing. The identified patient was the first to put a mark on the paper. She enthusiastically began working with a line (soon to be a lawn) across her side of the paper. Immediately, the mother rose, leaned across the paper, and began drawing the lines of a house on top of Kelly's line. (The mother's complaint had been that Kelly would not leave her alone, yet here was a demonstration that it was the mother who was unwilling to leave Kelly alone.) In broad strokes, the mother constructed a house on top of Kelly's lawn and began to color in the roof, her product dwarfing Kelly's efforts, which were now relegated to the thin strip of paper left on the bottom of the page. Perplexed, Kelly began to draw family figures in her remaining space. Mother and daughter certainly seemed to be in some sort of struggle with one another for space, but it was the mother, not Kelly, who initiated and maintained the struggle.

For the first few minutes, the father and two siblings hung back, watching this nonverbal sparring between Mrs. Harris and her daughter. When the mother finished her lines on the house in Kelly's area, she resumed her seat and began drawing flowers on her portion of the paper. At this point, Rona began to draw. Although described as resourceful and independent, she was watching her sister carefully and taking cues from her regarding subject matter. Rona began her own version of a house, family, and lawn scene, which became a copy of Kelly's work with few original touches. Steve continued to stare uncomfortably at the paper and intermittently drummed his crayon on the paper; beyond the few dots he produced, he drew nothing. The mother was visibly upset at his inactivity, drew some of her flowers in his direction, and motioned with her hand for him to join in. She succeeded only in obliterating his space and leaving him little drawing room. The father was also watching rather than participating. However, unlike his son, he eventually began to draw the form of a sailing ship. His lines were light and indistinct, and he became dreamily absorbed in his work, seemingly oblivious to the work of the rest of the family. The most diligent worker of all was Kelly, the child with "no initiative." By the time the drawing was complete, she had embellished her mother's house with walls, doors, windows, flowers, trees, sun, and people.

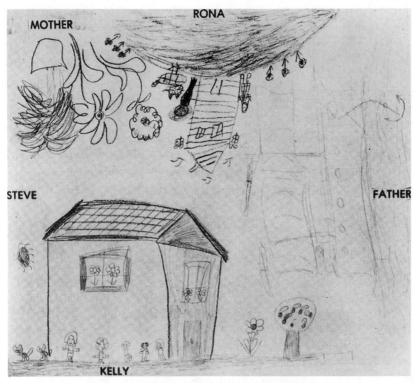

Figure 5.1. The conjoint drawing by the Harris family.

The pediatrician opened the post-drawing discussion.

Pediatrician:	Okay, now I would like each of you to come up with one word that describes how you felt about this task. What feelings did you have as you were participating in the drawing? We'll go around the table, and I'll start with you, Mrs. Harris.
Mother:	Frustrating, very frustrating.
Pediatrician:	Next, Steve.
Steve:	Silly.
Kelly:	Fun. I thought it was fun.
Father:	Interesting.

Rona:	I thought it was fun, too.
Mother:	(starting to laugh) That's so funny, Al, that you thought it was interesting . . . you over there on your sailboat or whatever it is, just doing your own thing, never mind what's happening with the rest of us . . . just like at home.
Pediatrician:	Would you tell him directly what you found frustrating about the experience?
Mother:	Well, that . . . for one thing. You seemed so removed over there, drawing that boat. That's like where you are most of the time, and I was hoping that somehow we could all get together and draw something . . . one picture, not separate ones. That was one part of my feelings. And then Steve—not drawing anything at all! I was very impatient there, wanting him to get going, and I could see that he wasn't going to.
Pediatrician:	Ask Steve what he was experiencing.
Mother:	I think I know.
Pediatrician:	Ask him anyhow.
Mother:	Well, what was happening with you?
Steve:	Well, at first I couldn't think of anything to draw, and then the space started getting filled up.
Mother:	(speaking for her son) And you decided that if you couldn't have all the space, then you weren't going to use any of it, right?
Steve:	Well . . . well . . . yeah.
Mother:	I knew it. And then I started getting frustrated about that. I knew that's what he was doing, and I couldn't say anything about it since we had to be silent.
Pediatrician:	It's hard not to speak out?
Mother:	Well, yes, I guess it is. They all tell me I have a big mouth. Right, gang? (The children all quickly agreed with mother's last comment.)
Pediatrician:	And I was wondering if you all noticed Kelly's independence and enthusiasm, her ability to work creatively and alone?

Father:	That's what I found so interesting—not my own drawing, Sally, but that Kelly was so clearly taking off on her own. I wouldn't have expected it.
Mother:	Well, she likes to draw, that's all.

The "how" or process of the drawing uncovered useful family data, much of it contrary to the earlier version of the "family problem" (i.e., Kelly's dependency and clinging). For example:

1. Kelly was capable of considerable independent activity. However, this activity was hardly validated in the family. It was summarily negated by the mother ("she likes to draw, that's all") and a surprise to the father.
2. The mother had loudly complained of perpetual infringement on her own space at home by Kelly. However, in this experience it was mother who intruded on her daughter's area.
3. Mother and father were at odds, specifically about the issue of involvement in family matters.
4. Steve was hardly the resourceful, independent, cooperative youngster that both parents had described.
5. Rona, for all the parental praise about her creativity and independence, was little more than Kelly's mimic.

All of this information, which proved accurate, could be used in subsequent sessions. The drawing had provided an effective entrance into the family system, enabling the pediatrician to glimpse what lay beyond the family's official version of themselves and their difficulties.

Family Sculpture

The family sculpture is another means for helping families interact, while avoiding what they are most comfortable doing—endlessly explaining their "problem." The technique borrows much from the field of psychodrama, and, similar to conjoint family drawing, it is largely a nonverbal task. Peggy Papp has been cited as the originator of the technique (8,9). A family sculpture is basically a physical arrangement of family members that expresses their relationship to one another at a particular moment. The technique of directing a family to produce such a sculpture in the doctor's office is best understood through a clinical example.

THE FRENCH FAMILY

Laura French, age 15, had anorexia nervosa. She recently entered the hospital where the diagnosis was confirmed and where she was now in the process of gaining weight before family treatment would continue through outpatient visits. During her hospitalization on the pediatric ward, her family agreed to begin family counseling by meeting Laura and her doctor in a room just off the pediatric ward. This was the first such session, and thus the pediatrician-interviewer and family were new to one another. Besides Laura and her parents, there were two other children, 19-year-old Anna and 6-year-old Joe.

As the interview began, the physician was struck by the general feeling of caution coming from the family. Concerns were discussed in such a constricted manner that the interviewer felt bogged down in the family's polite, careful chat. Nothing much was happening. At this point, the interviewer decided to risk injecting some liveliness into the session, hoping to relax the family, move beyond their protective veneer, and reveal something more of their family system. He began:

Pediatrician: Okay, I would like to do something different with this family. First of all, I would like everyone to stand up and push the chairs back. (He quickly rises and pushes his chair out of the way and assists others in doing the same.) Good. Now I am going to ask you to do what's called a family sculpture. Does anyone know what I'm talking about? No—okay, I will explain. I would like you to assume that everyone standing in the middle of the room is clay to be modeled. One of you is going to be the sculptor—Laura, I will begin with you. You are the first sculptor. Everyone will have a turn eventually. I would like you to consider that everyone in the family is made of clay and that you are going to mold them into a sculpture, a family grouping that will show something about how you see relationships in your family. Do you follow me so far?

Laura: Well, I'm not sure.

Pediatrician: Let me see how else to put it . . . well, you know that in your family, just as in other families, certain people are closer than others. I would like you to show me your version of that by physically taking, for instance, your mother, moving her body, her arms, her facial expression, her hands, whatever, into a position that says something about her place in the family and her closeness and distance relative to others in the family. You may move her wherever you feel she is in relation to you and others in the family. You may want some people to be touching others; you may want faces to look or not look in certain directions. You may want to arrange faces in certain expressions. And don't forget to include yourself in the sculpture.

Laura: (indicates, though tentatively, that she gets the idea)

Pediatrician: All right. I would like you to start now. Oh, one more thing. There is to be no talking with one another or with me while you are doing this. If you want someone to be smiling, don't tell them; move their facial muscles with your hands. Remember, no talking.

Laura: Well, I don't know if . . .

Pediatrician: Do the best you can. Give it a try.

Laura's sculpture did help the family and the interviewer move into a productive area for subsequent work. She placed her mother and father side by side, close together, and holding hands. Next to her father, on his left, she placed her younger brother, Joe. The two males were in friendly contact each with one arm around the other. Anna was placed kneeling on the floor in front of her parents, facing front, with her left hand extended to and touching Joe and her right hand stretched backwards into Mrs. French's hand. Anna's face was positioned looking over her right shoulder into her mother's face. Laura did not put herself into the picture. When the interviewer urged her to do so, she inserted herself standing in the middle of this small family circle. The final configuration then was a tiny enclosed circle: mother, father, brother, and sister—all touching. Inside, touching no one, was the identified patient. She indicated with a helpless gesture that she did not know what to do with her hands.

The interviewer amplified the arrangement by asking the family to transform the picture into a kinetic sculpture by saying, "Now, maintaining the positions in which Laura has placed you, I would like each of you to take just one step—in any direction . . . it doesn't matter where." They promptly, literally fell over one another. The interviewer was then able to introduce a specific concept to them: "Sometimes when families are tremendously close, as you are, there is little room for individual movement and growth. Any attempts at individual steps lead to inadvertent stepping on one another while no effective individual movement occurs." This metaphor developed into a major theme in the continuing work with Laura and her family.

Laura's sculpture suggested several family issues to explore:

The parents did not look at one another.
The mother's posture was directed toward her older daughter.
The identified patient, Laura, had no eye contact with anyone in the family.
Anna was in a particularly awkward position in the family, on her knees in front of the parents.

Although any one of these observations could have been used by the pediatrician in the beginning stages of working with the family, he chose one issue and returned to the others as time went on.

Family sculpture may be used in other ways besides the static configuration. The interviewer can introduce speech by asking the sculptor to give each family member a sentence to utter while in the designated position—something that would befit the person and the position. When sentences have been assigned to each individual (including the sculptor), the interviewer may request that the family in turn repeat their sentences while standing in position. Often a picture of family functioning emerges, and dialogues may develop out of the assigned sentences. For example, assume that a mother is placed with her hands on the sides of her head and this sentence given: "I can't stand it anymore." The father is positioned with legs apart and his hands on his hips, saying, "Well, what are you going to do about it?" The interviewer may ask other family members to drop away for the moment, encouraging the mother and father to have a conversation with one another, carrying their interchange beyond those initial statements.

An interviewer may ask each family member, while in assigned position, to assume that this is his or her permanent position in the family and in life. Each member is asked to describe how life would be if permanently in this position. Family members often report that their description of life in the assumed position closely matches a description of their actual existence. A mother, who was placed by the sculptor, her 14-year-old daughter, facing away from the family toward a corner of the room, declared: "I don't have to imagine that this is my permanent position. It is! I feel turned away, isolated, and out of it. I'm in that kitchen, and all I look at is a row of cupboards. I feel very lonely and isolated."

Family sculpture has proved useful as an informal maneuver to break the ice with anxious families. This technique is generally popular with children. Often, the children in a family who have not yet been selected as sculptors will ask directly for a turn. We think that one reason family sculpture appeals so to children, playfulness and adventurous novelty aside, is the sanctioned opportunity for children to literally push parents around. We generally give everyone in the family, including parents, an opportunity to sculpt the family. The first family member selected as sculptor may be chosen because he or she appears to be the most interested, the most open, the brightest, the least likely to sabotage efforts, or the most likely to "spill the beans." For every family member, parents included, the sculpture exercise is a time when touching is not just allowed but required. For families who have grown out of touch with one another, it may be the first such experience in months or years.

List of "Appreciations and Resentments"

The technique of writing a list of "appreciations and resentments" for encouraging family interaction in the interview is effective and quite easy to introduce. Virginia Satir often used it. Each family member is given paper and pencil, and everyone is asked to list five things he or she appreciates about each family member, including oneself. Following that, each person is to list five things resented about each family member, also including oneself. The family is given as much time as necessary, usually 20 to 30 minutes. When they have finished, the family members are encouraged to share their lists, discussing in detail with each person.

Several things are accomplished using this method. Initially, the task clearly sends the family a "let's get down to business" message from the interviewer. It allows every family member to organize thoughts privately and relieves fears of the identified patient because everyone, not just she, must participate. The technique gives permission for family members to appreciate and to resent, to feel two ways about others in the family. Families in trouble often polarize members, assigning them restricted roles (e.g., the good child, the bad child, the sympathetic parent, the insensitive parent). In addition, some families have unwritten taboos (e.g., no one is allowed to say anything critical of another family member, no one is permitted to verbalize positive feelings toward someone else). The writing task suggests that everyone in the family has attributes on both sides of the coin. Frequently, the parents require an adjustment in their thinking to first conceptualize, then write down, and finally discuss positive qualities in the identified patient. The task serves as a beginning lesson for all that they do have and are expected to have both positive and negative feelings for family members and themselves.

Discussing appreciated qualities allows the physician to teach family members the importance of effective validation. Discussing resented qualities provides for the expression of anger and frustration in a relatively safe environment. Particularly with the resentment comments, the physician must prevent the family's communication pattern from deteriorating into a tirade of blame and accusations. Family members should understand that they have a right to their feelings of anger and resentment, and that these feelings can be expressed in some form other than blame and personal attack. Re-framing (i.e., rephrasing a specific resentment in the form of a positive request) and the use of "I" statements are helpful in these situations.

Father:	(speaking to his wife) Number 3, Marion, on my resentment list, is that you're too unselfish—that goes for both of us.
Physician:	Be more specific.
Father:	Well, she . . .
Physician:	Be more specific, but tell Marion directly.
Father:	Well, you give 90% of your time and energy to the children. You and I only get 10%, if even that much.
Physician:	Rephrase your resentment in the form of a request of Marion, Elliott. Begin your sentence with the pronoun "I."
Father:	I don't like our never having time together.
Physician:	Tell you what, I'd like you to do it once again—this time tell Marion what you *would* like from her, not what you don't like.
Father:	I'd like us to have more time together, Marion.

In this illustration, the physician had to intervene four times in an effort to have Elliott transform his resentful statement into a specific request for which he takes responsibility. The statement of resentment, if unchanged, would either stifle further interchange or initiate a battle when Marion rises to her own defense. Elliott's specific request provides room for a nondefensive response from Marion. The work continues from this point, with the interviewer helping Marion to respond in a nonthreatening, nondefensive way and continuing to work with Elliott on making specific requests. How much time does Elliott want, when, and doing what?

The resentments that individuals list about themselves often indicate their desire for growth. For example, when someone writes: "I don't show my feelings," that person may articulate the issue in hopes that he can become less fearful and more open when expressing feelings. Listed self-resentments represent dissatisfying aspects of an individual's style that are permissible to reveal in such a safe format.

This technique of listing "appreciations and resentments" can supply a wealth of diagnostic and potentially therapeutic material, particularly in the areas of communication patterns, expression of feelings, and revelations of self-worth.

INTERVIEWER GOALS FOR AN INITIAL INTERVIEW

Although no two family interviews are the same, this does not mean that a family interview is a haphazard event or that it should be conducted by simply gathering the family together in a room, blindly hoping for the best. A successful interviewer has a tentative plan before the interview begins and continues to elaborate specific goals for the interview as it progresses and even as it ends. These specific goals originate from a study of and interaction with the family and are developed to help the family resolve the situation. Examples of such goals and plans are mentioned in the clinical examples presented throughout this book.

There is another level of goal planning that must occur, particularly during a first encounter with a family. This set of goals transcends the specific clinical problem presented, having little to do with why the family came. An interviewer needs to do the following:

1. Establish that he or she will be in charge of the interview
2. Develop a beginning formulation of the problem and a tentative treatment plan

3. Make the interview a "touching" experience for every family member
4. Ensure the family's return, if indicated

These goals can be applied to any clinical situation, even those more traditional medical interviews that do not include seeing an entire family.

Establishing Who Will Be in Charge

Although it seems obvious that the interviewer will be in charge of the family interview, the family does not always see it that way. As an interview begins, many of the difficulties reflect a basic power struggle between the family and the interviewer. Some of the clinical illustrations we have already discussed illustrate this power struggle:

"Oh no, my husband couldn't possibly come."
"I wonder if you and Harry could have a little talk together—just the two of you."
"Even if my husband can't come, perhaps I could come in alone, Doctor."
"You're not going to give her a shot, are you? She hates needles."

These are all efforts by at least part of the family to control the interview situation, and there are many others. A family may reveal its control manipulations through its general behavior in the session:

A child will not talk.
A parent will not be quiet.
A child will not sit still.
Siblings will not stop fighting.
A family member leaves the room.

A family may also demonstrate its intent to control through specific communication methods in the interview:

A family member speaks for someone else:
"Franklin won't talk, he hates doctors." After this prophecy and expectation, Franklin doesn't talk.
A family member uses generalizations:
"Gregory, why do you always become sullen and difficult the minute we bring this up?" Gregory, like Franklin, takes the cue and obliges with sullen and difficult behavior.
A family member attempts to mind read:

"I think what you really want to know, Doctor, is whether Frances and I are having problems. Isn't that it?"

A family member projects his own feelings onto others:

"The doctor is ashamed of you, Stacey."

A family member cross-examines:

"When was the last time I reminded you about that, Hal? When? Wasn't it only two nights ago, just as we were ready to go?"

A family member attacks and depreciates something that another person stands for:

"Well, Doc, I suppose you feel this family interview is going to tell us something. Well, OK, I guess you should know. After all, you're the doctor. By the way, are you an intern or a real doctor?"

A family member brings up the past:

"Doctor, I think it would probably help you to have a little background before we get started. Now 12 years ago, the child was only 3 months old, and my husband . . . "

A family member uses intimate knowledge against someone:

"Now, Gene, I know you didn't want me to tell the doctor this, but . . . "

The list could continue. Families are ingenious in their often extraordinary efforts to gain control of the session. Generally, the family is motivated by fear. They are simply frightened about their problem, exposure of the family, and the unknowns of the interviewer and the interview process. Exerting control is one way to hold on to the known.

No matter what the family's motivation, the physician must win this power struggle if the work is to be successful. A family interview in which the family exerts its control over the interviewer is an invitation to chaos. A clear example of this occurred with the Martins, the sort of family that we have come to recognize as an uproar family. Successful interviewing with an uproar family is helped by nerves of steel.

THE MARTIN FAMILY

The Martins asked for counseling help with their 10-year-old son, David, who had a learning disability and an explosive temper. Apparently, he was always in trouble, at home and school. His mother was worried and depressed, while his father traveled and was seldom home. There were three siblings: Michael, 12, Rebecca, 14, and Susan, 16. The entire family arrived a little early for the scheduled appointment, and their presence in the waiting room was immediately felt. The four children launched a joint assault on the furniture. Chairs, tables, and lamps were rearranged and magazines were rolled up and transformed into jousting rods, with which the children hit each other. The receptionist's effort to calm them was mildly successful, but within a few minutes, they were fighting again. In one corner of the waiting room, Mrs. Martin sat never looking up, trying hard to find meaning in an office copy of *Curious George Goes to the Circus*. Mr. Martin occasionally roared at the children from his vantage point beside the fish tank. However, he was no more successful than the receptionist. The physician gathered the group to begin the family interview and ushered them into the room. Before the doctor was in the interview room, one of the kids had turned off the tape recorder, another was holding his head under the office faucet getting a drink, and a third was pinching the fourth. Mrs. Martin slid into the nearest chair, shifting little from her previous posture in the waiting room; she was still carrying that book. She said nothing, while Mr. Martin roared at the children to behave. They did not heed.

Families such as the Martins, while perhaps entertaining to envision, are horrendous to work with in an interview. As long as they are controlling the interview process, nothing productive can happen in the encounter. This degree of frenzy and confusion may call for strong measures on the therapist's part. The therapist may refuse to proceed with them until order is restored, or he or she can direct the parents to bring their children into line, halting the interview until this has been accomplished (keep in mind that this step may take the entire session). This task may demonstrate the family's difficulties with clear communication around the issue of setting limits. The therapist may decide that the entire family cannot be interviewed together and can choose to interview subsystems in the family (e.g., parents alone, children alone, parents with certain children). Other family members are then excused from the room.

The Martins represent an extreme in the control issue between interviewer and family. Most families are not so flamboyant in their desire to control the situation. However, what these families lack in drama, they more than compensate for in subtlety and effectiveness. A family's control manipulations consist of behaviors that its members are using with one another daily, and each person has developed his own repertoire into a finely practiced skill. These same control manipulations are turned toward the interviewer who begins to enter their family system.

Control manipulations may be either active or passive in nature. Active manipulations are easier to identify and deal within an interview setting (Table 5.1). Passive manipulations require considerable interviewer vigilance to recognize and then avoid (Table 5.2).

An interviewer must be ready when any of these control manipulations are attempted, so that "the family members are in charge of themselves, while the interviewer is in charge of the session" (10). In order to accomplish this, we urge trainees to do whatever is required to provide for their own working comfort in the session, to take care of themselves. If interviewers pay attention to their own needs and the circumstances needed for productive work, they will likely be in control of the interview. Although this can mean different things for different interviewers and families, remember it is the interviewer's responsibility and not that of the family to determine the rules of the session. The interviewer may share these rules explicitly with the family at the outset or introduce rules as needed. Examples of rules often used in family interviews include:

No blaming is allowed.
One person at a time may talk.
The past is not to be discussed; discussion stays in the present.
The children may play with the available toys; they may not use them
    as weapons.
Individuals may not run around the room.
The room equipment is off limits.
Each person speaks for himself or herself. No one speaks for someone else.

The interviewer should direct the parents to establish and maintain order with their children. However, order in the session is ultimately the physician's responsibility. If the parents are unable to control their children, the physician must look to his or her own needs as a guide for the next step. If an 11-month-old child will not be quiet enough to allow a conversation with the rest of the family, the doctor should arrange for child care outside the interview room or terminate the session. Taking care of oneself means knowing under what conditions one is comfortable working and also under what conditions one is unwilling to continue.

Table 5.1. Control Through Active Manipulation

CHARACTER	ACTION
Judge	Blames
	Accuses
	Distrusts
	Says "I told you so"
Bully	Threatens
	Humiliates
	Argues
	Insults
	Is sarcastic
	Name calls
Calculator	Deceives
	Lies
	Tries to outwit
	Uses pressure tactics
	Blackmails
	Bribes
	Makes false promises
Dictator	Gives unilateral solutions
	Gives orders
	Suppresses
	Bosses

Developing a Beginning Formulation and Treatment Plan

The goal of developing a beginning formulation and treatment plan goes almost without saying. Trainees usually understand that figuring out what's going on in a family and helping the group learn what to do about it is the interviewer's job. In an initial visit with a family, a *beginning* formulation is required. Conclusions must be tentative because both diagnostic formulations and treatment plans are in flux while the family continues to provide information about its system. An interviewer will not have all the pieces of the puzzle by the end of the first interview. Family members may be withholding important information at first. Thus, puzzle pieces may be missing or the puzzle itself may change over time. Only a beginning construct is possible in the first session.

However, beginning formulations are important because they determine early therapeutic interventions. Intervention must happen quickly. Families seek the physician's assistance because they are in distress. If the physi-

Table 5.2. Control Through Passive Manipulation

CHARACTER	FORM OF MANIPULATION
Protector	Exaggerates her support of others Is nonjudgmental to a fault Is oversympathetic Spoils others Cares only for others and not for herself Says "I'm only doing it for your own good"
Nice guy	Exaggerates caring and loving Is too kind Is always aiming to please Never asks for what she wants herself Apologizes prematurely and unnecessarily Appeases and smooths over
Clinging vine	Wants to be taken care of Lets others do his work Cries Plays helpless and confused Demands attention Complains Is easily fooled
Weakling	Exaggerates sensitivity and is easily hurt Forgets Does not hear Is passively silent Gives up Worries Withdraws
Intellectualizer	Explains and rationalizes Stays with facts, not feelings Uses words to impress and create distance Quotes opinions and authorities

cian does not begin alleviating distress within the first session, the family will lose hope and might not return. We believe the family members should leave the session feeling that they have received something from the physician, and the physician should feel that he or she has given something of value to the family. The implementation of a beginning therapeutic plan is one means to make the family feel they are benefiting from the visit. The physician may propose a task for the family to do at home, may begin to challenge communication styles, or the physician may intervene in the family's structure and begin to disrupt accustomed coalitions. These efforts are evidence that intervention has begun, and the group will feel they are receiving something more than good listening.

It is critical to develop a tentative treatment plan and begin using it quickly. However, we hesitate suggesting this to physicians, particularly pediatricians. Because we are in the field of pediatrics, we are familiar with the pediatrician's well-developed impulse to offer *something* to patients quickly. Therefore, we would not like the pediatrician to use our suggestion (i.e., that families need to leave the first session feeling that they "received something") as support for a style that promotes "getting them in, getting it solved, getting them out." We often encounter this approach in the beginning family work of our pediatric resident trainees. In their zeal to help a child and the family, trainees often give advice and directive solutions long before the family is able to act on or even understand such advice.

Pediatrician:	You folks are just going to have to be more firm.
Mother:	Well, I . . .
Father:	That's what I keep telling her, Doc.
Mother:	But Frank, you don't understand
Pediatrician:	Fire-setting is a serious problem, Mrs. Anderson. Do you realize, Dwayne, you could have set the garage on fire!
Dwayne:	It was only a Coke bottle full of kerosene.
Pediatrician:	No matter. I want you to promise your parents right now you will not do that again—ever.
Dwayne:	(silence)
Pediatrician:	Now come on, Dwayne. Your parents and I can't leave today until this gets settled. Be reasonable. Think about what could have happened.
Father:	Sit up and listen to the doctor, Dwayne.
Mother:	He's so upset.

The advice itself may be accurate and the directive necessary. We daresay that such an approach may even be looked upon favorably as good medicine by certain administrators of managed care (those intent on reducing the complexities of medical care to a slogan: "treat 'em and street 'em"). But the advice-giving happens so fast and with such insensitive persistence that the family feels programmed rather than heard. Our experience has been that advice so offered is not followed, nor does the group return. Probably the resident's therapeutic urge to make things better and solve the problem in one fell swoop overtook his attention to our suggestion that the interview should be a "touching experience" for each family member.

Making the Interview a "Touching" Experience

Family members should leave the first interview feeling relieved because the physician has heard, understood, and acknowledged their distress. Such feelings of relief, of being touched, have a direct impact on their level of hopefulness regarding change, their willingness to work diligently on issues, and their desire to return for future sessions.

Facilitating these feelings in every family member is hard work for the interviewer, particularly if the family is large. However, the interviewer should spend sufficient time with each family member so that each can acknowledge: "This doctor is listening to me, seems interested in me, even understands some of what I am feeling inside." That awareness alone may be enough to bring individuals back for a second session.

The techniques for touching family members in this way are varied, depending on an interviewer's personal style for expressing empathy toward others. Regardless of style, an interviewer may be guided by this internal thought: "While this person is talking about _____, what is he or she experiencing inside?" When that question is answered, the next becomes: "How do I let him or her know that I see and can appreciate those feelings?" A similar mental process must be repeated with each person in the room. The actual touching process is straightforward and uncomplicated. For example, some acknowledgment regarding an individual's feelings should be expressed:

"Gee, that's tough."
"You look very worried."

"What an awful spot to be in."

"Your eyes look pleased as you tell me that."

"How frustrating."

"Are you feeling pretty helpless about that?"

These communications "touch" the feelings of the person and are the ways in which an interviewer signals an understanding of what that person is experiencing. These statements are essential for the family's development of trust in the interviewer. Ironically, until the family views the interviewer as someone who hears, they themselves will be unable to listen. Conversely, as the interviewer shows that he or she is listening, family members begin to listen—to the interviewer and to one another.

Ensuring the Family's Return

If an interviewer has been successful in beginning a therapeutic program with the family, and has been able to touch most of the members, the family will return, assuming that a return visit is indicated. Occasionally, a follow-up session will be needed; yet, the interviewer for various reasons was not able to offer a beginning treatment plan, nor effectively touch the necessary family members. Under these circumstances, it is probably best to acknowledge the situation in a statement such as the following:

Physician:	Our time is just about up, and I am feeling very frustrated. You must be feeling it even more. This family came in for some help, and you've not gotten to any solutions yet. I know from what you have said that you were hoping for some specific answers to come out of this session today. Frankly, I feel that you and I need more time to understand your difficulties. And frustrating as that may sound, I am asking that you come in again in 5 days so that you and I may continue working on the problem.

This sort of bridge at least demonstrates that the interviewer has heard the family's desire for instant answers.

ENDING THE INTERVIEW

Good endings, like good beginnings, require planning. We do not feel that an interview should simply ooze to a termination, nor should it end abruptly because, "Our time is up." Instead, a family interview should be led to a conclusion by the interviewer. Each interviewer must decide how much time will be required for the conclusion process. The following may need consideration:

1. Reviewing the presenting problem with the family
2. Offering a specific directive or task, short or long
3. Planning the next appointment time
4. Selecting the family cast for the next appointment
5. Discussing the expected duration of the therapy process
6. Settling fee issues
7. Providing the family time to recoup after a very unsettling session
8. Sharing reading material
9. Discussing what the family, physician, or both will do between sessions (e.g., contact school authorities)

The interviewer must allow sufficient time to settle important items such as those listed. We suggest silently reviewing the interview at the halfway point (e.g., at 30 minutes after beginning if the session is an hour) and planning how the interviewer would like to conclude. Frequently, bringing the interview to a satisfactory conclusion will take a quarter of the total session time. A good ending influences a family's return. As Minuchin states: "All therapeutic interventions must be made with the clear knowledge that the first rule of therapeutic strategy is to leave the family willing to come again for the next session" (11).

References

1. Minuchin S. Families and family therapy. Cambridge, MA: Harvard University Press, 1974:207.
2. Haley J. Problem-solving therapy. San Francisco: Jossey-Bass, 1987:17.
3. Haley, 23.
4. Wadeson H. Conjoint marital art therapy techniques. Psychiatry 1972;35:89.
5. Mosher L, Kwiatkowska H. Family art evaluation: use in families with schizophrenic twins. J Nerv Ment Dis 1971;153:165.
6. Rubin J, Magnussen M. Family art evaluation. Family Process 1974;13:185.

7. Bing E. The conjoint family drawing. Family Process 1970;9:173.
8. Papp P. Family sculpture in preventive work with well families. Family Process 1973;12:197.
9. Simon R. Sculpting the family. Family Process 1972;11:49.
10. Whitaker C. Personal communication. October, 1975.
11. Minuchin, 212.

chapter 6

Common Behavioral Problems

When observing someone else's child in a waiting room, trainees sometimes have admitted, "Whew, if that kid were mine, I would be going nuts about now!" Their discomfort may have been caused by the child taking "forever" to feel comfortable in the new situation or by the child's stubborn persistence. Yet, the parents were not particularly irritated by the behavior that the observer found troublesome. In the observer's household, this child would be considered a "problem." In the child's home, he was not a problem. In some way, his behavior meshed with that of his family and was not troubling. Conversely, occasionally a child has seemed particularly appealing to a clinician, while exasperating the family. The parents, far from appreciating the child's intense aggressive approach to life, for example, have become irritated with his behavior. Complaining and scolding, they have come in with concerns about their "problem" child to an interviewer charmed by this trait, willing to take the youngster home for keeps.

BEHAVIORAL INDIVIDUALITY IN CHILDREN

The work of Alexander Thomas, Stella Chess, and Herbert Birch has explored the phenomenon of behavioral individuality (1). Beginning in the 1950s with an extensive longitudinal study of children's individual behavior, their work provided documentation for two basic concepts.

1. Each child has his or her own specific, individual behavioral and temperamental style, detectable in the first week of life and perhaps persistent throughout the child's subsequent development. Such traits, present so early in life, appear to be a child's innate contributions to his or her environment and may often determine the reactions of a given child

to imposed parental and environmental influences. Thus, parenting approaches can take neither total credit nor total blame for many of a child's behavioral characteristics.

2. An understanding of children's behavior cannot be obtained through scrutiny of these specific temperamental characteristics alone, nor can such understanding occur by an exclusive focus on the parents and their influences on their children. Behavior becomes understandable only through the clarification of the interaction between a particular child and a particular set of parents.

Not only does the child screen his environment, he also influences it. Thus it is not alone the parents who influence the child, but the child who influences the parents. The child, by his own nature, "conditions" his environment at the same time that the social and cultural environment affects him. In short, there is a continual effect produced by the child on his world, as well as by his world upon him. (2)

Numerous excellent examples demonstrating the interaction of nature and nurture as an important determinant of children's behavior are found in the written work of these investigators. The following case study paraphrases one of those examples:

RALPH AND JERRY

Ralph and Jerry, from different families, were much alike as babies. In any new situation, their initial reaction was to back off quietly. With each new experience (e.g., first bath, first new food, a new person handling them), they either turned solemn or quietly refused to participate. Both boys would turn away from a new food or let it dribble out of their mouths. When older, each boy ran behind mother's back if a strange person greeted him. However, after tasting the new food over and over again, or seeing the new person many times, both children would gradually come to accept the innovation. Both boys took a long time to warm up.

By the time they were 5 years old, however, the two children behaved differently. Ralph was a well-adjusted member of his kindergarten group. He looked forward to going to school, greeted his playmates pleasantly, and visited back and forth with friends after school. Ralph's parents had come to understand early on that his hesitancy about accepting the unfamiliar needed to be honored.

They found that rushing him did not work, and they provided him with the necessary time and warming-up period in new situations.

Jerry's early functioning was much like Ralph's. His parents, too, did not rush him and did not care how long it took him to begin eating solid food or changing from four to three feedings a day. But his mother's attitude changed when she started to take Jerry to the neighborhood playground. He reacted to the new situation and strange faces by holding back and clinging, and she was sure that other mothers in the playground were blaming her for having such an "anxiously" timid baby. They probably were. Instead of holding him or giving him a familiar toy to play with until he warmed up to the new setting, she began to push Jerry insistently to play "like the other little boys." The more she pressured, the more he clung. Finally, she gave up taking him to the playground at all and avoided placing him in new situations if possible. When Jerry entered kindergarten, he cried and clung again. Before school each morning he clung to his mother, and he rarely spoke above a whisper in class. Jerry had become the anxious fearful child his mother dreaded.

From birth, both Ralph and Jerry were examples of what Chess and others refer to as the child who is "slow to warm up." This behavioral attribute was handled differently by the parents of each boy and illustrates how the mix of a child's own temperament and that of his parents determines many aspects of behavioral development and often whether or not a "behavioral problem" develops.

> *Normal and deviant development is at all times the result of a continuously evolving interaction between a child and his individual characteristics and significant features of his intrafamilial and extrafamilial environment. Temperament is only one attribute of the growing child—in its internal relations with abilities and motives and in its external relations with environmental opportunities and stresses. (3)*

This view has considerable common sense appeal and is reassuring to parents, providing them with some relief from the traditional finger of blame, which has declared that a child's behavior is "the parents' fault." Psychotherapy, from the 1930s to the 1980s, was particularly hard on mothers. A prominent therapist from that period, Dr. Hilde Bruch, empathized with the plight of parents:

> *Modern parent education . . . implies that parents are all responsible and*
> *must assume the role of playing preventive Fate for their children. . . .*
> *An unrelieved picture of model parental behavior, a contrived image of*
> *artificial perfection and happiness, is held up before parents who try*
> *valiantly to reach the ever receding ideal of "good parenthood," like dogs*
> *after a mechanical rabbit. (4)*

In this orientation, when problems in a child surface, a parent inevitably feels responsible.

Nine Categories of Child Behavior

Chess and her colleagues intended to alleviate the parental guilt that was imposed by approaches similar to Bruch's description. Their publication for parents, *Your Child Is a Person,* was subtitled, *A Psychological Approach to Parenthood Without Guilt.* We feel they succeeded in their purpose and have made a major contribution to the understanding of children's behavior.

They found that infants' behavior could be accurately classified under nine headings:

1. **Activity level.** Some babies were from early infancy onward much more active than others.
2. **Biological regularity.** Babies were found to differ significantly in the regularity of their biological functioning (e.g., feeding, bowel, and bladder function, crying).
3. **Approach or withdrawal as a characteristic response to a new situation.** Regarding the child's initial reaction to any new stimulus pattern, be it food, people, places, toys, or procedures, they found that some babies easily accepted these new experiences, whereas others pulled away.
4. **Adaptability to change in routine.** Some babies shifted easily and quickly with changing schedules. In general, they changed their behavior to fit in with the new routine the mother wanted to set. Others accommodated more slowly to change.
5. **Level of sensory threshold.** Babies with a high "sensory threshold" did not startle at loud noises or bright lights. They did not react to being wet or soiled. At the other extreme were babies who cried the moment they soiled. A slight sound would attract their attention; they would wake the moment the light was switched on.

6. **Positive or negative mood.** Some children cried when they woke up or were put down, and they just generally fussed. Others predominantly cooed, gurgled happily, and smiled.

7. **Intensity of response (in terms of the amount of physical energy displayed).** Some babies greeted hunger with loud, piercing cries. Others cried softly. These differences were often apparent in other aspects of their behavior as well. Some babies demonstrated tremendous energy in response to both painful and pleasurable activities, whereas others showed less energy and were more gentle and less vigorous.

8. **Distractibility.** Some babies seemed able to concentrate better than others on feeding or staring at a mobile, no matter what else was going on around them.

9. **Persistence and attention span.** Babies demonstrated great variation in the ability to continue an activity in the face of difficulties or to resume it after interruption.

The authors referred to the child's preponderant pattern of functioning in these nine categories as the child's temperament.

There is nothing mysterious about temperament. It merely represents a statement of the basic style which characterizes a person's behavior. Some students of behavior have divided psychological functioning into three parts which they call the what, the why, and the how. The what refers to the content of behavior, including intelligence, skills, aptitudes, and talents. The why relates to motivation, or the reasons for behaving in a given way. The how refers to temperament—the manner in which the what and the why are expressed. (5)

The usual variability shown by infants and children in these nine categories all reflect normal, healthy development. A child who is characteristically negative in his mood and intense in his response to situations is not necessarily abnormal. He may not have many friends at the park, but his behavior may simply be a reflection of his temperament, and one temperamental style is not better or more normal than another; styles are simply different, with some easier for parents to manage than others.

The "Difficult" Child

In 7 to 10% of babies (according to these investigators), a child did show a specific selection of behaviors from the nine categories, which won him the dubious title of "a difficult child" (6). Such a child, partly because of his temperamental style, was more at risk for the onset of behavioral problems than his temperamentally different peers. This child demonstrated irregularity in biological functions, particularly during the newborn period. He did not establish definite hunger and sleeping patterns. He did not have regular bowel movements, and he tended to have withdrawal reactions to new stimuli and situations. In addition, this child was not easily adaptable, and almost every change in his routine involved a struggle and his own high intensity of response.

Even though this temperamental pattern may have smoothed out somewhat as this child grew older, such behavior as an infant was particularly troublesome, particularly for a new mother who might easily, yet erroneously, assume from the above collection of behaviors that something was drastically wrong with her parenting. The combination of irregularity, slow adaptability, withdrawal reactions, high intensity of response, and predominantly negative mood was often perplexing to handle. However, even in children with this temperamental style, the authors stressed that they could find no evidence that mothers or fathers of these "difficult" babies were responsible for the child's mode of behavior.

The "Easy" Child

The authors described another category called the "easy" child. Temperamentally this child was regular in his biological functions, was moderately active, adapted well to change, seemed always happy, was not particularly intense, yet was not distractible and could persist long enough to complete a task. He was almost always charming, seen as easily adaptable and wanting to please. The combination conjures up notions of a parent's dream, but that was not always the case. Chess and her colleagues cited one example of a "model" child who stimulated her parents to accept indiscriminately the child's every move. The result was a child who, by age 3 years, knew how to be charming but did not work and play well with others. Those outside the immediate family found her "babyish and immature." Her social style had not progressed much beyond that of infancy.

We see behavioral individuality as an important variable for the clinician to consider when working with families concerning common behavioral problems. Recognizing a child's temperamental pattern as it differs from that of the parents and assisting the parents to understand and work more effectively with their child's pattern can be important in working with families.

Chess and her co-workers reported the case of a mother who had failed to wean or toilet train her 3-year-old daughter or even leave her alone with anyone else for an evening because she "didn't believe in making issues over the crucial steps in development" (7). When it came time for preschool, she realized that her daughter must be toilet trained to be accepted. The mother became panicky and asked for help from Dr. Chess. The child's temperamental pattern was found to be one of biological irregularity, mild intensity of response, and easy adaptability. It seemed to the authors that, given these characteristics, if her mother had set a schedule for her, she would have been a model child rather than a whiner around whose demands the whole family danced. The therapists believed that she could still be toilet-trained by firm scheduling and consistent management. The mother was desperate and agreed. By the time school began, the child was trained. In this case, an understanding of the child's behavioral pattern suggested the appropriate solutions for both the doctor and the parents.

As we prepared this edition of our text, we learned that *Your Child Is A Person* is no longer in print. That small volume was an integral part of our thinking and teaching for decades. Although written primarily for parents, the book was recommended by us to trainees and families. Finding that it was no longer available was like losing an old friend. We were pleased to find an excellent replacement text for trainees by Carey and McDevitt called *Coping with Children's Temperament: A Guide for Professionals* (8). This text includes a review of all the original material that we have found timeless and useful, with the addition of current developments in the field of behavioral individuality. This volume provides a succinct distillation of 40 years of thought by those interested in the realm of children's temperament. It is a somewhat less satisfactory reference, acknowledged by the authors themselves, for parents and families to use. There are other books that we have recommended to parents (9,10,11); however, we will continue to hold onto our dog-eared copies of *Your Child Is A Person*.

FREQUENT BEHAVIOR PROBLEMS

In pediatric practice, behavior problems, such as temper tantrums and discipline problems, are extremely common and often do not disappear as quickly as everyone might wish. They tend to be extremely persistent. The child's pediatrician is often the *first* professional to be consulted in such situations. In addition to "discipline problems," parents regularly seek pediatric advice concerning any of the behavioral symptoms in Table 6.1.

Some might find it appealing to proceed in cookbook fashion with separate recommendations for working in each category in Table 6.1. However, this approach becomes impossible because there is no single correct strategy to use for the child who refuses to sleep at night, or for the child who eats too much. Defining a child's symptoms alone may not determine the necessary therapeutic approach. A clinician may determine this path better by helping family members become aware of their particular system of communication and interaction, because it is often this pattern (along with differences in neurodevelopmental maturation and behavioral individuality) that underlies the development symptoms. Figure out the family system, its meaning and purpose, and one will frequently determine the problem and its resolution.

Remember an earlier example from chapter 1: Joan Locksley's symptom was that she did not sleep. However, it would have made little difference (in terms of the pediatrician's treatment) if her grandmother had complained that Joan would not eat. In both cases, the pediatrician would be correct to proceed by helping the family understand and alter its existing system, structure, and pattern of behavior. The same is true in the case of Jennifer Maloney (chapter 3) and her symptoms of "night terrors," school avoidance, and enuresis. It was the family system of communication regarding unspoken feelings that required change, not just the symptom. Recognition of the specific purpose of a symptom is important in family work. It will often suggest an intervention, such as which task to assign the family. Symptoms *should* be discussed in an interview. Families come to the physician for specific help with a specific problem; they are offended if the symptom seems brushed aside and not discussed. A refusal to consider their stated problem may send them packing and understandably so. However, it is rare that a focus solely on the symptom will be sufficient to dictate a course of treatment.

Instead of illustrating each symptom listed in Table 6.1, we have selected one symptom (i.e., "she just won't mind") to demonstrate the use of family treatment in common pediatric behavior problems, discussing in detail

Table 6.1. Common Behavioral Problems

PROBLEM	SYMPTOM
"Minding" and discipline	The child —does not mind/obey —steals —lies —sets fires
Sleep	The child —will not sleep in his or her own bed alone —has nightmares —will not go to bed
Eating	The child —eats too much —does not eat enough —does not eat the right foods
School	The child —has failing grades —will not go to school —does not behave in school
Getting along with others	The child —fights with other children —will not play with other children —does not get along with adults or authority figures —is scared of children, adults, or dogs

our clinical work with a family who sought help. Although the specifics of this family's situation are unique to them, the principles used by the pediatrician apply in many other clinical encounters, with the same or a different common behavioral complaint.

THE THOMAS FAMILY

A fellow pediatrician, Dr. Tom Jones, called asking to refer a family to one of the authors. He knew of our interest in using family approaches with pediatric problems and often asked for such assistance. Dr. Jones indicated that the family was concerned about their 4-year-old son who "won't mind." He followed up his call with this letter:

I am sending Andrew Thomas and his parents to you for consulta-
tion regarding his behavior. This nearly 4-year-old child is a happy,
alert, quite verbal youngster who has seemed quite advanced for his
years. He is the Thomas's only child. There have been relatively few
medical problems except for an episode some months ago of what
seems to have been ketotic hypoglycemia, which was appropriately
treated with IV glucose and responded well to dietary changes; he
has had no further episodes since then. The parents are both profes-
sional dancers who lead a somewhat busy life. At the current time
they are very frustrated about his behavior, that is, his unwilling-
ness to accept any limits or to "behave." They are wondering if he is
abnormal in any way—developmentally and emotionally. I would
appreciate your comments regarding Andy and the family situation.

With best personal regards,
Thomas Jones, MD

Mrs. Thomas subsequently called for an appointment and readily accepted the stipulation that the entire family come for the first interview. The pediatrician kept the call brief and did not encourage her to discuss in detail the family's concerns. For the most part, she complied. She sounded frustrated and amused by her son's obstinacy, saying with a laugh, "He's such a little devil, Dr. Anderson. I just don't know what to do with him." The physician heard both sides of her message but chose not to comment on the discrepancy. He acknowledged her frustration and filed his observation of the double-level message for future use.

The First Session

The family and pediatrician met as scheduled 1 week after the initial call. The family arrived 15 minutes late for their first appointment, and their entrance reminded the doctor of a processional, with Andy leading the group. Although he was only 4 years old, he seemed to swagger into the office. When the physician greeted him, Andy gave him a long, careful look, then headed for the toys in the office, remarking, "Ooh Mom, look at the toys!" He settled himself on the rug and began to explore the array of play materials kept for such purposes—all of this before his parents were quite in the room. They were following closely behind, however—Mrs. Thomas, breathless, held out her hand, "Hello Dr. Anderson, I'm Carla. Sorry we're late, got held up in traffic. This is my husband, Rod . . . and Andy . . . Say hello to the doctor, dear, yes aren't those nice toys! Oh! (spilling her purse as she shook hands with the doctor) Isn't that the limit, how clumsy!" Mr. Thomas brought up the rear of the procession. He too was breathless, sweeping up after his wife and maneuvering the group into the office.

The family's appearance was interesting. Andy was lithe and handsome, wearing new clothes. Dr. Tom Jones said that the parents were both dancers, and they seemed ready for a performance of some sort even now. The father was tall and solidly built, dressed in a shirt open to the navel. His pants were tucked into knee-length boots, and he was wearing a necklace. The mother's dramatic makeup and flamboyant hair style suggested the appearance of Raggedy Ann. The interviewer relaxed, thinking that no matter what happened, this session would be lively.

Mrs. Thomas completed the retrieval of her purse contents and sat down. Her husband shook the physician's hand and took a seat beside his wife. Andy continued to play.

Physician:	I spoke with Dr. Jones on the phone; however, I don't have very much of the story. What help would this family like from me?
Father:	We're not sure if we even have a problem, but we thought—
Mother:	Oh we do, at least I do. Andy is just really a handful.
Physician:	Explain, Mrs. Thomas.
Mother:	What do you do, Dr. Anderson, with a child who refuses to stay in his seat belt in the car—while you're driving on the middle of the freeway!
Physician:	(acknowledging the feeling that he hears in her tone of voice) That sounds frightening. How have you handled the situation?
Andy:	(coming over to his mother and putting a toy in her lap) How does this work, Mom?
Mother:	(allowing the interview to be interrupted) It's a puzzle, dear; you put the green piece right in that little slot. No, not like that. Here. 'll show you. There, that's it. Now the red one. Where do you think that goes? Gooooood. Isn't that a fun puzzle? Maybe we could get one like that sometime.
Andy:	(returning to toy shelf and depositing a second item in his mother's lap) Show me this one; show me!
Mother:	All right—why Andy, this is exactly like the one at preschool. You know how that one goes.

Father:	Don't interrupt your mother, son. She and the doctor were talking.
Mother:	He's just so excited by all these toys. You little dickens—are you bringing me another one? Mother's going to run out of lap room.

This bit of dialogue already displayed many useful facts.

1. The family was lively; their entrance suggested they were also somewhat disorganized.
2. Andy literally led the way in this family, during and after their entrance.
3. The mother and father were not in agreement regarding the need for concern, nor were they united in their way of guiding their son.
4. The mother suggested that it was she who felt helpless with her son.
5. The mother allowed and even encouraged Andy to control with interruptions in this situation; she made no attempt to assert her own needs.
6. The father spoke for his wife in correcting their son, suggesting that the father too saw her as unable to take care of her own needs in exchanges with Andy.
7. The father was disregarded by both his wife and Andy for his efforts.

The interviewer could proceed in several ways. He could encourage the mother to set some limits on Andy's interruptions, pointing out her subtle encouragement of Andy's interruptions through her enthusiasm and interest. He could mention her readiness to drop her own needs and train of thought in the face of Andy's maneuvers. The father's speaking for his wife could be challenged by introducing the rule that each person speaks only for himself or herself. The interviewer could ask each parent to share his or her feelings as this family scene is being played out, or both parents could be asked to talk together about what was happening in the office.

The physician chose none of these options maybe because it was so early in the interview, he felt the need for more time to watch their system unfolding. He encouraged them to continue.

Physician:	You were mentioning difficulty with Andy in the seat belt . . .
Mother:	Oh yes, well, it's not just that. He simply won't mind. Is that normal for 4-year-olds? I've heard about the terrible twos, but should it go on this long? It seems as though *everything* is a hassle. Getting dressed in the morning, Rod and I both have to leave very early in the morning for the studio. Andy knows that—it's really a tight schedule in the morning. Get-

	ting him to the nursery school and all. He knows how to dress himself pretty well, don't you honey?
Andy:	(sets his jaw and vigorously shakes his head no)
Mother:	Well, he does. When he wants, he does it fast—all but the socks and shoes. And I help him with that; I don't mind. I get him up in plenty of time . . . 30 minutes later, I come and everything is still where I left it, and he's playing on the floor in his pajamas. Doesn't ever do that on Sundays—just weekdays, when he *knows* we have to get going. And I come unglued—there's no doubt about it. Ask Rod—he has to rescue both of us when I blow! That's when he comes in. First of all I have a really short fuse . . . Rod will tell you that! (laughs and slaps her husband's knee)
Father:	(smiling) Things do go smoother in the morning if I can get Carla to just either stay cool or stay out of it. *I* don't really have that much trouble with Andy. If she would just . . .
Physician:	(interrupting) This sounds like a message for Carla. Would you tell her that directly now? I'll listen along.
Father:	She's heard it before. I'm like a broken record on that one. Isn't that right, hon?
Physician:	Perhaps, but it doesn't sound like you've ever gotten anywhere with it and that must be very frustrating. Do it once again, now.
Father:	(turning to his wife) Well, you know, if you would just let me handle Andy's getting dressed in the morning . . .

Having facilitated the start of direct communication between the parents, the physician now had two choices. He could encourage the parents' dialogue and begin to work on their communication style, or he could forego a focus on communication for now and point out that the family's actions seemed to suggest that Carla was inadequate as a parent. He was about the choose the latter method when Andy, true to form, changed the course of the interview. The interviewer had momentarily lost track of the boy, who had tired of the toys and had meandered to the other side of the room. He proceeded to strip all the way down to his underpants, looking and smiling specifically at his mother as he did so. The interviewer noted that his mother returned the smile; she even laughed. Mr. Thomas shifted his legs nervously but said nothing about what was happening. Every now and then, the mother would turn toward Andy, smile, and then return her gaze to her husband and the interviewer.

An interviewer might feel frustrated were this child's provocations seen solely as interruptions to the flow of the interview and the adult conversation. They were far more significant: the child's important contribution to a disclosure of the family system. Andy's behavior was helping the family play out their problem in front of the physician. At that moment, both parents were talking about Andy's getting dressed in the morning. Their talk was mostly "just words," whereas their child's behavior was a more powerful demonstration of the family dilemma. Through discussion and action, the problem was revealed: Andy's clever manipulations stimulated mixed messages (approval and disapproval) from his mother, and mixed messages from his mother stimulated Andy's clever manipulations. The two had developed their own dance with one another. While Andy was becoming more powerful in his ability to control family situations, his mother was growing less competent in her mothering. The physician also suspected that the father augmented the notion of the mother's incompetence by succeeding in situations that had given his wife trouble and by criticizing her approaches with Andy.

The interviewer resolved to use the unfolding situation to help Mrs. Thomas be effective with her son immediately. Through this process, she might also reveal what feelings were immobilizing her with Andy. The physician asked her to take action now, simultaneously coaching her to change the dysfunctional aspects of her communication with Andy. He also determined to keep Mr. Thomas from "rescuing," criticizing, or showing her up with his own parenting prowess.

While Andy was doing exercises (nude except for his underpants), the interviewer began:

Physician:	(to parents) Tell me what you're feeling right at this moment.
Father:	(shakes his head in exasperation)
Mother:	(whispering, as though she did not want Andy to hear) You want to know what I'm feeling? Huh? I wish that kid would put his clothes back on. I am so embarrassed.
Physician:	OK, make it happen, Mrs. Thomas (pushing his chair back out of the action).
Mother:	Andy, it's chilly in the doctor's office.
Andy:	I don't care.
Mother:	You might catch a cold.

Andy:	No, I won't.
Mother:	You might (teasing in her voice).
Andy:	I don't care.
Mother:	(turning back to the physician) See?
Physician:	Make it happen, now (motioning for her to continue).
Mother:	Andy, wouldn't you like to put your clothes back on?
Andy:	(shakes his head no)
Physician:	Are you really giving him a choice?
Mother:	Well . . . no, not really.
Physician:	You want him to get dressed now?
Mother:	Yes, I'm about to boil. I've never been so embarrassed.
Physician:	Well, stop smiling, and make it happen now.
Mother:	Andy, put your clothes on.
Andy:	I don't want to. Can I get a drink?
Mother:	(sputter)
Physician:	Do whatever you need to do, Mrs. Thomas to have him get his clothes on *now* . . . if that's what you want.
Mother:	(She drops her pleasant expression and gets out of her chair, moving toward Andy and his pile of laundry. She is deadly serious. Her strong voice reflects her feeling and expectations.) I want you to put those clothes on . . . right now.
Andy:	(He starts to cry and starts to put on his clothes. His sobbing and stomping increase but do not interfere with his dressing himself right down to his socks, which ordinarily his mother helps him with. Finally, he stops crying and approaches his parents.) Can I leave my shoes off until we go?

Mother and father both nodded agreement, and Mrs. Thomas fell back into her chair. The whole episode had taken about 15 minutes. Andy now played quietly, and he occasionally sat in his mother's or his father's lap. He was not provocative, nor did he interrupt again.

Physician:	I think we need to talk about what just happened. I'm won-

	dering how that experience was for each of you . . . Mrs. Thomas?
Mother:	Hard, really hard. I'm absolutely exhausted. At home it would have been different.
Physician:	In what way?
Mother:	I would have walked away from the whole thing, but I might have given him a swat before I did.
Father:	Or you would have been screaming at him, and I would have come running.
Physician:	That brings up a point, Mr. Thomas. I was admiring your silence throughout what happened. I was wondering how it was for you to sit and watch but not be involved yourself. (The interviewer hoped recognizing the father's silence would facilitate a sharing of his feelings and expectations regarding the episode.)
Father:	Very . . . uncomfortable, I guess . . . I guess I was expecting my wife to fail. I think I really was.
Physician:	All right. Again I would like you to say that directly to your wife—with two changes: take the "I guess" out of your statement and put the whole thing in the present tense.
Father:	(turning to his wife and nodding to show that he understands the interviewer's directions) Well, hon, that's right; I did expect that you couldn't do it.
Physician:	Good, now once more and put it in the present tense.
Father:	(to his wife) I do expect you to fail with Andy?
Physician:	How does that sound?
Father:	It sounds terrible, awful. No, that's not right . . . I don't want her to be a failure with our son.
Physician:	And yet your behavior . . . ?
Father:	(after a long pause) Yeah, I have been doing that—sort of waiting and predicting that I'll have to bail her . . .
Physician:	(points to Mrs. Thomas)

Father:	Predicting that I'll have to bail *you* out with Andy.
Physician:	And is that the way you want it to be?
Father:	Heck, no. I don't want to bail her . . . *you* out. I want you to bail yourself out if you need to.
Physician:	What do you say to that, Mrs. Thomas?
Mother:	Well, I . . .
Physician:	Say it to your husband, not me.
Mother:	I'm not sure I'm up to it. I'd like to, but . . .
Physician:	Hold it . . . sorry to keep interrupting . . . about that word, "but"; it has a way of canceling out everything that has just preceded it. Would you in fact like to be able to manage Andy successfully on your own?
Mother:	Oh yes.
Physician:	OK, then begin again: "I would like to, *and* . . . "
Mother:	I would like to . . . and . . . I'm scared.
Physician:	Tell your husband, scared of what?
Mother:	I'm not sure. But something really clicked in the middle of all that a few minutes ago. When you asked me, Dr. Anderson, if I was giving Andy a choice. Well, I realized that I do that all the time at home. I can hear myself over and over again: "Don't you think you're tired Andy? . . . Wouldn't you like to finish your soup? . . . Wouldn't you like a nice bath?" Of course he mostly says no . . . and then I'm livid. What do I do then? That's when I start screaming usually.
Physician:	So if it isn't a choice, don't make it a question (failing to notice that he had allowed the issue of Mrs. Thomas' fear to slip away).
Mother:	Absolutely, now how do I remember that?
Physician:	Now you're trying to trap *me* into seeing you as incompetent. It won't work. I won't buy it. As a matter of fact, I think you've been selling yourself short for a long time regarding your talents as a mother.

Mother:	(smiles as though she has been caught, nods, and falls silent)
Physician:	Are you clear about what was effective in what you did just now with Andy?
Mother:	Well—this changing questions to statements for one thing.
Physician:	And what else?
Mother:	Ummmmm, getting serious, I think.
Physician:	Right. You let him know that you meant business.
Mother:	Uh-huh
Physician:	How?
Mother:	You told me to stop smiling.
Physician:	Had you been aware that you do that *a lot* with Andy?
Mother:	What do you mean?
Physician:	Smiling . . .
Mother:	He's so cute . . .
Physician:	Do you see any consequences for smiling at him when he misbehaves and when you want to get something serious across?
Mother:	Well, sometimes I just enjoy him—even his antics . . .
Physician:	Are you aware that you let him know that you enjoy his antics and that you are encouraging him? He gets a mixed message from you when your voice and face don't match or when what you want and what you say are two different things. He pays a lot of attention to your smiling encouragement.
Mother:	I just find him so delightful—even when he's acting up sometimes. You mean I'm not even supposed to enjoy my child? Well, I don't know . . . and actually I'm not sure that kids, especially as young as Andy, are as perceptive as you are suggesting. Do you think he really watches my facial expressions that closely?

The interview continued for another few minutes, and, for the moment, Mrs. Thomas was not going to buy the doctor's premise about double-level messages.

There was more work to do, but the session was almost over. With Andy asleep in his father's lap, the physician asked the parents if they would like to return. Both parents said yes, volunteered that the session had been helpful, and made a return appointment. As an extension of their behavior in the interview, the physician gave each parent an assignment: the mother was to concentrate on turning questions into statements with Andy without worrying about doing anything else differently with him, and the father was to focus on developing the ability to stay out of issues between Andy and his mother.

The Second Session

In 2 weeks, the family returned. Unfortunately, Andy did not come; he was sick with chickenpox. Mrs. Thomas had called the day before to let the physician know that Andy was ill, but the physician decided to proceed with the session because he had some specific issues from the initial visit that could be pursued without Andy. His pre-interview thoughts about the Thomases were organized in this way:

1. Had each parent been successful in their assigned task? If not, that issue would need to be discussed.
2. The mother said that getting Andy to put his clothes on in the office had exhausted her. She also mentioned that she was frightened of managing him alone without a rescue from her husband. What was behind all of that?
3. What was standing in the way of her recognizing the obvious double-level messages that she repeatedly offered her son?
4. Aside from father's too available helpfulness, the physician knew very little about him. He wanted to shine a brighter light on Mr. Thomas during the second session.

There could have been a fifth item on this list; however, the interviewer was unaware of it at the time, not realizing until later that his efforts in the initial interview to promote direct dialogue between the two parents had largely failed. He had encouraged their talking to each other; however, a quick review of the transcript shows that no matter what the verbal direction to the parents had been, the interchange proceeded mostly in a doctor-mother-doctor-mother sequence. An appropriate fifth concern might have been: what was standing in the parents' way of direct communication, and how could the interviewer move himself out of their dialogue more effectively?

With these thoughts in mind, the interviewer asked the parents to start the session, giving them the responsibility for bringing up their own concerns and indicating that he expected them to develop their own resources for using the time. The physician began by saying, "How would you like to use the time today?" For a moment, neither parent spoke. They were both looking pleased. Remembering Mrs. Thomas's counterfeit smile of the previous session, the interviewer was not sure how to interpret their expressions. He waited.

Father:	I did it . . . we all did it. (triumphant)
Physician:	Good . . . did what?
Father:	Our assignment.
Physician:	Ahhh. I see. OK, I would like you to talk about your own assignment, Rod, and Carla will talk about hers.
Father:	I was able to stay out of the middle with those two this week. Of course, it helped that everything was working OK . . . I didn't need to come in.
Physician:	How are you feeling about that?
Father:	Ummmmm . . . in a way like 200 pounds is off my back. Oh, sorry, Carla—you know what I mean. (Both break up at the metaphor, especially in light of their profession, and that they are dance partners.) But I am serious . . . I feel . . .
Physician:	To your wife, Rod. Say it to her.
Father:	I feel tremendously relieved. I had not realized how much I ran around poised and ready to break up anything out of line between you and Andy.
Mother:	Well, I really depended on you for that. You are a tremendous help. My temper is—well, you know—I flare really quickly. Sometimes it scares me, I think I always have in the back of my head, "Rod will get us cooled down."

The interview was going well. Of course, the mother was sloppy in her use of pronouns (e.g., "it," "us"), but the physician said nothing because he was beginning to hear about the success of their assignments, at least from Mr. Thomas, and the mother had yet to be heard from. More importantly, she was voluntarily returning to the theme of feeling "scared" in encounters with Andy. The interviewer had intended to reintroduce that issue, but now he would not have to. However, he would make it his responsibility to see that the mother's fear, when upset with Andy, did not get lost this time.

Physician:	And what if he doesn't?

Mother:	What do you mean?
Physician:	What do you fear might happen if Rod doesn't rescue you?
Mother:	(long pause and then in a very soft voice) My temper is something fierce. . . . (another long pause and then tears)
Father:	(He moves for the tissues and begins to stuff three into his wife's hand. The physician shakes his head no, and the father stops. The physician takes the box and puts it down within her easy reach but not in her lap.)

The interviewer's behavior in this situation did not stem from insensitivity or the inability to afford tissues. Dr. Alan Leveton, our psychiatric consultant, observed that an offer of tissues to someone in tears often has the effect of drying up that person's expression of sadness and driving the painful feeling inside where it remains unavailable. Providing tissues may say, "I see your pain." Unfortunately, it may also say, "Stop crying." It is sometimes true that the offerer hopes for a drying up because of his or her own discomfort with the display of such strong emotion. With this family, the offer was another example of Rod offering "help" to Carla at a time when "helping" might not be helpful. The box of tissues was kept available so that Mrs. Thomas could be in charge of her own flow of tears.

Father:	What is it, hon?
Mother:	(banging her fist on her knee and continuing to cry softly) I remember how it was with my own father—he had such a mean temper. I hated him. I don't want to do that with Andy, and when he ticks me off, it's right there in a flash . . . I'm so angry I can't stand it. With my own parents it was hit first and talk about it later—except we never talked about it later. It was all so . . . strict. We were never allowed anything, and I mean anything. That house was run like a military school. And the belt was always kept where my brother and I could see it. I used to get so angry, but I wouldn't ever let them know. That was the only way I could feel like I won anything—I wouldn't let them—well, actually it was him, my father—I wouldn't let him know how he got to me. And I also decided—by the time I was 13—that with my kids it would be different. I wanted them to have spunk, not to feel beaten down . . . I also said I wouldn't treat them like he did

us . . . (long sigh and then cries aloud again) and here I am doing exactly the same! . . . that's what terrifies me.

Father: You never told me about your dad.

Mother: No—but didn't it seem strange that I never mentioned him much?

Father: Mmm. I just didn't realize (joins wife in thoughtful silence).

Through the mother's breaking down, the origin of her explosive and ready temper seemed obvious. Also, her double-level messages to Andy were explainable as one method for validating and encouraging his "spunk." She revealed her fear: that she, like her father, would allow her anger to get out of control and then physically abuse her son. She had unwittingly encouraged spunk in her child to the point that she was now terrified by her own angry reaction to his show of that very behavior.

Mother: (after an extended silence) Well, what I didn't say was that these 2 weeks since we saw you have been phenomenal. I did look out for questions to Andy that weren't really questions. And I don't know—something has changed somehow. We just didn't get into all those hassles.

Physician: And so how are you feeling?

Mother: I guess like Rod . . . relieved. And I don't really understand how it has all happened I just know that we're—that I am not having the same problems as I was 2 weeks ago. Is it going to last? I keep asking myself.

Physician: Probably not is my guess. This is probably some sort of temporary change. You all are too good at doing things the old way.

Mother: Doctor, are you being sarcastic? (teasing tone in her voice)

Physician: I'm just saying, be prepared for things to work around back to the old system.

Father: I hope not.

Physician: Well, that will be up to you. I would like to see you again.

The physician's prediction of a reversal was not sarcastic banter. He was aware that reported progress in the family had been rapid, and sometimes returning to previous behavior can happen just as quickly. When this occurs, the family may lose confidence in its ability to change and in the physician's expertise. With his suggestion that a relapse was likely, the physician was cushioning their possible fall and protecting himself. He was using Haley's suggestion of encouraging a relapse in order to prevent one. He also suggested with his final comment that they themselves had control and were responsible for their own future behavior.

The Thomases were enthusiastic about returning. The entire family was about to leave town for a month, so the third appointment was set up for shortly after their return.

The Third Session

All three family members attended the third session. They were still pleased with themselves and with the change occurring within their family over the 6-week period. Carla was feeling effective and successful with her son. Although Andy still continued to be provocative at times, his mother did not respond by ignoring his provocations or approving of his behavior until she could tolerate it no longer. On one or two occasions when the old pattern threatened to return, Rod, hearing bickering between Andy and his mother, shouted from wherever he was, "I'm not coming in. Settle it yourselves." That seemed enough to "call the system," and Carla was then able to take the cue and focus on what she needed to do to prevent an escalation. She was pleased to realize that she had control of her own angry feelings and could manage them.

Physician:	I've been somewhat concerned about all that unfinished business with your father.
Mother:	I've been concerned about it all my life, but . . .
Physician:	But?
Mother:	And . . . and, I think I don't want to get into it right now.
Physician:	That's up to you. What's your objection?
Mother:	Maybe sometime but not now. I do have a handle on what to do with Andy—and it's been going OK. Not easy. This is not easy, my setting limits with him. But I'm working on it. And I think I want to leave it there for now.
Physician:	OK by me.

The Fourth Session

In 4 weeks, Carla called to cancel their next appointment. She said that nothing was wrong; in fact, things were progressing well enough that she and Rod had decided another appointment was unnecessary. The pediatrician encouraged them to continue the work on their own and said that he would be delighted to see them in the future if they wished.

Nine months later Carla called and asked for an appointment. The parents came in without Andy. They were quick to state that their visit was prompted by something different than their concern 9 months ago. Setting limits with Andy was going reasonably well. Now, they were disturbed by an incident that had occurred 10 days previous to the visit. Rod saw Andy and another 4-year-old playing "doctor" with each other, undressed. The parents discussed their concerns about how to handle such an episode. They had actually managed the situation well with no shaming or blaming; both parents had encouraged Andy's questions about his body, responding to the questions accurately and matter-of-factly. Their main need was assurance that exploratory sex play in 4-year-old and 5-year-old children does happen and that they had handled the situation appropriately. The physician felt he could reassure them on both counts. Neither he nor they brought up the old issue, still unresolved, of Carla's feelings toward her father.

The physician never saw the family again after that fourth session. However, he did hear from their referring pediatrician that both Andy and the family continued to do well.

Loose Ends

Work with the Thomas family was brief. After only four sessions, only three of which were devoted to the initial presenting problem, the work was incomplete. First, Mrs. Thomas's issues with her father were never resolved. Without some direct psychological intervention, these issues might resurface, influencing her parenting behavior as before. The second loose end was whether the family fully understood the impact of double-level messages. Was the mother aware of her role in encouraging the undesirable behavior about which she complained? Should the interviewer have returned to that topic? Finally, because changes occurred in the family's behavior so rapidly, the physician might question the permanence of such change. In our own training, we learned that cases such as these should take longer to unravel and resolve. Current managed care recommendations aside, anything less than in-depth psychological exploration has traditionally been seen as poor work.

However, the family came to the pediatrician with a specific problem, and that problem disappeared or at least changed enough that the family felt comfortable handling their business on their own. They indicated that they had received what they came for and that they did not wish to proceed further. Generally, an interviewer should respect and be comfortable with a family's desire to stop because, despite what the interviewer may feel, the family will probably terminate the interviews anyway. Ending on good terms is excellent preparation for their return in the future. If the interviewer suggests that they are running away or avoiding, the family may skulk out of the office feeling scolded, not returning even when things get worse. Accepting a family's wish to end sessions leaves them in charge of the pace at which they want to face life's problems. The Thomases did return later, and all indications were that they would feel comfortable about returning again should the situation warrant.

The use of double-level messages was never explicitly acknowledged by the family as a significant mischief-maker in their interactions. However, the changes in the family, particularly in Mrs. Thomas's increasing effectiveness with Andy, strongly suggest that she did accept the message offered about her discrepant communication and that she corrected it. Even in the course of defensive nonlistening, patients and clients sometimes hear what the interviewer is saying.

Concerning the rapid change, the family did move quickly. They also demonstrated that the changes they produced lasted for 2 weeks, then 4 weeks, and were sustained 9 months later. The last follow-up through Dr. Jones was approximately 3 years after the family's initial family appointment. At that point, the family was functioning well.

We have never seen a family in which loose ends have not dangled at the last session. There is always the feeling that some issue has not been clarified or worked through, whether the work went well or badly or if the termination was the family's idea or that of the interviewer. We have come to accept that a feeling of unfinished business is a "given" of the termination process with families, not a sign of failure. Although the interviewer's work stops at some arbitrary point, the family's work does not.

Implementing Direct Communication

In 1972, Randall Foster noted that many parents in his family therapy practice made one striking omission in dealing with their "problem behavior" children (12). These parents reported that they had done "everything" (e.g., punished, spanked, deprived, talked; threatened reform school, the police, foster placement; promised gifts or money) in an effort to change the child's behavior. What was lacking from their lists, however, was the simple fact of telling the child to change. No parent said to the child directly, "Stop it now," or "Do it now." Mrs. Thomas illustrated this in her approach to the undressed Andy. She used many ploys, all indirect, to entice him to get dressed. Andy did not respond until she gave him the simple command, "I want you to put those clothes on . . . right now!"

Foster's hypothesis is that such a direct communication does not flow from parent to child because the parents doubt their child's ability to do what they are requesting. Many of his interventions with families are based on his findings that children do what their parents tell them to do when:

1. The parents perceive the child is able to do it.
2. The child sees himself able to do it.
3. The child hears the parents' clear demand to do it.

These three ingredients developed for the Thomas family in that first interview and were made possible by the inclusion of one additional step. Before Mrs. Thomas's successful demand of Andrew, she was given a similar command by the pediatrician (i.e., "Make it happen now."). This command carried the following assumption: "I trust your ability, Mrs. Thomas, to make it happen now, or I would not be asking you to do it." Thus, we should add one item to the three proposed by Foster: children will do what their parents tell them to do when the parents trust their own abilities to make such a clear demand. Just as the parents must communicate faith in the child's competence, so too must the interviewer show that he or she trusts the basic parenting abilities of the mother and father.

Useful Concepts for Family Interviewing

We selected the illustration of the Thomas family for several reasons. Their common pediatric behavioral complaint responded to brief, successful intervention through family interviewing by a pediatrician in clinical practice. In addition, they offered an opportunity to demonstrate several of the ideas presented in earlier chapters (Table 6.2).

Table 6.2. Examples of Family Interviewing Concepts

CONCEPT	EXAMPLE
A. Family homeostasis, family system	The family was, for instance, organized around Mr. Thomas's persistent rescue of Andy and his wife from herself. The family balanced itself in this way.
B. Communication style	
1. Content and process	There were many examples: most striking was Andy's acting out through silent undressing while the parents were engaged in a verbal dialogue with one another.
2. Functional communication	*Father:* "Hell, no. I don't want to bail her . . . *you* out. I want you to bail yourself out if you need to."
3. Dysfunctional communication	*Father:* "Well, you know, if you would just let me handle Andy's getting dressed in the morning . . . "
a. False assumptions in communication	*Father:* "She's heard it before. I'm like a broken record on that one."
b. Double-level messages	Almost too many too count. Noteworthy was Mrs. Thomas's continuing smile toward Andy as she confided, "I wish the hell that kid would put his clothes back on."
4. Parental validation	The lack of appropriate parental validation for mother in her own growing up was now seriously hampering her validation of her son. Also, there was little validation of Andy by his parents in the session when he would do well.
5. Use of pronoun "I"	The parents were encouraged to use "I need," "I feel," and so on in the session and directed to talk to one another rather than about each other.
C. Family structure	
1. Subsystems	Mrs. Thomas and Andy had a fairly well-defined (though conflictual) subsystem that alternately included (at home during angry outbursts) and excluded (in the office when Mr. Thomas attempted to set limits with Andy) her husband.
2. Joining through tracking	*Doctor:* "You were mentioning difficulty with Andy in the seat belt . . . "

continued

Table 6.2. Examples of Family Interviewing Concepts

CONCEPT	EXAMPLE
3. Restructuring	
a. Actualizing family transactions	The interviewer insisted that the parents talk directly to one another
b. Marking boundaries	The interviewer decided to keep Mr. Thomas out of the interaction between his wife and Andy in the office, thus delineating the boundary around mother and child so that Mrs. Thomas might experience success with her son.
c. Escalating stress	*Doctor:* "Make it happen now."
d. Assigning tasks	Each parent was given a specific job to work on at home at the close of the first interview.
e. Utilizing "symptoms" and here and now behavior	Making use of Andy's provocative undressing rather than considering it just an interruption.
f. Support	The interviewer's acknowledgment of feelings of frustration for both parents. Also the following: *Doctor:* "Now you're trying to trap me into seeing you as incompetent. It won't work. I won't buy it. As a matter of fact I think you've been selling yourself short for a long time regarding your talents as a mother."
D. Repetitive family sequence	Andy provoked mother. Mother encouraged his provocation. Andy went too far. Mother exploded. Father entered. Father took over and calmed the situation. Mother was shown to be a failure. Father left. Andy provoked his mother. And so on.
E. Encouraging a relapse in order to prevent one and helping the family to an awareness of its own responsibility in change	In response to mother's query, "Will the changes last?", the response: "Probably not in my guess. This is probably some sort of temporary change." Also: "That (the permanence of change) will be up to you."
F. Unfinished business	Mrs. Thomas's relationship with her father in the past.
G. The stages of an initial interview	The session proceeded through the opening stages to a discussion of the family's

continued

Table 6.2. Examples of Family Interviewing Concepts

CONCEPT	EXAMPLE
	concerns, to an interactional stage, and to an ending.
H. Four goals of an initial interview	*First,* the interviewer early established that he would be in charge when he said to father: "That sounds like a message for Carla. Would you tell her that directly now." *Second,* he also developed a formulation of the problem (see "family sequence" and "double-level message"). *Third,* family members were touched. The interviewer touched Mrs. Thomas when he recognized her embarrassment with Andy and helped her to act on that and feel successful about herself as a mother. The interviewer touched Mr. Thomas by responding to his obvious discomfort at standing by and watching the scene unfold. Andy's changed behavior in the interview was an indication that he too had been touched. *Fourth,* the family did return.

CONFRONTATION

The use of confrontation with families is essential. We strongly agree with published reports that indicate a direct, positive correlation between positive patient change and a high degree of confrontation used by the therapist (13,14,15). In our view, family counseling is an active process in which the interviewer must *do* something to facilitate family change. Passive listening alone seems to us an inefficient, often ineffectual device, which bores both the family and the interviewer. However, listening coupled with active confrontation appears to stimulate movement, encouraging change in a family.

Types of Confrontation

There are several confrontation techniques. The directive to Mrs. Thomas regarding Andy's putting his clothes back on (i.e., "Make it happen now") was an *encouragement to act.* This confrontation method relies on the therapist's encouragement of, and faith in, the patient and family to act in a manner satisfying to them, specifically discouraging a defeatist, passive attitude.

A second type of confrontation was used with Mrs. Thomas when the interviewer said, "As a matter of fact, I think you've been selling yourself short for a long time regarding your talents as a mother." This is a *confrontation of strength,* which focuses on a patient's constructive resources and demonstrated indications of strength.

The third method, a *didactic confrontation,* is probably the most familiar technique. Using didactic confrontation, the therapist directly clarifies a patient's misinformation or lack of information. In chapter 3, the therapist didactically confronted Jennifer Maloney's parents when he told them that Mr. Maloney was crucial to the survival of his wife and family and that only he could help to solve this family problem.

A fourth type of confrontation, an *experiential confrontation,* refers to a therapist's commenting on discrepancies that occur in the session. For example, a therapist who points out a double-level message or requests clarification of unexpressed feelings is using experiential confrontation (e.g., "My words just now made you look very sad. I don't understand; would you explain?").

Characteristics for Successful Confrontation

The term confronting does not mean that the interviewer insults family members, is rude, or walks over their feelings. On the contrary, confrontation of this sort without regard for the patient is usually counterproductive. Confrontation and regard for the feelings of the family are both necessary. One study documented that it was not just the use of confrontation, but the type of therapist (i.e., the "highly facilitative therapist") using these confrontation techniques that was directly related to positive patient improvement (16). In this study, a highly facilitative therapist was defined as a therapist who offered patients significantly higher levels of the following:

1. Empathy, in which the therapist communicated an accurate understanding of the patient's feelings
2. Positive regard, in which the therapist communicated his deep caring and respect for the patient
3. Genuineness, in which the therapist was freely himself in the relationship with the patient
4. Concreteness, in which the therapist insisted on direct exploration of the patient's specific feelings and experiences, rather than allowing vague, general discussion.

Therapists who rated significantly higher in possessing these four qualities were shown to confront their patients significantly more often than others and were judged to facilitate greater positive change in their patients.

The qualities of accurate empathy, positive regard, genuineness, and concreteness seem to us to be those attributes that encourage a touching experience between a therapist and a patient. We agree that these are essential qualities for successful work with families. Ultimately, good interviewing is a process of both touching *and* confronting the family, with the therapist balancing each aspect in a way that encourages and supports the family's change.

COMMON FAMILY TYPES

Just as there is no single prototype of the child who will not mind, there is no one type of family producing this complaint. The concept of family typology, although appealing, has never worked out. A physician cannot generalize about the family of a child by looking at that child's problem. For example, there is no more a typical bedwetter's family than there is a typical bedwetter. Also, we find it offensive to depersonalize children by labeling them as a symptom (i.e., a diabetic, an epileptic, a bedwetter). Complicated systems such as children and families cannot be reduced to labels.

However, certain families are alike. After some family interviews, each of us has said, "I've experienced this family before. Maybe the family's concern was different then, but I distinctly recall facing a similar family system in a previous situation." In these cases, the common link between two families was how the members of each group behaved toward each other and the interviewer, despite the initial family complaint. In our experience, there are at least six repetitive family configurations: the enmeshed family (to be discussed in chapter 9), the uproar family, the reasonable family, the silent family, the blaming family, and the intellectualizing family.

The Uproar Family

The Martin family in chapter 5 is an example of an uproar family. This type of family is easily identified and can be difficult to treat. Often, the "uproar" precedes the initial visit in the form of frequent phone calls, several appointment changes, difficulty with the nurse or receptionist, and chaos in the waiting area. The children seem out of control, moving or talking excessively. The parents may sit by silently, may make frantic but useless attempts to bring order, or may themselves be out of control. Physicians can assume that the parents of this family are in some way encouraging their children's behavior.

In this situation, the interviewer's first priority is to establish rules of behavior for the interview. The therapist makes room for himself or herself in order to carry on business. This task takes precedence over any discussion of the chief complaint, which may actually be behavior stemming from a lack of control. The interviewer may use control measures including turning the situation over to the parents; telling family members to settle down, sit down, be quiet, do not interrupt, and talk one at a time; or actually terminating the interview until order is established. When a therapist feels like a member of a crowd scene in a disaster film, an uproar family is probably in the room. Reinforcements in the form of a cotherapist can be useful with uproar families because these families frequently benefit from the combined energies of two interviewers.

The Reasonable Family

Mother:	Marvin is such a good boy, really, Doctor. We just don't understand what's been getting into him, do we, dear?
Marvin:	(sulks)
Father:	We wouldn't want you to think Marvin is always like this. He's shy around strangers. It's all right, son. The doctor is going to help us. Don't be upset.
Mother:	Mommy gets upset sometimes too, Marvin—you know, in the middle of the night when you want Mommy to sleep with you. Well, Daddy wakes up too, and he's so busy and tired; he needs his sleep.
Father:	It's you I'm worried about, Martha. You can't sleep on that hard mattress of his.
Mother:	Nonsense. I can sleep anywhere, Leon.

Father:	Well, you certainly don't look very rested in the morning.
Mother:	(lip trembling) Leon, I've only missed fixing your breakfast on two occasions.
Father:	Now don't get upset, Martha. I wasn't taking about that. Let's not get upset. Nothing is solved by arguing. Actually, Doctor, we're very proud, Martha and I—we don't fight. In fact, I don't remember that we've ever had one fight in over 8 years of marriage, have we, dear?
Mother:	(blowing her nose) No. Marvin, I'm sure the doctor would like you to sit on that chair like a big boy. Now be reasonable, darling. We're only doing this for your own good.
Father:	There must be a reason for Marvin's seeming to need his mother each night. Should we be concerned, or are we just making a mountain out of a molehill? We're willing to do whatever you suggest; you're the doctor.

Although some of the roles assigned in this family may seem unreasonable (e.g., the mother is clearly expected to fix father's breakfast daily), the dialogue reveals interesting communication highlights. Both the mother and father insist on the use of collective pronouns (e.g., "we," "we're," "let's"). The father speaks for mother, and the mother speaks for Marvin and the interviewer as well. The family's collective style avoids responsibility for each person's own thoughts, words, and feelings, while at the same time assuming to know the thoughts, words, and feelings of others.

However, this family is so reasonable in the discussion. Each family member—often including the identified patient (although in this case, not)—seems nice, fair, reasonable, unemotional, and perpetually looking out for the best interests of others. The family may be so convincing in its reasonable stance that the interviewer erroneously concludes that the family is a model of togetherness. In such a situation, the novice interviewer may then question the need for any sort of family interview or counseling. At other times, the family overdoes their rationality to the point of becoming a caricature of caring and solicitude. These families usually see the physician as the sole authority, directly asking his or her advice and vowing to follow these suggestions.

Open disagreement is a missing dimension in the reasonable family's conversation. Because there are no disagreements, the interviewer has few entries for intervention. Interviewing these families is a frustrating experience because there is no direct conflict with which to work.

The specific approach to such a family depends, of course, on the family and their circumstance. However, some general guidelines may be helpful. Although these techniques have been recommended when interviewing any family, they may be particularly important in helping a reasonable family.

1. Get the family to talk to each other rather than reporting to the interviewer "about" each other. Instead of becoming trapped on the receiving end of reasonable statements, watch how family members use reasonableness with each other.
2. Listen particularly for any hint of interpersonal conflict, which is usually hidden. Work to encourage its open expression. For example:

Mother:	(lip trembling) Leon, I've only missed fixing your breakfast on two occasions.
Father:	Now don't get upset, Martha. I wasn't talking about that. Let's not get upset. Nothing is solved by arguing.
Physician:	Leon, would you tell Martha what you see on her face right at this moment?
Father:	Well, uh . . . she's a little upset.
Physician:	Ask her if you're reading her correctly.
Father:	Well, are you?
Mother:	Yes. But it's nothing. I'm all right now.
Physician:	Not so fast. Your tears are nothing?
Mother:	Well . . .
Physician:	Leon, see if you can talk further with Martha; find out what her tears are about.

Do not be dismayed if it does not go this smoothly. Leon and Martha could easily conspire to defeat the interviewer's suggestions:

Father:	Now don't get upset, Martha. I wasn't talking about that. Let's not get upset. Nothing is solved by arguing.
Physician:	Hold it, Leon. Would you tell Martha what you see on her face at this moment?
Father:	(ignoring the doctor's request) I don't think she's really upset. Martha understands that I don't mind cold cereal once in a while.
Mother:	(quickly pulling herself together) Leon is really very good in the kitchen.
Physician:	(confused as to how things slipped from the expression on Martha's face to a discussion of Leon's culinary skills in the short space of 30 seconds) Well . . .
Father:	Oh, sure, I can even fix eggs if I have to. But now back to this sleeping problem Marvin is having. Do you think . . . (removing the focus from himself back on to Marvin)

The interviewer simply has to try again. With any type of family, our pediatric residents often exit an interview feeling frustrated that they missed an opportunity to address a specific aspect of the family's system. We reassure trainees that because families demonstrate repetitive sequences in their behavior, family members will continue to present their same sequences over and over until the interviewer becomes aware of the pattern. We would be confident in telling the therapist working with Leon and Martha not to worry. There will be many future demonstrations of the same dance step: the suggestion of conflict, followed by a quick coverup, indicating that each is denying his or her own needs and feelings. The therapist can prepare to confront the family when this repetition occurs.

3. Concentrate on increasing each family member's use of the pronoun "I." The interviewer may say, "Martha, would you tell Leon what you are feeling at this moment? Start your sentence with 'I.'"
4. Be cautious of dispensing quick advice and answers, even when the fam-

ily directly asks for or demands this. Although the request may seem reasonable and the family members may appear attentive, they are usually most reasonable of all in their eventual disregard or sabotage of the advice given.

The Silent Family

Silent families are a challenge. Typically, the children have vocabularies limited to "I don't know" and "Uh-huh." The mother waits for the physician's lead, and the father says, "I came because she told me I had to." Opening pleasantries are followed by a deafening silence, with all eyes on the interviewer. Often, a pact of silence by the family reflects their collective fear regarding the interview process. In this situation, the interviewer can spend time discussing the family's individual and mutual anxiety and their expectations of the doctor, rather than forging ahead with a premature disclosure of the chief complaint. Such a discussion can be introduced in several ways. The interviewer may say:

- "Before we get down to what problems bring you here, tell me what each of you is experiencing as you sit in this office today. Henry, I'll start with you."
- "I am feeling uncomfortable. The family looks very ill at ease. Tell me what worries you about being here today."
- "I would like each of you to write down two 'good' things and two 'bad' things that you feel might happen here today."
- "I tend to feel that my own family concerns are pretty private matters. I wonder if this is a private family, also? If so, maybe we need to talk about that before getting started. I recognize that some family matters may be hard to discuss."

Directly challenging a silent family member to talk about the "problem" usually intensifies the atmosphere of strained discomfort. The preceding suggestions have the advantage of approaching the family about their fears and expectations in the session rather than encouraging their defensive stance.

Some families are nonverbal in their interactional style even outside the office. These families often respond well to a nonverbal task, such as conjoint family drawing or family sculpture (see chapter 5).

The Blaming Family

In blaming families, someone is always under attack, whether it be a child, a parent, or the interviewer.

Mother:	Harvey, I said sit up!
Father:	She's on him all the time, Doc.
Mother:	Well, if you'd be on him a little more, I wouldn't have to. I saw this program on television about a father who—
Father:	Don't bring television into it, Ethel. That's all you ever talk about.
Harvey:	It was a good show. Mom and I—
Father:	Don't interrupt, Harvey.
Harvey:	You never listen to me. (sticks his tongue out)
Mother:	Harvey, don't talk to your father like that.
Father:	Stay out of it, Ethel. I'll handle him. Isn't that right, Doc? When my own kid sasses me, shouldn't I handle it?
Physician:	That is—
Father:	I don't know what we're coming here for; it's not helping.
Mother:	You're never willing to stick with something for more than 5 minutes. Harvey, I'm not going to tell you again, sit up!

This family is only a few insults away from becoming an uproar family. They are escalating into that position by blaming: something is always someone else's fault. In this situation, the strategies an interviewer uses are those that encourage a focus on communicating feelings without blame.

Mother:	Well, if you'd be on him a little more, I wouldn't have to. I saw this program on television—
Physician:	Hold it, Ethel. That's an important message you just gave

	your husband. Tell him again, and this time find a way to say it that doesn't blame him.
Mother:	(She sputters and indicates that she doesn't know how.)
Physician:	That's a tough spot, having something that important to say and not quite knowing how to say it. What is it that you would like to get across to Mel?
Mother:	I don't know . . . I guess that I feel everything is on my shoulders.
Physician:	Ah, then that's what he needs to hear now. Tell him that.
Mother:	Yeah, why do I have to do it all?
Father:	You—
Physician:	Hold it. Back up, Ethel. Start your sentence with, "I feel."
Mother:	(after a long pause) I feel all the responsibility is mine.
Father:	Who asked you to take it all?
Physician:	Mel, is it hard not to answer Ethel with a defense?
Father:	Well, she insinuates that I don't do anything.
Physician:	And that leaves you feeling how?
Father:	I don't know . . . sore, and like she doesn't notice what I am doing.
Physician:	What a dilemma for you both. Ethel, you're feeling overwhelmed, and Mel, you feel unappreciated. There ought to be another way to air those feelings and settle them, aside from attacking each other. That must be frustrating for both of you.
Father:	It sure doesn't get us anywhere. (This is the first positive comment in 10 minutes.)
Mother:	Well, if you'd just listen more to what I'm saying. You never . . .

Then it's back to blaming. The interviewer can persist, slow them down again, and continue to urge their expression of feelings other than through attack and blame. The interviewer needs to be careful that the interventions are balanced so that individuals do not feel that the physician is taking sides. In many ways, treating the blaming family amounts to a "gentling" process, in which the interviewer helps the family to realize that feelings other than blame and defensiveness can be safely exposed and communicated.

The Intellectualizing Family

The intellectualizing family attempts to beat the interviewer at his own game. Physicians are experienced at restricting communication to facts and rational thought. When a whole family decides to function with one another in this way, the result can be staggering.

Mike:	I don't see why I can't stay up until 10.
Father:	(rather than declaring his own desires on the subject, he offers an outside source) I think authorities pretty well agree, Mike, that the sleep a child gets before midnight is the most important.
Mother:	(siding with her son against her husband) But what about that article I showed you in Family Circle? It made a lot of sense to me. It said that a child knows his own sleep need and will regulate himself.
Father:	Well, Helen, I hardly think Family Circle compares to that piece in the Scientific American.
Mother:	The Family Circle study was done at the Gesell Institute, Arnold. Oh, well, I suppose you're right.
Mike:	None of the other kids have to go to bed at 9:30.
Mother:	Other kids don't concern us, Mike. Their parents aren't as responsible as your father and I.

Father:	When you have children of your own, son, I think you'll understand what we mean.
Mike:	I'm the only kid in the ninth grade who can't stay up until at least 10.
Mother:	Now, that just isn't true. I was talking to Connie Harris's mother, and she . . .
Mike:	I tell you, I feel like a freak. And besides, Connie Harris is in the eighth grade.
Father:	Think of how much fresher you are each day for school, Mike.
Mike:	I even get teased about being a baby.
Mother:	We think you should be able to rise above that, Mike. They probably tease you because they're jealous of your good grades. And if their parents would set some bedtime limits for them, maybe their grades would show it, too. Did you ever think of that?

This family could go on endlessly. The parents have certainly not exhausted their store of good and rational reasons why children should be in bed by 9:30. Whether the interviewer agrees with the parents or not, something important has not occurred: neither parent has acknowledged his or her own feelings or Mike's. Nor has Mike been given the opportunity to hear the feelings and expectations of his parents. Feelings have simply not been expressed, and for each individual the communication has been a recitation of rationalizations supported by authority, a conversation "from the neck up."

In order to break such a family's intellectualizing habits, the physician must help the family members shift to statements of feeling. The interviewer's responsibility is to pry the family away from their defensive rationalizations with content and direct them toward an understanding of their defensive process.

Mike:	None of the other kids have to go to bed at 9:30.
Mother:	Other kids don't concern—
Physician:	Stop just a minute. Mike, you say that none of the other kids have to go to bed by 9:30. How does that make you feel?
Mike:	I feel like a freak.
Physician:	I would like you to share your feelings about that with each of your parents.
Mike:	(to his mother) I do. I positively feel like a freak with other kids my age.
Physician:	Virginia, what do you hear in your son's voice and words.
Mother:	He just needs—
Physician:	No, stop. I want you for this moment to listen to his feelings and let him know that you hear him.
Mother:	I see that . . . he's upset.
Physician:	Ask him why he is upset.
Mother:	Upset about what, Mike?
Mike:	I feel humiliated with the kids at school.
Mother:	Now, Mike, that's silly.
Physician:	See if you can listen to his feelings without judging. Were you aware that he was feeling humiliated with his friends?
Mother:	Well . . . no; I just thought . . .
Physician:	What are you feeling right now, Virginia? Tell Mike.
Mother:	Well, I don't think he should feel that way.
Physician:	And yet somehow he does. And what feelings does that trigger off inside you?
Mother:	Just awful.

Physician: Tell Mike, starting your sentence with "I feel." I think it is important for you and Mike to share your feelings now, that's all ... just feelings. Talk together, you two, about what's happening on your insides at this moment.

As in previous examples, the interviewer must be willing to persist and repeat his efforts. All families, no matter what their type, are practiced and committed to their behavioral style. They will not relinquish it easily, even though that style may be responsible for their distress. Fearful of critical judgment from others, they also do not respect their own feelings and needs. Therefore, these families cannot express feelings without expecting blame in return. Helping them develop new and different expectations through the interview experiences is the interviewer's goal.

References

1. Chess S, Thomas A, Birch HG, et al. Behavioral individuality in early childhood. New York: New York University Press, 1963.
2. Chess S, Thomas A, Birch HG, et al. Your child is a person: a psychological approach to parenthood without guilt. New York: The Viking Press, 1972:21.
3. Chess S, Thomas A. Temperamental individuality from childhood to adolescence. J Am Acad Child Psychiatry 1977;16:218.
4. Chess, Thomas, Birch, et al. Your child is a person, 5–6.
5. Chess, Thomas, Birch, et al. Your child is a person, 32.
6. Chess, Thomas, Birch, et al. Your child is a person.
7. Chess, Thomas, Birch, et al. Your child is a person, 47.
8. Carey W, McDevitt S. Coping with children's temperament: A guide for professionals. New York: Basic Books, 1995.
9. Chess S, Thomas A. Know your child. New York: Basic Books, 1987.
10. Turecki S, Tonner L. The difficult child. Revised edition. New York: Bantam Books, 1989.
11. Budd L. Living with the active alert child: Groundbreaking strategies for parents. Revised and enlarged ed. Seattle: Parenting Press, 1993.
12. Foster R. Parental communication as a determinant of child behavior. Am J Psychotherapy 1971;25:579.
13. Berenson B, Mitchell KM, Laney R. Level of therapist functioning: types of confrontation. J Clin Psychiatry 1968;24:111.

14. Bergin A, Garfield S, eds. Handbook of psychotherapy and behavior change. New York: John Wiley & Sons, 1961.
15. Mitchell K, Berenson B. Differential use of confrontation by high and low facilitative therapists. J Nerv Ment Dis 1971;153:165.
16. Mitchell, Berenson, 165.

chapter **7**

Chronic Conditions

Mother:	You forgot? Well, you can't forget, that's all there is to it. This is what I'm up against, Doctor. I've told him hundreds of times that this is his only job. I don't ask him to do anything else around the house. I get no support.
Father:	Evelyn, I think you're being too hard on the boy. After all, he's only 13.
Mother:	(to Frankie) I give up on asking you to do anything anymore!
Frankie:	You say that, but you won't do it.
Father:	Don't speak to your mother that way.
Frankie:	Well, why not? You do.
Father:	Now that's about enough out of you, young man.
Mother:	Will you get off Frankie's back? That's all the two of you do is fight
Father:	You're a good one to talk.
Mother:	Look, Jerome, how are we going to teach this boy to be responsible for himself if he won't do the one job we have asked him to do? One of us has to have some expectations for Frankie. And he's certainly not getting any from you.
Father:	Like I say, Evelyn. You're too hard. You can't expect the boy to be an adult overnight.

Jerome, Evelyn, and Frankie are involved in a round robin with a topic we find familiar: teaching responsibility to children. Families often en-

171

counter difficulty with this issue. This particular family's trouble is related in part to a repeating sequence of behavior.

1. Feeling alone in her parenting, the mother takes a unilateral stand regarding the expectations of her son.
2. The mother feels undermined by her husband, unknowingly setting herself up to be so treated.
3. The son enters with anger, provoking each parent.
4. The parents attack each other.
5. The son withdraws, unnoticed. The issue of responsibility falls from view.
6. Parental fighting takes precedence, leading to increased feelings of alienation.
7. Subsequently, the mother, feeling isolated in her parenting, again takes a unilateral stand regarding the expectations of her son.

If this family were discussing Frankie's not taking out the garbage, forgetting to brush his teeth, or letting homework slide, the same seven-step sequence might unfold. However, they are not discussing these issues. Frankie has chronic renal disease and is currently in relapse. He has been "forgetting" to take his steroid medication. The stakes are higher than those resulting from unfinished homework. Continued forgetting could be, if not fatal, certainly serious. Appropriate medical management of Frankie and his renal disease requires that he take medication consistently. Because the family's repeating sequence of dysfunctional behavior around responsibility issues stands in the way of Frankie's compliance, medical management must include alterations of this sequence.

In this chapter, we consider the child who requires care first and foremost because of a presenting physical symptom. When a child is diagnosed with seizure disorder, diabetes mellitus, or attention deficit hyperactivity disorder, the family is deeply affected. These families also have specific systems, communication patterns, and repetitive sequences of behavior that are inextricably woven through the child's illness. The physician responsible for the care of a chronically ill child must pay attention to both the illness and the family's interaction around it.

However, the clinician does not need a new hypothesis for working with the family of a chronically ill child. In our experience, the hypotheses that we have previously summarized, regarding how families in general function, are appropriate to understanding specifically how the members of a family with a chronically ill child interact. Our trainees are occasionally surprised after observing us interview the family of a child with a brain tumor, noting that our clinical approach has not differed from that used in family interviews regarding "garden variety" behavioral complaints. We explain that principles of family interviewing transcend specific clinical issues and are applicable across a wide spectrum of pediatric problems, both behavioral *and* physical.

PRESENTING THE DIAGNOSIS

One of the most difficult tasks for a health care provider is to tell parents that their child has developed a serious medical condition that the youngster may carry throughout life. The child will *never* be quite the same as before the illness. Specific examples in which such news must be communicated are listed in Table 7.1. In few of these examples does the disease kill the patient outright; rather, the patient lives a substantially altered life. The child may die months or years after the diagnosis; the family is plunged into a protracted course along with the ailing child. It is a cruel detour from the mainstream of life for all involved. Frequently, the child's physician is the first to inform the family of this chronic condition, a pronouncement that is always devastating for the family and may be so for the messenger as well.

Table 7.1. Chronic Conditions Affecting Children

DISORDERS	EXAMPLES
Blood dyscrasias	Sickle cell anemia, hemophilia
Central nervous system disorders	Seizures, cerebral palsy
Congenital and acquired heart disease	Pulmonary stenosis, rheumatic heart disease
Metabolic disorders	Phenylketonuria, diabetes mellitus
Pulmonary conditions	Asthma, cystic fibrosis
Gastrointestinal disorders	Inflammatory bowel disease, short bowel syndrome
Immune disorders	HIV infections, rheumatoid arthritis
Sensory defects	Blindness, deafness
Physical defects	Ambiguous genitalia, hypothyroidism

When discussing the management of chronic conditions with our trainees, we typically begin at the point when the reality of the diagnosis must be faced for the first time. The following transcript reflects the conversation between a pediatric resident, Dr. Elliott, and the family of a child in her care. As the interview begins, the family knows only that their 20-month-old child has not been well. He eats listlessly, has gained weight poorly, and seems to have had a "bad cold" for the past several weeks. He was hospitalized 2 days before this dialogue occurred when the cold progressed into pneumonitis. Tests have been performed, but no results have been discussed. The resident knows that the sweat chlorides were highly elevated and that the child has cystic fibrosis. Both the resident and parents are dreading this meeting.

Physician:	Hi, Mr. and Mrs. Nichols. Let's sit down. Any trouble finding a place to park? No? Well, I'm surprised. The parking around here is murder. What's that? Oh, Eddie, is doing much better. Have you been in to see him yet? He's still in the tent but breathing quite nicely. He's even been able to take some clear liquids. I wanted to go over his tests with you.
Mother:	He looks so pale, Dr. Elliott.
Father:	Jean's been so upset since Eddie was admitted, Doctor. Come on, hon, let's hear what the doctor has to say.
Physician:	Well, she's right. Eddie is pale. However, the vascular system is a very wonderful system. At the moment, most of Eddie's problem is in his lungs and with his breathing. His arteries and veins in that area are working overtime, and some of the blood normally going out to his skin and giving him good color is now being shunted to his lungs and breathing apparatus.
Mother:	He just looks so pale.
Physician:	You mustn't worry, Mrs. Nichols. His skin doesn't need his red blood corpuscles now. Red blood cells are the body's main carrier of oxygen. Eddie's skin doesn't need so much oxygen right now, but his vital organs—heart, lungs, brain—do. It is really the body's way of utilizing reserves in an emergency.

Father:	You told us yesterday that his blood count was up. Doesn't that mean that he has too much blood somehow?
Physician:	No, Mr. Nichols. That was his white blood count. We all have two kinds of cells—well, three if you count platelets—red, white, and platelets. Now Eddie's white count is up above 17,000—that's because of the infections. But his red cells are if anything a little low, around 2.5 million. I know this must be confusing. Perhaps if I give you some normal figures for white and red counts and draw you a picture of a typical red cell and a typical white cell . . .
Mother:	So ghastly white, he looks awful (anxiety rising).
Father:	Geez, Jean, aren't you listening to what the woman's been saying?
Physician:	That's all right, Mr. Nichols. Let's see how else I can explain . . .

Not surprisingly, finding alternate explanations comes easy to this physician. Not only must the Nichols family endure the stress of their son's serious illness, they must also withstand Dr. Elliott's kindly explanations—and she has not even gotten to the diagnosis yet.

This interview does not have to go so badly. There are some useful guidelines to follow when presenting to parents a diagnosis of serious, chronic illness in their child. We teach our trainees to respect the event, share the diagnosis quickly, attend to the feelings of those present, keep medical facts to a minimum, withstand—even encourage—silence, and avoid running away.

Respecting the Event

A terrible business will occur in this interview. A lifetime sentence is about to be declared on Eddie Nichols. The physician knows this, and the parents fear it. Although we wish this could go without saying, news of this sort is not delivered on the telephone, in the hallway, in the elevator, or in the hospital cafeteria. The physician should not reveal the diagnosis in a waiting area peopled by other anxious parents, nor should he or she deliver the news while standing or on the run. The news calls for time, privacy, and a place with as much physical comfort as possible. We prefer that all parental figures be present, and that older siblings (depending on the parents' wishes), particularly those older than 10 years of age, also attend.

Whether or not the patient attends the initial interview around the diagnosis depends on the child's age, the parents' wishes, and the physician's degree of comfort with handling both the patient and the parents simultaneously. Many physicians prefer to talk first with the parents and designated siblings, excluding the patient. In addition to sharing the diagnosis, the physician may use a portion of this time to help the family plan how and what they will tell their sick child later. At a second interview, the parents can describe the diagnosis to their child in their own words, using the physician for support and information as the situation warrants. This format encourages an experience that is personal and relatively private, with the physician there to help as needed.

With the Nichols family, Dr. Elliott has been careful in arranging the interview. Eddie is too young to be included, and there are no siblings. The physician has set aside time to see both parents, and they are meeting in a quiet, private room off the pediatric ward.

Sharing the Diagnosis Quickly

Here, Dr. Elliott has gotten herself into trouble. As mentioned, she knows what must be discussed, and the parents fear it. The anticipation of that discussion by both parties accounts for the uncomfortable dialogue reported previously. Each person has entered the room feeling alone, with a unique set of worries. Dr. Elliott may be thinking, "Your son has a terrible disease for which there is no cure. Why do I have to be the one to tell you this?" Mrs. Nichols fears the worst: "My son is going to die, I know it. That's what his paleness means—he looks like death. And that's what those tests are going to show. I don't want to hear about them—and yet I do. I can't even think clearly." Mr. Nichols is also anxious: "My wife is so embarrassing in her upset state. What will the doctor think of us? I'll have to stay calm. And what is wrong with our son? It must be bad. Do I really want to know about Eddie's tests?"

Because little of this is explicitly stated, the conversation takes on an "as if" quality, resembling an enactment. Mrs. Nichols talks as if "pale" is the issue. It is not; pale is a metaphor for death in her mind. Death is unspeakable, but pale is not. Dr. Elliott cannot know this of course; she has not been told. But she might assume that any parent in this interview situation is terrified. Such feelings require noticing and acknowledging. However, neither Dr. Elliott nor Mr. Nichols attends to the mother's feelings or behavior (i.e., process). Instead, both respond only to her words (i.e., content). Mr. Nichols at first chides his wife for her preoccupation with their son's pale appearance and becomes more openly critical of her with time. The physician, ostensibly listening to her patient, chooses to focus on Mrs. Nichol's words rather than her feelings by launching into an inappropriate discussion of the causes of pallor in acute illness. Dr. Elliott has failed to remember that medical exposition is not the reason for holding this interview. Delaying the diagnosis—even in the name of caring concern and "helping parents to understand"—prolongs their pain. For many parents, the longer the physician delays, the greater their fears. The enormity of their child's medical condition becomes directly proportional to the time required for disclosure (e.g., "It must be really bad if the doctor is taking this long to tell us.").

In this interview, the physician's misdirection is unknowingly encouraged by Mrs. Nichols' inability to express her fear. Detailed talk about blood cells forestalls approaching the larger issue she dreads. In this situation, we would encourage an interviewer to move quickly into a discussion of the diagnosis with the parents. The unapproachable must be approached, and, if need be, the physician must lead the family there. If the diagnosis is known and if the interview is being held for the purpose of relaying that information, a reasonably rapid declaration is important.

Attending to Feelings

This "diagnosis" interview does not differ from any other family interview. The interviewer has a responsibility to acknowledge and touch the feelings that are spoken, shown, or suggested by each family member. As mentioned, it was Dr. Elliott's failure to acknowledge Mrs. Nichols' worry that precipitated her lengthy blood cell discourse, delaying a discussion of the diagnosis. The following dialogue would have been more direct.

Physician:	I wanted to go over his tests with you.
Mother:	He looks so pale, Dr. Elliott.
Father:	Jean's been so upset since Eddie was admitted, Doctor. Come on, hon, let's hear what the doctor has to say.

Physician:	Actually, you both look pretty worried. Me, too. What's most worrisome about Eddie's looking pale?
Mother:	Oh, I don't know. He just looks so sick, so awfully sick.
Physician:	He has been—very ill. Have there been times when you wondered if he was going to make it?
Mother:	(nods yes)
Father:	Don't worry about us, Doc. What about Eddie? You said you had some tests back.
Physician:	I do. And I'm concerned about both of you as well as Eddie. The first thing I want you both to hear is that Eddie is not going to die. His pneumonia is under control. (Both parents express relief.) Eddie is going to get over this pneumonia, but our tests show that the reason for his pneumonia is very serious. Eddie has a condition called cystic fibrosis.

In this discussion, the physician is juggling two transactions—leading the parents quickly to the diagnosis, while inserting and legitimizing attention to feelings. The simultaneity is important. Occasionally, our trainees ignore the diagnosis in their zeal to put into practice newly learned concepts regarding the discussion of feeling with parents. Recognizing the importance of "feelings" and excited about the techniques for encouraging patients to talk about emotions, the resident may focus so closely on feelings that the following occurs:

Physician:	Before we get down to business, Eddie's condition, I need to know how each of you is feeling.
Mother:	We want to know about Eddie, Doctor.
Father:	Yes, have you gotten those tests back yet?
Physician:	In just a minute, Mr. Nichols. You look really worried.
Father:	Damn right, I'm worried. Neither Jean nor I have slept in days. This business is hell.
Physician:	I'm sure it's been hard. You sound angry, too. I think we need to talk about that a little bit.

Father:	Hells bells, woman—I don't want to talk about my anger. What's wrong with Eddie?

Although this interviewer is persistent, she is delaying a discussion of the diagnosis through dogged determination to "get feelings out on the table." This resident, like Dr. Elliott, has lost sight of the purpose of this interview. The family has not come for psychotherapy. They have come for concise, understandable, diagnostic information regarding their child. Therefore, it is information, delivered while acknowledging the parents' feelings, that must be offered. Information alone is not sufficient; neither is an exclusive, forced focus on feelings. If either method is used in isolation, it transforms the experience into a caricature of decent medical care.

Keeping Medical Facts to a Minimum

Dr. Elliott's interview with the Nichols is not over with the announcement of the diagnosis. However, in some sense, the session has ended for the family. Families have reported to us that when the diagnosis of a serious, chronic illness was explicitly verbalized, all subsequent talk became a blur. Their minds could not move beyond the enormity of the diagnosis. When parents realize that their child has a serious condition, a protective barrier often descends, preventing the assimilation of additional medical facts. This barrier does not mean that the parents are silent. On the contrary, most parents inundate the physician with a multitude of questions, some of which are unanswerable.

Physician:	Eddie has cystic fibrosis. (There is a pause. Both parents are visibly shaken.)
Father:	What does that mean? Where did he get it? I've heard of it, but I don't know anything about it.
Mother:	It's that awful lung disease, Harvey. Remember that family down the street in Petaluma—their two boys?

Father:	Eddie's not like them. They were much older . . . and they were . . . invalids. I don't even think they could get out of bed. Eddie's not like that. Before this pneumonia, he was fine.
Mother:	What does it mean, Dr. Elliott? What do we do now? Is there some treatment Eddie has to have? Isn't there some medicine? (She begins to cry.)
Physician:	Well, that is . . .
Father:	What my wife is trying to ask is how do we get him over it? Can they do operations for this sort of thing? He is going to get over it?
Physician:	He *is* going to recover from this bout of pneumonia. But the difficult news that I must tell you is that he will very likely continue to have difficulties with recurrent lung infections.
Mother:	For how long?
Physician:	Probably for the rest of his life.
Mother:	(crushed) Why?
Physician:	For an answer to that, I need to talk with you in some detail about cystic fibrosis, what it is, and what we can do about it.

The physician may proceed at this point with a discussion of cystic fibrosis, or she may not. If the physician does continue, she would do well to understand that much of what she says, though correct and important, will probably not be understood or remembered. The prior announcement was simply too staggering. Sometimes, we have found it more useful to acknowledge the blow directly, rather than proceeding with questions and answers.

| Physician: | I do need to talk with you in some detail about cystic fibrosis. At the moment, I am aware that I have just hit you with very serious news about Eddie, and I wonder if you can hear much more in the way of information right now. |
| Mother: | I feel numb. |

Father:	(shakes his head and wipes his eye)
Physician:	(after purposely allowing a silence to intervene) You are going to have a thousand questions. You've already asked me several that are very important. I would like to answer all of them as well as possible. Yet you are both really stunned. Let me give you some time. Just hearing what I've said so far is enough for anyone to withstand. I would like to meet with you again at a time convenient for you, later this afternoon or tonight, and we can begin to go over your questions one by one. How would that be for you?
Mother:	I can't think, yet I have a million questions.
Father:	Is he . . . is he . . . ever (with tears) going to come home?
Physician:	(sensing father's fears) Absolutely. What are you frightened of, Mr. Nichols?
Father:	. . . that he's going to die here in the hospital.
Physician:	(placing his hand on Mr. Nichols' arm) I thought so. Eddie *is* going to recover from his pneumonia, and I feel certain that he will be home with you in just a few more days. Do you believe me?
Father:	I don't know. I don't know anything. (He breaks down completely. He and his wife cry and comfort one another. The physician does *not* leave immediately.)

We support Dr. Elliott's decision to avoid being led into a detailed discussion of prognosis, possible complications, the use of specific medications and therapies, the purchasing of specialized equipment, genetic implications, and etiology *at this time.* These issues must be explored at some point, but we question such an exploration so close to the diagnostic announcement.

The moments after sharing a diagnosis are crucial in an interview. The parents are often desperate and insistent in their questioning, and most physicians are far more comfortable answering questions than dealing with the grief, anger, and despair behind the parents' questions. Some questions, of course, must be answered immediately, but others can wait. Persistently questioning parents and a persistently answering physician result in an interview that may seem medically sophisticated but is humanly a disaster. The parents may leave such an interview feeling overwhelmed by the news and alienated by the physician's "clinical and unfeeling" approach. The physician may think that he or she has done a good job because every question was answered. If the physician also feels self-congratulatory because he or she never answered a question with "I don't know," then the interview was assuredly not well done; the need to preserve the myth of medical omniscience had overridden sensitivity for the unfolding of a human tragedy.

Using Silence

Silence in interviews is often under used, particularly when sharing a diagnosis. Too frequently silence is viewed as awkward, a sign that the interview is not going well, and something to overcome. Both the family and the interviewer sometimes make efforts to fill up the silent spaces in an interview. However, when used skillfully, silence can be an asset to the interviewer.

When delivering bad news to a family, a physician does not need to supply facts, words of solace, or explanations immediately. The physician might as readily encourage silence to allow a momentary turning inward for the family members so they can recognize their own feelings and reactions. This flood of emotions will prevent attentive listening to subsequent issues in the interview. Also, encouraging silence is a way of giving permission for each family member to look inward. Silence is the interviewer's way of saying, "I expect that this news is a hard blow, and that you are reeling from it. I consider you and your feelings important enough that I will keep still and not rush past your emotions with words and talk." Dr. Elliott illustrated the judicious use of silence in another clinical situation.

Physician:	Yes, it is serious. It's hemophilia.
Mother:	(gasps and then buries her head in her hands)
Father:	But, Doctor, how could it . . .
Physician:	(placing her hand on the father's shoulder) For just a moment, stay with your inside thoughts and feelings.

> (A silence fills the room, and then the dialogue reopens.)
>
> Mother: (sobbing) It seems so unfair. First Edgar and now John—both our sons. I can't bear that.
>
> Father: (He takes his wife's hand. They talk comfortingly together.)

In this situation, the use of silence to focus on feelings has avoided a question and answer sequence between the father and the physician. In the place of such a sequence, mutual support between the mother and father was facilitated and encouraged. Such mutual support between spouses will be needed repeatedly for optimal management of their boys with this serious, chronic illness.

Avoiding the Urge to Run Away

It is expected that not only the parent but every physician anticipating an interview of this sort will enter it with strong approach-avoidance feelings. How the physician handles these feelings is crucial and may vary. Some physicians may even avoid the session completely by canceling the session, by asking another member of the medical team to do the job, or by attempting the interview over the telephone with only one parent. Other less glaring avoidance maneuvers include conducting the interview in a detached manner that ignores the family's feeling, using too much complicated medical information, presenting too hopeful a picture, or quickly presenting the diagnosis and then "ducking out" with the excuse that "an emergency has come up." In each case, the physician is avoiding the acknowledgment of deep feelings—the family's *and* the physician's. The impulse to put distance between oneself and painful emotions is understandable, but there is no more important emergency than that of two parents potentially overwhelmed by information that the physician has just delivered. We urge physicians to "screw your courage to the sticking place" and remain (unless the family asks to be alone), offering silent strength and support.

SUBSEQUENT QUESTIONS

Paul Steinhauer and colleagues have said that the family of a child with chronic illness initially comes to the physician with specific questions in

Table 7.2. Preconceived Parental Questions and Answers in Children's Chronic Illness

QUESTIONS	ANTICIPATED ANSWERS
What is the matter?	Nothing serious
What caused the condition?	No one, certainly not parents
What can the physician do to help?	Everything necessary
What can parents do to help?	Everything necessary
How long will the condition last?	Almost no time at all
Will the child be completely cured?	Yes, of course

mind (1). We agree that a family arrives at the interview with such questions and often with their own set of idealized answers (Table 7.2).

Trouble occurs when the family hears the physician respond with less ideal answers, which is usually the case. Often, the child's condition is serious, it may have been genetically transmitted, medicine may have little to offer for treatment, parents may be powerless to change the situation, and the illness may be lifelong, without hope of a cure. When any of these situations is true, family dilemmas will occur. If all of these answers are true, significant family stress is assured. A family approach and the use of conjoint family interviews can become an important piece of the comprehensive medical care for such a child and the family.

GRIEVING

Sharing the diagnosis and answering subsequent question is just the beginning of what these families endure. Family members move away from the moment of diagnosis, rapidly or slowly, only to be faced with an array of questions, problems, and unexpected events. Although circumstances vary, one task looms large for nearly every family—the task of grieving.

For many chronic conditions, death is not in the immediate picture. Why then does grieving need attention? For many chronically ill children, the staggering fact is not that the child will die but that he or she will live very differently than envisioned by the parents or the child. It is this loss of a "normal" child and a "normal" life for which the family grieves. They mourn the hopes and dreams surrounding the (now broken) promise of that child's growth and future. This mourning is appropriate and important; it is the family's way of saying good-bye to an ideal that is no longer possible.

The circumstances of a child's chronic illness require substantial alterations in the family's pattern. A refusal to let go of the old hopes may hinder the parents' efforts to face the situation, rendering them unable to help their child cope with the illness. The Morenos illustrate the dilemmas facing the family of a child with a chronic handicap, demonstrating that when the necessity of mourning is not appreciated but denied, a family can get itself into serious trouble.

THE MORENO FAMILY

Kathy Moreno was diagnosed with diabetes 2 years ago when she was 10 years old. Now 12 years old and in the sixth grade, Kathy was doing reasonably well with diabetes control until 6 months ago, when ketoacidosis began to crop up several times, requiring hospitalization twice. At home, she still had not progressed to the point of administering her own insulin (although she was competent to do so), and dietary management remained almost exclusively in her mother's hands. On this particular visit, her pediatrician was seeing her for something other than diabetes, or so he thought. Because of the mother's concerns on the telephone, the pediatrician had asked the whole family for an interview. The family consisted of Ray Moreno, 35, a police officer, his wife Ann, 31, a clerk in a local department store, and their two children, Kathy, the identified patient, and Lee, a 2-year-old boy. Lee did not attend the interview; his mother had left him at home with a sitter.

The family entered the office all at once, with the mother tightly grasping 12-year-old Kathy with one hand, swinging her into a chair as if she were a much younger child. The mother motioned with a nod the chair in which she wished her husband to sit. He did so and then slouched. The picture was that of a controlling, busy, exasperated mother with two errant children, a preteen and an adolescent. No one looked happy. The mother sat down alone on one side of the room, with the father and Kathy lined up facing her.

After initial introductions and a brief social interchange, the pediatrician asked how he might help this family. Mrs. Moreno unleashed an angry storm:

Mother: Stealing! That's what it is, stealing! Now don't look away, Kathy. There's no other word for it. I don't understand. We give her everything—it's not as though she's wanting for anything. Am I wrong? Well, am I? That man there (indicating her husband) works the equivalent of two jobs, and I

	work, too. We do it for just that reason, so that our children and our family can have the things they want. And this is the thanks we get—stealing. . . . I can't believe it, in my own family!
Pediatrician:	You're *really* upset, Mrs. Moreno.
Mother:	Well, that's something that I can't tolerate for 1 minute—dishonesty. We've worked so hard for our kids, and . . . (her words trail off).
Pediatrician:	And what?
Mother:	Oh, I don't know. I'm sure part of this right now is pressure from his family (again pointing to her husband).
Father:	Well, that's always there, Ann. We always have that to deal with. That's not new.
Mother:	We always have that to deal with? What's this "we?" I'm the one who has to manage your parents. You know that, and I do too.

So much was happening so fast that the pediatrician felt inundated by the mother's flood of feeling. The chief complaint was Kathy's stealing, and yet that concern was becoming supplanted by some sort of family difficulty with another generation in the father's family. A glance at Kathy decided the direction the interviewer would take. She was looking increasingly frightened and embarrassed. The pediatrician chose to engage her:

Pediatrician:	Kathy, it's pretty hard, I imagine, to be sitting here right now.
Kathy:	Uh-huh.
Pediatrician:	What are you feeling?
Kathy:	(very glum) Mom's right. It is stealing. (She looks up briefly at her father.)
Father:	It's all right, Kathy. That's what we're here for. We have to talk about it.
Mother:	You'd better believe it. And tell him *all* about it while you're at it. Tell him everything you've been doing.
Father:	I don't think anything is served by that sort of thing, Ann.
Mother:	Look, Ray, I'm the one who had to face some of *your*

	coworkers at *our* front door and explain to them how come *my* daughter has been stealing. I don't understand why you're not more embarrassed about it. It was the most humiliating experience I have ever had.
Pediatrician:	And the hurt of that humiliation is still with you.
Mother:	Doctor, I don't think I will ever forget it. Ever.
Pediatrician:	And it's so big that you find it hard to forgive Kathy right now.
Mother:	Well . . .
Pediatrician:	You still have too much anger inside?
Mother:	Oh, I am still *furious*. I know it's probably wrong, but—
Pediatrician:	Just a minute. I can understand that if you are still feeling so angry, then forgiveness seems some way off just now. You know, you don't have to apologize for your anger. You were placed in an embarrassing position.
Mother:	I was. Indeed, I was.
Pediatrician:	I understand. For a minute, I would like to talk a little more to Kathy about what's been going on.

By taking the time to validate mother's feelings and communicate that she had a right to her anger, the interviewer "touched" Mrs. Moreno. She visibly relaxed and allowed the interviewer to proceed with her daughter.

Pediatrician:	Kathy, even though it's hard to talk about, I need to know— what have you been stealing?
Kathy:	(barely audible) Money.

Kathy explained that she had been stealing as much as $20, usually from her mother's purse and occasionally from her aunt. Ten days before, she had entered a friend's house while the family was out and had taken $27 from that family's piggy bank. It was this incident that brought the police and eventually the scene that the mother had described, during which she had to face some of her husband's fellow police officers and account for her daughter's behavior.

Pediatrician:	(Kathy seemed willing to discuss the episode further.) Tell me what you do with the money.
Mother:	(breaking her laudatory silence) Candy! Candy! Candy! This child has the worst sweet tooth you ever saw. She

can spend $10 on candy bars alone and then go back a day later and buy a box of cupcakes! And, of course, she's not supposed to have much of that at all nowadays. But that's where all the money has gone. And her urine, of course, is always four plus these days. Now tell the truth, Kathy, isn't that so?

Kathy: (nods in agreement)

Mother: And I've been over and over it. I don't know why she can't understand how that wrecks her diet and how damaging sweets are for someone with diabetes. Maybe she'll listen to you. She sure doesn't listen to me.

Father: Kathy just won't consider the seriousness of her condition, Doctor. I thought those two hospitalizations might even be good—a way of showing her what can happen. But nothing seems to make any difference. She almost seems to be defying us now around this diabetes thing.

Pediatrician: So both you and your wife are feeling exasperated on that score.

Father: Absolutely. But, well, it probably isn't as much a problem for me. I'm not there as much as the wife. She's the one who has to find the candy wrapper under the bed.

Mother: You can say that again. I've preached at her until I'm blue in the face. And him (pointing to her husband), he's never home for the bad times. He can't understand why I get so upset. And I tell him, "Ray, if you were only home . . . "

Pediatrician: Well, I would like you and your husband to talk to Kathy now about those things you'd like her to know and remember about her diabetes.

Mother: But, I've . . .

Pediatrician: Already done it 27 times? I'm sure you have. I would like you to do it once more, this time in front of me, and now I will help you get your message across.

Mother: I hardly know where to start.

Father: Well, I tell her . . .

Pediatrician: Tell her now.

Father:	Like I've told you, Kathy, having diabetes is nothing to be ashamed of. You are normal, completely normal, and there's nothing to be embarrassed about. Haven't we always tried to tell her, Ann, that she is normal?
Mother:	Absolutely. Why, her friends don't even know she has it. I don't think they have to know anything about it. You just have to watch what you eat and when they ask you about it, just tell them that you think good eating is important for everyone's health. And it is, you know. You wouldn't be lying to them. There's no reason why you can't do everything all other kids do, anything at all. You just have to be careful about certain foods. The fact that you take insulin is nobody's business. As far as anyone else is concerned, you are completely normal. We haven't even told Ray's parents—your own grandparents, Kathy—that you have diabetes. And they don't suspect a thing. So you see how normal you are—your own grandparents don't even realize.

Mrs. Moreno explained that the reason they had not disclosed Kathy's diabetes to her husband's parents was to save them worry. Mr. Moreno's father had been diabetic for 25 years, with serious complications—failing eyesight and most recently the amputation of his right foot. Kathy paled at the mention of the amputation. So did the pediatrician, who also noted that Mrs. Moreno frequently referred to her in-laws in the interview with an edge of icy exasperation in her tone.

Many themes were beginning to emerge, including the obvious connection between the presenting complaint of stealing and Kathy's diagnosis of diabetes, the continuing "presence" of paternal grandparents in the mother's thoughts and words, the mother's exasperation with the father's frequent absence from family crises, and the dogged determination of both parents to promote the notion of Kathy as "normal." The connection between these issues was not yet clear. At the moment, the mixed messages around normality were repetitive and glaring. Kathy could probably hear the contradiction: having diabetes is normal, but let's keep it a secret. Hoping to connect with Kathy, the pediatrician decided to pursue this discrepancy and help the parents understand the confusing information they were giving to their daughter:

Pediatrician:	(to both parents) You use the word "normal" often in describing Kathy and her diabetes. She does have diabetes. Is that, strictly speaking, normal?
Mother:	(a little shocked) I don't know what you mean. We have

worked very hard in these past 2 years to make Kathy understand that she is no different from anyone else.

Pediatrician: Yet, isn't she different?

Mother: Well, not really. I mean, that is . . . she just has a type of medical problem. But that shouldn't stand in her way. We have never wanted it to interfere with her leading a perfectly normal life. And that's what we've tried to tell her.

Pediatrician: I hear you. I'm beginning to wonder, Mrs. Moreno, if you haven't been working *too* hard at telling her that. (He pauses.) Kathy, what's it like for you to have diabetes?

Kathy: Awful, I just hate it.

Mother: Well, it wouldn't be so bad if you'd just follow a few rules.

Pediatrician: Wait, Mrs. Moreno. Kathy, I want you to think of all the worst parts of having diabetes, all the things you hate the most. Wait, don't tell me—just think about all of them for a few moments. Make a list in your head.

Mother: (while Kathy is looking thoughtful) Doctor, do you think it is wise to discuss such negative things in front of Kathy? We have tried so hard to have her see the positive side.

Pediatrician: You deserve a lot of credit for encouraging her positive attitude. Facing the negative side of her illness is not easy, not for Kathy nor for you as parents. But I think it will need to be faced by Kathy and by you, if she is to cope adequately with diabetes for the rest of her life.

Mother: (silent)

Pediatrician: (when Kathy nods she is ready) All right. Now I would like you to tell your mother and father. But, before you begin, turn your chair so that you and your mom are facing one another and be very sure that you are looking at one another. You must catch her eyes. Take her hand as well.

Kathy: (holding her mother's hand) I *hate* not being able to eat what I want, especially sweet things . . . I *hate* shots and testing my urine . . . I don't like . . . (at this point her voice cracks and she is close to tears) having always to be so careful . . . of *everything*.

The pediatrician noticed that Mrs. Moreno had tears streaming down her cheeks as she listened intently to Kathy's words. Mr. Moreno's eyes were also teary. The pediatrician's intuitive hunch to lead the interview in this direction had been important and useful. (We have come to regard hunches with great respect in our own family interviewing work.)

Pediatrician: Tell your mother, Kathy, that there are many times when you don't *feel* normal.

Kathy: (now openly crying) I don't—I never feel normal! Yet you and Daddy are always saying that. If I'm so normal, how come I can't eat sugar? How come those shots—every day? How come the hospital? How come this bracelet?

All the bitterness and anger had left Mrs. Moreno's face, replaced by an expression of profound sorrow. She reached out and took her daughter's other hand.

Mother: I'm going to tell you something I've never said, Kathy. I hate it, too, all of it. From the first day that you got sick and the doctor said it was diabetes—I never went back to see that man, ever again. That's why we switched doctors—it wasn't anything that he did really. It was just that he was the one who gave us the news, and I could never forgive him for that. He dashed my hopes for you, and all I could see was your grandfather with his lifetime of problems. I was determined that I would prove him wrong—your life would *not* change. Your father went along with me, and I decided then and there that you would be treated absolutely normally, so that nothing for you would be different. And . . . (now sobbing) it's all a mess.

It was no wonder then, as the father had said, that "Kathy just won't consider the seriousness of her condition." Both parents, clinging to their own dreams of a "normal" Kathy, refused to acknowledge the seriousness of her condition, and through this denial they communicated to Kathy dangerous messages that she too could deny the reality of her diagnosis. Yet when she followed their lead and joined in the denial, she was scolded for her behavior, and she sometimes became ill. These issues were discussed in the session when Kathy declared that she felt she could never win. If she talked about her illness, particularly if she complained, she learned that both parents, especially her mother, would become angry and berate her for feeling sorry for herself and not acting grownup. A lecture about her "normality" would follow. If she took this lecture seriously, considered herself normal and in so doing disregarded her diabetes, that brought its own problems: ketoacidosis and more lectures, this time about irresponsible behavior.

Until both parents could accept the reality of Kathy's diabetes, she would continue to have confusion about her own approach to her illness. The pediatrician decided to encourage the parents to claim, perhaps for the first time, their own negative feelings around the issue. If they could openly discuss diabetes, with all its ramifications, then perhaps their daughter would no longer have to sneak and steal. The parents' dream for a normal child would have to fade so that new, more appropriate plans might develop.

Kathy and her mother were still holding hands; more importantly, they were listening to one another.

Pediatrician:	Mrs. Moreno, put your own tears into words right now, so that Kathy can understand what you are feeling.
Mother:	I . . . I . . . I . . . feel so stupid, crying like this. It isn't like me.
Pediatrician:	I agree, it's not like you. Your tears have been a missing, but very important, element. (Then, to Kathy) Were you aware that your mother had such deep feelings regarding your diabetes?
Kathy:	(indicates no) She just always seems mad.
Pediatrician:	So perhaps, Mrs. Moreno, it's important that Kathy understand that you feel more than anger about her diabetes. Wait a minute. No "perhaps" about it . . . it is important. Tell her now what you are feeling inside.
Mother:	I feel . . . as though we've been in a bad dream for 2 years, Kathy. I keep waiting for it to end, and it doesn't. I ache for you . . . and even sometimes I . . . (she doesn't finish.)
Pediatrician:	Keep going, Mrs. Moreno.
Mother:	I can't . . . it's so selfish.
Pediatrician:	Your "self" is very important and deserves to be heard.
Mother:	Sometimes I feel sorry for . . . me. But what right have I to feel that way? She's the one who has it, not me. Anyway, that's what I tell myself.
Pediatrician:	You can't give yourself permission to feel sad, angry, and cheated that your daughter became ill?

Mother:	I shouldn't. No.
Pediatrician:	Where in the world did you get that idea?
Mother:	(returning to her store of bitterness) Ask him. (She points to Ray.)

The interviewer found himself peeling off successive layers of an onion. The outermost layer was stealing, which became stealing sweets, which became Kathy's denial of her illness, which became mother's denial of Kathy's illness, which became the. . . . But the pediatrician had not yet gotten to the father, and the omission was beginning to trouble him. It now seemed that Mr. Moreno's role in the unfolding drama would be revealed. That left only his parents in the wings. The pediatrician had not forgotten them either. All in good time, he hoped, although glancing at the clock, he was dismayed to see only 10 minutes remaining.

Pediatrician:	It sounds like something that the two of you need to talk about, rather than Mr. Moreno and I.
Mother:	(feeling hopeless) It's no use. (There was a long silence.)
Father:	What my wife is referring to . . .
Pediatrician:	Say it directly to her, Mr. Moreno.
Mother:	What I mean is I'm not supposed to complain, and you know it. You and your precious parents. Sometimes I feel like I married three people—you and your mother and father. So I don't complain. I make it a point.
Father:	No, not in words you don't.
Mother:	What's that supposed to mean?
Father:	No matter what I say, you jump down my throat . . . like right now.
Mother:	(beginning to cry again) What am I supposed to do, Ray? What am I supposed to do? I'm not supposed to mention Kathy has diabetes since that would worry your parents, "and they have enough to worry about already." And you tell me that the guilt would just kill your father if he ever found out that his disease had been passed on. Or you tell me that I'm the strong one, that your parents count on me to be a rock, that they depend on me for everything. But what about me, Ray? Who can I depend on? Who's my rock? When does my time come? (There is deep silence as Mrs. Moreno sobs.)

Pediatrician:	Be her rock, right now.
Father:	Er . . . that is, uh . . .
Pediatrician:	Comfort your wife.

The pediatrician was suggesting several changes in this family's customary structure. The mother, not Kathy, was moved openly into the position of "needing." Kathy was shifted to the periphery of the action, an unusual and probably welcome position for her. And the father was encouraged to be the strong, competent force in the trio. Implied in the pediatrician's command was that the father had that capacity and could do the job.

He did. Rising from his chair, he moved to his wife and put his arms around her, holding her close and saying in words that no interviewer could improve on: "It's all right. I'm here." He no longer looked or acted like a scolded teen; he seemed a grownup now.

The final 10 minutes of the interview had passed, but they had been put to good use. An additional 5 or 10 minutes was spent drying tears, commenting on what had just taken place, and making plans to meet again in 2 weeks. The parents both look drained. They left with the father still keeping his arm around his wife. Kathy looked relieved.

The Moreno family did return in 2 weeks. The work was not finished. Considerable time was spent in five succeeding sessions on having Mr. Moreno make some choices between his present family and his parents. With support, he began to separate more from his parents, taking a stand in favor of his wife and children. Similarly, Mrs. Moreno used the encouragement to step down from her controlling position, where she was seen as always capable, no matter what the demands. Although she had complained bitterly of being placed in that position by others, she kept herself there as well and gave it up grudgingly at first. However, as Mr. Moreno began to attend increasingly to the unmet needs of his wife, she became less bitter and more willing to accept help from others. Even Kathy noticed the change. As for Kathy, there were no subsequent stealing incidents. In the ensuing 2 years during which the pediatrician followed Kathy's case, there was only one episode of ketoacidosis, caused by an intercurrent infection, unrelated to any dietary indiscretion.

Adhering to a rigid style of denial, this family previously had no avenues for discussion of the child's disease. Any "difference" attributable to the disease was disallowed. Consequently, Kathy, as is often the case for youngsters with chronic diseases, felt ashamed of her condition and isolated, certain that she was a disappointment to her parents. The Morenos needed to grieve the calamity of Kathy's diabetes, face it realistically, and move on. They did that. Of course the work was not that simple, involving several issues throughout three generations. However, the result was that Kathy developed a more realistic appraisal of her situation with diabetes, permitting her and the family a more adaptive coping style for the vicissitudes of her medical problem. Helping the family to grieve, face the reality of diabetes, and put aside old unworkable dreams was facilitated by the pediatrician's attention to and alteration of family structure, communication pattern, sequence, and system. This family beautifully illustrates our view that chronic illness is an important family affair. Appropriate medical treatment of chronic conditions in children always deserves inclusion of the family in ongoing care.

Families with a chronically ill child must face many other issues, aside from grieving their loss. Those issues have been discussed by other writers, such as Chancellor and Luben, who outlined the coping problems of families having a child with cystic fibrosis (2). Although the authors limited themselves to this particular patient population, their comments apply to most families with a chronically ill child, regardless of the specific condition. In our experience with such families, major dilemmas have centered in the following areas.

Isolation

Many families have reported that their child's illness has alienated them from situations and others outside the immediate family. Energies that were devoted to social relationships are diverted inward toward the ill child and managing the grief reaction of each family member. Facing a diagnosis of serious, perhaps lifelong, illness brings inescapable feelings of anger, guilt, and frustration. With such feelings, parents, the ill child, and often siblings may withdraw from outside contacts, weakening social relationships. The chronic sorrow induced by the child's illness is also uncomfortable for outsiders, causing friends to stay away "out of consideration" or because they "just don't know what to say." This aversion only compounds the problem; not only are family members pulling inward, their social contacts are pulling away. A caregiver may be helpful in assisting the family to resolve this issue, putting them in touch with other families in the same situation, encouraging their participation in support groups or another setting in which the family can begin to feel less cut off from the rest of the world.

Discipline

With inevitably heightened feelings of sadness, fear, guilt, and anger, parents of a chronically ill child find their discipline notions in disarray. On the one hand, they worry about the child's ability to tolerate the frustrations surrounding consistent limit setting. On the other hand, they fear crippling their child with overindulgence and permissive behavior on their part. The danger lies in parents' overreacting at either extreme. Parents who fear that their child will use illness to manipulate and exploit may become overzealous in their determination to set limits. They and the child then become caught in a battle over rules far more rigorous than any they had previously experienced. Conversely, some parents, particularly those in whom guilt has taken a serious foothold, are immobilized when it comes to setting appropriate limits with their ill child. Concerned primarily with the child's vulnerability or uncertain future and "not wanting to make the situation worse," these parents abdicate a position of responsible authority with their child. Even for parents not represented by either extreme, the subject of discipline for their sick child and the siblings can be a dilemma and often requires discussion.

Family Relationships

Often when a child becomes seriously ill, the machinery of the family stops. Previous routines are curtailed, and the focus falls exclusively on the sick child. In addition, the family's mobility may be limited, particularly if the sick child requires special equipment for outings or if certain environments are found to be hazardous or inaccessible. These changes are felt by siblings who suddenly find their lives altered for reasons that seemingly have little to do with them directly. Parents are no longer as accessible, and even when available, they seem different—short tempered, preoccupied with worry about the sick family member. Because they may experience this lack of attention without understanding the reasons, siblings may assume incorrectly that they are no longer loved by their parents.

Parents may not only spend less time with their well children, but also with each other. They become so caught up in the care of the ill child that their own marital relationship is neglected. One parent may single-handedly take on the child's illness as a "career" to the exclusion of all other relationships, interests, and people. Anyone other than the child and his or her disease may be considered an irrelevant interruption, including the spouse. In these cases, communication difficulties between husband and wife are inevitable. The feelings involved are often those that are considered unspeakable so that each family member begins contributing to a conspiracy of silence. When a person feels angry, ashamed, guilty, selfish, jealous, neglected, vengeful, sad, or despairing toward or because of a very ill child, then that person often swallows their emotions and tries to get on with life. The sad culmination of this decision is that each family member walks around with a burdensome load of uncomfortable feelings and no place to share them, as illustrated by the Moreno family.

Financial Burdens

For many families with a chronically ill child, particularly if hospitalizations and medical equipment are required, the financial responsibility can be staggering. In those families experiencing guilt around the issue of the child's illness, this may be a taboo topic because "how, with Mary so ill, can we possibly allow ourselves to worry about how much it is all costing?" Such an attitude can have serious consequences. Extended hospitalization these days can completely wipe out a family's financial worth. To avoid this, parents must be realistic from the outset about their own economic limits, including the constraints of their medical insurer, if they have one.

Physicians, particularly now with the advent of managed care, must take the lead in helping families face financial issues surrounding their chronically ill child. Physicians must struggle over what procedure or medication will be allowed by an insurance contract—a concept that sometimes works against the physician's desire, the patient's interest, and, worst of all, optimal medical care. Physicians also will assist a family by understanding its financial limits. Beyond insurance infighting between caregiver and a particular insurer, physicians need to attend to the impact of costs in a larger sense on the life of the family. For example, there is usually less money available for trips and family activities. Siblings may complain that "we don't ever get to go to the movies anymore, not since Mary got sick," for which they may receive a tongue-lashing from a parent who is already feeling regretful about that very fact.

Misunderstandings

Medical jargon and terminology are particularly troublesome for the families of chronically sick children. Since the child's condition is often lifelong and may involve the entire family for ongoing care, unnecessarily complex medical terms used by medical staff are just one more frustrating hassle for family members. Families want explanations from physicians to be simple and understandable. It is a reasonable request because medical clarity can only enhance parents' understanding and care for their own child.

Parents' Emotional Concerns

Parents with a chronically ill child worry. They fret about the child's physical appearance, emotional state, anxieties, and feelings of inferiority. They ask themselves and each other how to cope with such problems. Parents wonder if they are giving enough to the sick child and to the other children. They worry about having more children. Parents suffer from the thoughtless comments others make to and about their sick child. Having seen the disease previously in a childhood friend or a neighbor may cause them to worry that their child will have the same dreadful course. Parents particularly worry about their capacity to help their child with these problems, and they often need considerable help from the physician with these and other worries.

Hope for a Cure

Even for parents who accept the hard facts of a particular illness, its course, and prognosis, a kernel of hope usually remains—hope that a cure will be found in their child's lifetime. Although sometimes irrational and highly improbable, hope is essential in helping parents withstand difficult present circumstances, allowing them to begin some future planning. As one parent stated, regarding her teenager with systemic lupus erythematosus: "You can't live thinking they're going to die every minute. You do that at first. Then you learn to live for their life, not for their death." Hope for an eventual cure is an important factor in nourishing day-to-day hopes, fostering the pursuit of limited goals, such as attending school for a full day, getting a driver's license, or successfully managing an overnight trip. Hope springs from sources other than finding a cure. Some parents derive hope and satisfaction from fully acknowledging the child's condition and moving on to help the child find a meaningful daily existence in their permanently altered life.

Parental Guilt Regarding Transmission

Even with diseases not clearly transmitted genetically, parents still feel guilty about having "given this to my child." The physician should assume this feeling is present in *every* parent of a child with chronic illness, even if not stated directly by the parents. Unfortunately, undergoing a medical history interview can activate these feelings in parents. Even before a diagnosis is made, when parents know only that something is seriously wrong with their child, they are subjected to a medical interview. The physician, doing her or his job, asks about the details of conception, pregnancy, and delivery. For some parents, one conclusion is inescapable: "The doctor is looking for the cause of my child's condition in something I have passed on or something I did to my child." Even without this line of questioning, some parents would still feel guilty. It is unfortunate that one aspect of traditional medical practice seems destined to augment such an uncomfortable feeling in parents. The physician can help by bringing parental feelings out into the open rather than leaving them hidden and unspoken. Parental guilt, particularly in diseases that are transmitted genetically, will not vanish with one discussion and some reassurances. Alleviation of such feelings requires considerable time, from months to years. The physician can initiate this process and should be willing to persist, working toward a resolution of the family's guilt.

Fear of Death

Just as parental guilt is present where it is not warranted, likewise the fear of death seems to be ubiquitous in families of chronically ill children, even when the disease is not fatal. Again, the physician should assume that the fear of death is present in every situation, even when not verbalized. Death may be the most taboo topic of all, and a conspiracy of silence can be particularly upheld around this fear. Physicians may also assume that if the fear is alive in one family member, it is probably felt at some level by every family member, even if never discussed (e.g., if a parent is fearful of a child's death, the child probably is frightened too). Such fears may need to be discussed with the family.

Treatment Regimen

A family's focus on treatment depends largely on the specific condition. Families of children with chronic lung disease, for example, can be preoccupied with the working of oxygen tanks, compressors, motors, and nebulizers. For families facing other diseases (e.g., seizures), the focus can be much simpler, limited to a single medication or combination of drugs. In either case, when the family becomes actively engaged in the treatment of their sick child, they will have questions. Again the issue of medical terminology arises. Family members need to know what to do and how to do it. Their feelings regarding specific treatments also need consideration because without parental understanding and acceptance of the prescribed treatments, even the best planned regimen will fail.

Another aspect of treatment deserves mention. Depending on age, it can be helpful for the child to participate in care to develop a sense of responsibility and competence. Occasionally, parents thwart such participation in an effort to protect their child, taking on themselves the total responsibility for care. This is particularly the case when one parent adopts the child's illness as a career. Excluding the child from any responsibility for maintenance of his or her own health must be altered and can be done in the context of a family interview.

For all of the issues listed above, judicious family interviews by the individual providing medical care may be helpful. We recommend family interviews when any of the statements in Table 7.3 are volunteered by a family member. In family interviews surrounding these complaints, we explore the family's communication style, structure, system, and sequences of behavior, as discussed in previous chapters. Meeting with the family together affords an unparalleled opportunity to evaluate and assist in the family components of a child's chronic condition. The interview may allow a physician to observe a family's level of acceptance and understanding of the child's illness, help a family with its grief reaction, and evaluate the involvement and feelings of siblings. The interviewing physician might be able to clarify misunderstandings surrounding the medical management of the child or help the family broach formerly unspeakable topics, from death, to anger, to exhaustion. A mutual support network may be formed among family members, and the physician may provide the necessary emotional support when the family falters and feels done in by the mean trick life has played. When a child suffers a chronic illness, it is a family matter. Attention must be paid.

Table 7.3. Statements Indicating a Family Interview May Be Useful

STATEMENT	ISSUE
"We feel so alone; there's no one to talk to about this problem."	Isolation
"He just won't stay in his tent, and you said it was essential."	Discipline
"We just never get out anymore; no baby sitter could do the job."	Family relationships
"There's just never any money anymore to do things."	Financial burdens
"I don't know how we're supposed to do that. And also, what in hell does phlebotomy mean? Isn't that some sort of illegal brain operation?"	Misunderstandings
"She just seems to be giving up, Doc."	Parents' emotional concerns
"Sometimes I think I just can't hope any longer. It's been so long."	Hope for a cure
"I read that article about diethylstilbesterol. Just what could than mean for Mary's situation? I took that medication, you know."	Parental guilt about transmission
"He's been having trouble breathing at night but wouldn't tell us for days. He said he didn't want us to worry."	Fear of death
"Harvey seems awfully young to be giving himself his own shots. Are you sure he's ready to do that, Doctor?"	Treatment regimen

References

1. Steinhauer P, Mushin D, Ray-Grant Q. Psychological aspects of chronic illness. Pediatr Clin North Am 1974;21:825.
2. Chancellor B, Luben H. Conferences with parents of children with cystic fibrosis. Social Casework 1972;53:140.

c h a p t e r **8**

Hospitalized Children

Most of the clinical examples shared to this point are from our work with pediatric outpatients. We conduct family interviews with hospitalized children as well. On our pediatric ward, these interviews usually concern issues relating to a child's complex medical condition, reflecting the character of our pediatric inpatient population at the University of California, San Francisco. Because our hospital functions as a referral center for northern California and beyond, the patient population consists primarily of critically ill children with serious, complicated, and often chronic conditions. This makes our facility similar to many other university teaching hospitals throughout the United States. Children hospitalized for primary care are seldom seen. Tertiary care is the order of the day. During one 4-month interval, for example, we conducted family interviews surrounding the following diagnoses:

Chronic headaches
Ulcerative colitis
Cystic fibrosis
Failure to thrive
Chronic renal disease
Hypothyroidism
Hypoglycemia
Tuberous sclerosis
Microcephaly with mental retardation
Achondroplasia
Chronic abdominal pain
Intractable vomiting
Psychomotor seizures

Tourette's syndrome

Anorexia nervosa

Family interviewing by a pediatrician has proven useful in these situations, and we assume that family interviewing would also be helpful in settings that handle more common pediatric problems, with interviews conducted by a member of the primary care team.

Family interviews with pediatric inpatients can serve many purposes. We have used family interviews to do the following:

1. Clarify a diagnostic dilemma
2. Help pediatric staff understand (and therefore work more effectively with) a family's in-hospital behavior
3. Initiate ongoing family counseling when indicated
4. Share diagnostic findings and treatment plans with the family
5. Provide support to a family that has asked for help
6. Prepare a child and family for a proposed surgical procedure

CLARIFYING A DIAGNOSTIC DILEMMA

Family interviews on our pediatric ward are usually requested for one purpose: assistance in reaching a diagnosis for a child with unexplained, confusing symptoms. One diagnostic session, lasting 1–2 hours, with the family has often served and may be incorporated into an inpatient diagnostic assessment just as readily as other investigative studies (e.g., radiographs, blood tests). A diagnostic family interview becomes an especially important tool when there is concern for the influence of behavioral components on the child's health. Because we have been called so often for help in this way, we will illustrate the use of family interviews with hospitalized children from one such experience, Jason Douglas, age 12 years.

THE DOUGLAS FAMILY

Jason had experienced headaches since he was 6 years old. These headaches were severe, occurring as often as twice a month and sometimes lasting an entire day. They were so painful that Jason would be disabled, forced to stay in bed, immobile until the pain lifted. Analgesics had little effect. His parents had never felt that he was malingering or "putting on." He was always genuinely upset when an attack appeared, hating to curtail life and activities. In school, Jason had always been a hard worker and straight-A student. He was active and talented in sports. Boy Scouts took considerable time, and he was very involved in the youth program at church. He was immensely popular, and his parents described him as "almost a model child . . . just a totally normal, delightful boy."

Jason's father was a banker and his mother, a housewife. The family lived in a well-to-do suburb of a large Texas city. Extensive medical evaluations had been done at a university medical center there on several occasions, both inpatient and outpatient. Thorough studies had failed to disclose any medical reason for his continuing severe bouts of headaches. Still, the parents continued to search for answers. They changed physicians, had Jason undergo allergy testing, altered his diet, and read voluminously on the subject of pediatric neurology. Desperate, they took the advice of Mrs. Douglas's brother who lived in San Francisco and had recently urged them to see a particular pediatric neurologist at the University of California Medical Center. The family moved in temporarily with their relatives in San Francisco and made arrangements for Jason's hospitalization and evaluation by the pediatric neurologist recommended to them.

By the time Jason had been in the hospital for 5 days, only one or two of his laboratory tests were still incomplete. The diagnostic efforts so far had yielded no new findings, nor did they suggest a diagnosis. The family was frustrated, as were the medical staff. The team asked us to see the family in consultation, explaining to the family that the discussion was a part of Jason's comprehensive diagnostic evaluation and that the discussion would be led by a pediatrician who specialized in helping families of children with puzzling diagnostic problems.

"Just as long as we're not seeing a psychiatrist," was the father's reply. He indicated that physicians in Texas had suggested that Jason's difficulty "might be emotional," but both parents had considered that possibility absurd. A consultation held previously with a child psychiatrist in Texas, along with complete neuropsychological assessment by a psychologist, had supported the parents' view. According to Mrs. Douglas, these consultants declared that Jason did not have psychological problems. "And so we really prefer not to go through that again . . . it would be such a waste."

The pediatric resident agreed that he would not want to duplicate that study. He explained that this interview would be somewhat different, particularly because the meeting would include Jason with his parents and a pediatrician would be in charge. The family agreed reluctantly.

Performing the first (and sometimes only) diagnostic interview with the family of a hospitalized child is similar to performing any initial family interview (see chapter 5). There are some additional features to consider when the initial interview is, as in this case, a single episode for diagnostic purposes, concerning a hospitalized child with a medical condition.

Family Reluctance

First of all, our experience has been that resistance by the hospitalized child's family is higher than that of outpatient families. Winning the family over to a family view and facilitating their support rather than their anxious reluctance requires considerable work by the interviewer. The anxious reluctance may come from the fear and stress of the hospitalization itself, an experience decidedly outside the norm for most families. Also, hospitalization generally signifies the seriousness of a child's condition. Being on a pediatric ward reinforces the parents' belief that the child's problem is medical rather than emotional. For many parents then, the hospitalization denotes that their child is seriously ill and has a medical problem. A family interview may sound too "psychological" for the situation. Families may get defensive, wondering, "Are they suggesting we have psychological problems?" In addition, the family may have a long-standing worry (and well-practiced denial) that psychological issues are indeed involved, particularly in situations when the child's complaint *is* psychosomatic. This apprehension and denial feeds a family's reluctance to enter the unknown and "dangerous" environment of a family interview.

Thus, the reluctance of the Douglas family did not surprise us. Approaching such a family requires a delicate touch with considerable sensitivity for and acknowledgment of family apprehensions. How the subject of a family interview is introduced becomes important. On our own pediatric inpatient service, this introduction and preparation usually is done by the pediatric resident. Mentioning that the interview will be conducted by a behavioral pediatrician might help, because often, even now, there can be considerable reluctance for a psychiatric consultation, particularly when the stated problem is thought to be physical. Stating (as was done with the Douglas family) that the procedure is considered an integral part of the patient's total diagnostic evaluation may also reduce anxiety. If the referring house officer has established a good relationship with the family, further reassurance may result from mentioning that he or she will also be attending the interview. The family may want particular members of their child's medical team to be present as well, in which case that should be arranged, facilitating the family's comfort. Explaining the role of the interviewer as one who specializes in helping families of children with confusing diagnostic problems or chronic illness may be reassuring.

If siblings at home are invited, the family may ask why those members are being asked to attend. The physician might reply that because the patient's medical condition has had an impact on the entire family, everyone's input during this one family meeting will be useful. Even so, acknowledging the inconvenience of assembling everyone when this means missing school, leaving work, and traveling distances should not be overlooked.

Interview Goals

In our previous discussion of the four goals of an initial family interview, the final goal was ensuring the family's return. Follow-up visits are often not an option with family interviews on pediatric wards such as ours. The family usually has traveled from hundreds of miles away, hospitalization is short, and the patient's time is filled with a multitude of tests and procedures. One session may be all that geography, time, and the HMO permit . . . a fact at odds with the family's often heightened apprehension about the interview. Ideally, apprehension should be handled by a gentle, slow pace during the interview process, but such leisure may not be possible, in which case the interviewer's goals become amended.

1. Establishing that she/he will be in charge of the interview
2. Working quickly to establish a diagnostic formulation
3. Making the interview a "touching" experience for every family member
4. Making recommendations for follow-up
5. Facilitating the family's acceptance of treatment recommendations

This is a tall order for a single interview, and sometimes we find it impossible to achieve. Goals 4 and 5 may require subsequent interviews when one is suggesting ongoing counseling of some type to take place in a community many hundreds of miles away. However, there are times when the entire process can be accomplished in one interview, as with the Douglas family.

▶ The Douglas interview was held in a conference room off the pediatric ward. Jason, both parents, the interviewer, and the pediatric ward resident attended. An older sister remained home in Texas with relatives. The family was an attractive group. Jason was in pajamas but even so gave the appearance of having been organized for the event. The interviewer had never seen a child in bedclothes who seemed so fully dressed. He mirrored his parents in that there was not a trace of casualness in their dress or manner. The family was "squeaky clean." The father was first into the room, taking the lead by introducing himself and the rest of the family. Next was Mrs. Douglas; she was equally forthright in her greeting and impeccably dressed.

Jason entered last. He shook everyone's hand and sat between his parents. The family was very polite, and they looked nervous. A brief period of social talk about the hospital, their trip, and finding their way around San Francisco did not change their anxious look. The interviewer moved on to the subject at hand.

Pediatrician:	This business of Jason's headaches has really been a long-term problem. I imagine that you must all be feeling very frustrated by this time.
Jason and Father:	(nod vigorous agreement)
Mother:	We're almost used to it, aren't we, Jason—it's been going on for so long.
Pediatrician:	I would like to spend some time today discussing the problem with you. It has certainly dominated this family's life for the past several years.
Father:	Six years, Doctor.
Mother:	I don't think it's been that long.
Father:	Oh yes, it has. Jason was in the first grade. It was the year we lived in St. Louis.
Mother:	Well, you can't really count that, Merrill. Jason was having allergies at that time. It wasn't until a year or so later that the headaches, as they are now, came on. Isn't that right, son?
Jason:	I . . . I think so. I'm not sure.
Mother:	I'm certain it is. You just don't remember. Well anyway, it's a small point. What were you asking us, Doctor?

The family had already said much about themselves. Their need for properness, decorum, and control was well displayed in their appearance. Father and son seemed willing to acknowledge feelings of frustration in their situation. However, Mrs. Douglas was sidestepping feelings of any sort. She also suggested, with her controlling behavior, that she considered her account of things the proper one, correcting her husband and speaking for her son. Jason complied, knuckling under to her control.

As the family continued to talk about Jason's problem and its chronicity, the interviewer filed these observations about the family's interaction and kept the focus on a mostly medical discussion of all that the family had experienced together since the trouble began several years ago. Even so, he already had, from his own prior experience and that of others on our staff, a tentative hypothesis waiting to be tested: children's chronic headaches, those not caused by a space-occupying lesion or other medical calamity, have often seemed to us associated with a great reluctance on the patient's part to show anger supported by vigorous, unspoken family rules forbidding its direct expression. However, a beginning hypothesis must be just that, a place to begin. Although attractive as an organizing factor, to get an interview off the ground and begin inquiry, it must yield to change or be discarded should the family's story not fit. The interviewer was beginning his work with this hypothesis, mindful of the theme of anger, watching for its appearance or its conspicuous absence. He had even opened the session with an invitation for them to acknowledge possible frustration. As noted, Mrs. Douglas was admitting to no such emotion. Her husband and son did, but they were having difficulty getting a word in edgewise.

As the discussion continued, Mr. and Mrs. Douglas praised Jason, extolling his achievements. The picture was that of a bright, talented, athletic, gregarious young man who never complained and had his 12-year-old world by the tail. They were very proud of him. Once again, the interviewer offered them an opportunity to declare angry feelings about the subject of Jason's disabling headaches.

Pediatrician:	How maddening for all of you to have Jason's busy life and accomplishments so frequently interrupted by his headaches.
Father:	Yes, sometimes I feel . . .
Jason:	If only . . .
Mother:	(quickly) We just do the best we can. Jason is the greatest little patient in the world. Wouldn't you say that, Merrill? (without waiting for an answer) He is absolutely a wonder, Doctor. There are times I can tell the pain is really getting

to him. But not one complaint out of him . . . ever. (She reaches over and pats her son's knee.)

The pediatrician noted again that attempts to acknowledge frustration by Mr. Douglas and his son were minimized by Mrs. Douglas in a controlling sweep that praised silent adaptability and denial as the way to cope.

Pediatrician: Jason, you were saying, "If only . . . " Finish that sentence.

Jason: If only . . . if only we knew what was causing them.

Father: You can say that again. This whole business has gotten very old. And no one seems to have any answers, or at least any correct answers.

Pediatrician: What answers have you had from doctors along the way? How have they explained Jason's headaches?

Father: Brain tumor, migraine, seizure equivalent cerebrovascular abnormality, allergies, sinusitis, and others.

Pediatrician: None of those has turned out to be the case with Jason. And the whole business just keeps dragging on. That must be tremendously aggravating. Generally, when a family is confronted with such a continuing question—and no answer—everyone begins to have his own ideas about what might be going on, logical or illogical, rational or irrational. Now, I realize you don't know what's been causing Jason's difficulty, or you wouldn't be here now. But I would like each of you to share with me what you've occasionally *thought* might be causing his headaches over the years, as you've tried to make sense out of this business. I'll start with you, Jason. You've been experiencing these headaches for a long time. What have you yourself thought might be causing them? Your answer may be quite different from what the doctors have told you, but that's all right. I am interested in your own ideas about this situation.

Jason: Well . . . (he hesitates for a considerable time)

Pediatrician: Even your wildest thoughts. What in the world could be behind these headaches? (The interviewer was not expecting the answer given, but he was very grateful.)

Jason: (Becoming somber) Sometimes I think I worry too much.

Mother:	Worry? Why, Jason, whatever do you have to worry about? That's nonsense. (Mrs. Douglas was yet again rushing in with denial and imposition of her own view.)
Pediatrician:	What do you see on your son's face right now, Mrs. Douglas?
Mother:	Nervous; he's just a little nervous about this meeting. That's all.
Pediatrician:	Ummm, is that what you're feeling, Jason?
Jason:	Yes, I guess so.

Jason's feelings were heading underground, covered by the surface layer of agreement with his mother. The interviewer was concerned that he might now lose the moment for making contact with Jason around the issue of worry.

Mother:	Jason and I have a very special relationship. I usually know what's going on with him. I can tell when he's upset; he shares everything with me. I have always encouraged him to be completely open with me. Isn't that right, Jason? Don't we tell one another our problems? I guess I would know if you had any sort of worries. (turning to the doctor) But you know, this boy is amazing. No matter what he has to do, he doesn't complain. Jason is the eternal optimist.
Pediatrician:	Ask him if he ever has some private inside worries.
Mother:	You don't, do you, son? (Her question so phrased was actually a disguised command, ordering him to agree with her. Perhaps encouraged by the pediatrician's directive, he did not this time.)
Jason:	Sometimes I do.
Mother:	But they're not anything serious. (She uses a period, not a question mark, in her voice.)
Pediatrician:	Wait, ask him instead to share his worries with you.
Mother:	Well, of course, that's what I always want you to do. You know that.
Pediatrician:	Ask him to . . . now.
Mother:	What is it, Jason? Tell me.

Jason:	Sometimes . . . I worry . . . about the kids at school.
Father:	What do you mean?
Jason:	I don't think they respect me.
Mother:	Jason, darling, don't be silly. They all look up to you.
Pediatrician:	Ask him instead, Mrs. Douglas, what leads him to feel as he does.
Mother:	Well?

At each turn Jason's mother was there with a disclaimer for his feelings, insisting in a reassuring tone that he didn't or shouldn't have the feelings he was for the first time struggling to articulate. The pediatrician realized that he would have to continue to encourage Mrs. Douglas to *ask* her son questions, rather than allowing her to close him down by declaring her own version of his feelings.

Jason answered his mother with a story about his best friend, Mark. The two of them were apparently very much alike, both "popular" boys in the class and in the entire school. Both he and Mark had been candidates for the school's prestigious annual citizenship award. Mark won the prize, not Jason. Tears welled up in his eyes as he spoke:

Jason:	I am happy that he won it. Really, I am. He deserved it. And besides he's my best friend. But now all the kids seem to pick him for their teams and stuff; they don't seem to respect me anymore . . . and . . . Mark, he doesn't seem as nice as he used to be. I know he really deserved that award; he should have gotten it, but . . . (Falling silent he pounds his fist on the arm of the chair, he continues to have tears in his eyes and is obviously exerting effort so as not to sob.)
Pediatrician:	What feelings do you see in your son right now, Mrs. Douglas?
Mother:	(avoiding an answer) I remember this whole business, Jason. I was so proud of how you handled that situation when Mark won the award instead of you. Remember, you didn't let it bother you at all. Remember that I told you that?
Pediatrician:	(aware that mother has avoided facing her son's feelings) What do you see on his face?

Mother:	(She shakes her head, indicating that words will not come, appears very sad, and looks directly into her son's eyes.)

It was a moment of real contact finally between these two. There was silence in the room. Mr. Douglas had been listening intently, saying little.

Pediatrician:	How about you, Mr. Douglas? What do you see going on with your son right now?
Father:	I see a great deal of sadness and anger. I had no idea that he was so upset.
Pediatrician:	Check that out with him. Find out if you are reading him correctly.
Father:	Am I?
Jason:	(nods yes)
Pediatrician:	See if you can find out what his feelings are about.
Father:	I know.
Pediatrician:	But don't assume. Ask him.
Father:	I don't think he'll tell me. He's embarrassed.

Using different, equally effective means, it was now the father who was cutting off Jason's expression of feelings. By making assumptions about his son's feeling (e.g., "I know" and "he's embarrassed"), he was discouraging Jason's own disclosure. His prediction ("I don't think he'll tell me") was a page from mother's book of disguised commands, a message that Jason could hear as, "Don't tell me." Both parents were discouraging any openness Jason might venture regarding the expression of serious thoughts, negative feelings.

Pediatrician:	Ask him anyway.
Father:	Your are embarrassed, aren't you (like his wife, using wording to program a preferred answer)
Jason:	(looking down, no answer)
Pediatrician:	Mr. Douglas, try this one: "Jason, tell me about your anger."
Father:	(laughs) OK, tell me about your anger.
Jason:	I don't know . . . if . . . I thought . . . (finally) I wish that I won.
Father:	Is that what you're angry about?

Jason:	(nods yes) Mostly at myself.
Pediatrician:	And partly at Mark, too?
Jason:	I shouldn't be, but . . .
Father:	You are.
Jason:	A little.
Pediatrician:	Tell your father, "I *am* angry at myself and at Mark about that award."
Jason:	(to his father) I do feel a little mad mostly at myself that I didn't win . . . some too at Mark.

The pediatrician noted that Jason needed to soften his expression of anger. Nonetheless, it was a beginning; the interviewer did not confront or comment.

Father:	(now obviously touched by what is taking place) This is all very hard. I guess I see things differently than my wife. For me, Jason is not one to show his feelings. That's why I am amazed right now. I had no idea. I never know when he's mad. In fact I didn't think he got mad. And he certainly doesn't come to me with what's on his mind. We have *never* actually talked like this before. And I've never been really clear about what's going on inside with Jason. He's just always been very good-natured.
Mother:	(having composed herself, was back in stride) Actually none of us, I guess you would have to say, ever gets really angry. There's so much anger in the world . . . and we really don't need to have anger for one another. We can almost always settle things without getting mad.
Pediatrician:	I see. Yet when Jason gets angry, sad, upset—as we all do, *as Jason is right now*—I wonder, how is he able to show you these feelings? How can he let you know? Can he let you see?
Father:	Well, I certainly see what he's feeling about this Mark situation right now. (pause) Now I'm thinking: is it that Jason generally doesn't show his feelings, or is it perhaps that I haven't been looking?
Pediatrician:	Ask him.

Father:	(turning to his son) Well, I'm ashamed to say that I know I haven't been looking very much, but . . . how about it, son, do you keep things inside?
Jason:	Most of the time.
Father:	Why, Jason, shy?
Jason:	(after a silence) I can't talk to either you or Mom. (voice cracking) I don't want to worry you or make you not proud . . . of me.
Father:	(says nothing and continues to look with concern toward his son)
Pediatrician:	What are you experiencing right now, Mr. Douglas?
Father:	Well, now I'm remembering all sorts of things . . . like last summer. (He went on. Last summer had been difficult. In addition to headaches, Jason had developed severe "rectal spasm" [with diarrhea, cramps, and weight loss] before going off to summer camp.) What was that about, Jason? How many other things do you do to please us or not worry us? Did you want to go to camp . . . for yourself . . . or for us? I remember I couldn't figure it out at the time.
Mother:	Now, Merrill, really . . .
Father:	Don't interrupt, Dorothy. We need to talk about that, son.
Jason:	It . . . was sort of a combination . . . I knew you wanted me to go, and I did, too . . . but . . .
Father:	But what?
Jason:	(becoming tearful again, holds them back) I was worried about getting headaches there, but I knew you had paid all that money for me to go.

The pediatrician noticed it was mother now who was looking on silently. Even though still controlled, she appeared moved by her son's words. And she was not rushing in to disavow Jason's feelings. She was tolerating the boy's disclosure both for him and for herself. When she did speak, she had let down her guard at last.

Mother:	(sadly) I wish you had told us these things.

Jason:	I couldn't . . . (long pause) You don't listen.
Pediatrician:	Is there a part of you that would like your parents to listen?
Jason:	Sure.
Pediatrician:	I would like you to tell them that now, each one of them.
Jason:	Huh?
Doctor:	Go ahead, say it to each of them, here. Say this sentence to each of your parents: "I would like you to listen to my feelings."

Jason complied. His mother responded with a meaningful assenting nod, no words. Mr. Douglas said, "I want to do that, Jason" and squeezed his son's hand.

Here the interviewer used a strategy common in our work with families. He gathered the words that he felt needed to be said and heard within the family and asked the appropriate family member to deliver them aloud. When effective and tolerated by the family, this formulation moves the interview along, often dramatically. Occasionally, but not often in our experience, the person asked to deliver the statement will balk at "having words put in my mouth." At those times, an apology by the interviewer for having assumed too much too fast may be in order. The words, however, will still hover in the air and may subtly influence subsequent movement in the interview.

The pediatrician asked the family to discuss what they had learned about themselves in the meeting. Both parents acknowledged feeling deeply touched by their conversation with their son, recognizing with regret that there had been too little genuine openness. Jason felt both relieved and guilty—relieved at sharing and guilty that he had somehow disappointed his parents. The pediatrician supported the family by observing that everyone in the family needed some help with "uncorking" their feelings. They all agreed. Mrs. Douglas then voiced a fear that may also have been a threat: "That (uncorking) could be dangerous if I ever started!" Then she laughed bitterly. She allowed a trace of anger to flash across her face and looked directly at her husband. He turned away. The pediatrician noticed this but made no comment. Enough had taken place in this meeting; little time was left, and it seemed wrong to open more issues that might not be settled in this session. The interviewer saw the interchange as the mother's indication that ongoing counseling work was long overdue and that each family member would need to learn new ways of talking and behaving.

With the time remaining, the interviewer began to discuss finding a resource for continuing the work now begun, which was no small task because they were in San Francisco and seeking to find help in Texas. He urged that some of the work should include them as a family unit; therefore, family therapy was a clear recommendation. However, he knew of no resources for them in Texas. Fortunately, Mr. Douglas had some connection to the university medical center near their home. He was even aware of a specific family therapist in the department of psychiatry there. To the interviewer's surprise (Mr. Douglas had originally said he hoped the interviewer was not a psychiatrist), the father declared his willingness to follow through with a referral for family therapy.

Interestingly, the family did not ask further questions about Jason's headaches or diagnosis in the interview, and the meeting ended shortly. The pediatrician reviewed his work with the pediatric resident who had attended and Jason's pediatric neurologist. The few remaining medical test results were returned the next day; they were completely normal. A final conference was held the day of discharge with Jason, his parents, and the pediatric neurology staff. The pediatrician-interviewer was unable to attend. Both staff and family agreed that Jason's headaches now seemed related to stress and worry. By this time, Mr. Douglas had already contacted the family therapist in Texas and made an initial appointment.

A note came to the interviewer from Mr. Douglas about 8 months after the family's interview. He wanted to say that Jason's headaches were much less frequent, although he still had occasional attacks. There had been two episodes in the 8-month period since hospitalization. Mr. and Mrs. Douglas were now in marital therapy. Jason did not attend the sessions anymore. The father closed by thanking the pediatrician for pointing the family in a "new direction."

HELPING THE PEDIATRIC STAFF UNDERSTAND FAMILY BEHAVIOR

Most pediatric wards have a hectic pace with many stressors, not just for the sick child and his family, but for the staff as well. Nurses, physicians, social workers, recreational therapists, technicians, aides, clerks, and housekeeping staff must work with one another closely, often around crises. They must also encounter children and families in all varieties, some of whom will be seen as difficult. The patient and parents bring their own anxieties to the hospitalization, a formidable event for all concerned. When understandably stressed staff must work with an understandably stressed family, the resulting chemistry is often less than ideal. When this happens, mutual frustration and distrust develop and can compromise the patient care.

In such situations, a family interview may be advantageous, particularly if it can help an offended medical staff to become "curious rather than furious" with a family (1). Providing insights into the purpose and origin of a family's perceived difficult behavior may help staff to transcend feelings of irritation and allow them to work more effectively with the family. A family interview can be an effective tool for highlighting such insights, particularly if selected pediatric staff members are invited to attend as participant observers.

THE DEMARTINO FAMILY

Tracy DeMartino, age 4 years, was ill with chronic renal disease, renal failure, and hypertension. Around-the-clock medications, many injections, and other treatments were needed. Her father was with her constantly, and he was adamant about being present during the administration of any medication. Because our pediatric ward has for years provided living-in arrangements for parents, the staff is accustomed to the presence of parents, particularly those with young children. However, there seemed something different about Mr. De-Martino's stay. The staff felt it was less that he wanted to reassure, support, and comfort his daughter and more that he distrusted the personnel. Ward staff in turn were offended and intimidated, troubled by the father's scrutiny and apparent disapproval. With time, no one was eager to be assigned Tracy as a patient. Her care was a dreaded experiences for nurses, house staff, and particularly medical students who felt the father's disapproval most keenly. The following interchange occurred between the father and a fourth-year medical student surrounding the subject of a proposed venipuncture.

Student: Hello, Mr. DeMartino. I'm Robert Garfield, a medical student. I'm working with Dr. Carter to take care of Tracy.

Father:	What is that syringe for?
Student:	Tracy has to have a little blood test.
Father:	I haven't seen you before. Are you new on the case?
Student:	Well . . . Tracy has been my patient since Tuesday. I came on the service two days ago.
Father:	Well, how come I haven't seen you?
Student:	(by now on the defensive, feeling intimidated) Well, we've had a lot of conferences, and it took some time also to get oriented to the ward and that sort of thing.
Father:	Well, where is Dr. Carter? He's supposed to be the one in charge.
Student:	He's on rounds right now.
Father:	What did you say you were? An intern . . . or are you a real doctor?
Student:	I'm a doctor in training, a medical student.
Father:	Well, I'm not going to allow any of that. There is to be no practicing on my daughter. I don't know what this blood test is, but Dr. Carter is going to do it if anyone is. He's in charge. You tell him I want to talk to him.
Student:	I don't think he can be interrupted . . .
Father:	There will be *no* blood test. (He draws the curtain around his daughter's bed.)

After several episodes between the father and various ward staff, a family interview was held with the parents and Tracy, offered to the family as a way to use their input for improving Tracy's care. In addition the interviewer (one of us), a nurse and medical student from the ward also attended. In the course of the discussion, Mr. DeMartino's behavior became understandable. He told of his own father's death in a hospital in Italy 3 years ago from an inadvertent administration of the wrong medication. He had not told any of the staff of this incident.

Things improved considerably afterward. Mr. DeMartino continued to watch closely; now the staff encouraged him and even went to find him first before approaching Tracy's bedside with an anticipated treatment.

INITIATION OF ONGOING FAMILY COUNSELING

If Jason Douglas, the child with the headaches discussed earlier, lived in the San Francisco area, we would have suggested that the family enter family therapy with us, using that first interview on the pediatric ward to initiate that process. Many families hospitalized on our pediatric ward do live close by, so the inpatient family interview consultation is a logical introduction to continuing work after discharge. One of our pediatric residents referred to this as the "get-'em-into-treatment" interview, and, although the phrase may be offensive, it is true the family needs to be led to accept a referral for ongoing counseling. Some families accept a recommendation easily, some with difficulty, and some not at all. In our experience, the crisis of hospitalization has sometimes facilitated a family's agreement to move into family work. It almost seems that the anxiety surrounding the event of hospitalization has destabilized family defenses, allowing family members to take chances in a way they might not have done otherwise. Continuing family work is permitted into their thinking during this moment of crisis and is agreed on.

Even when an initial inpatient family interview cannot extend into ongoing sessions with the same interviewer, the physician may use the consultation, as we did with Jason and his family, to lead the group into continuing family counseling elsewhere. To do so, interviewers must have some knowledge of resources, both locally and regionally. We have made it our business to become well informed about family counseling facilities in northern California and have generally been able to recommend such persons to our hospitalized local families. (Texas is another story for us; we were relieved that Mr. Douglas was able to effect his own referral for his family.) We urge that physicians learn not only *how* to make a referral for ongoing family counseling, but also *to whom* one can refer in one's own area.

SHARING DIAGNOSTIC FINDINGS

Sharing diagnostic information has already been discussed in some detail in chapter 7. Eddie Nichols was an inpatient with cystic fibrosis. His situation was used to illustrate that when sharing initial diagnostic news with families, a physician must respect the event, share the diagnosis quickly, attend to the feelings of those present, keep medical facts to a minimum, withstand silence, and avoid running away. These rules are useful in any encounter with a family concerning diagnostic and therapeutic considerations. Our suggestion that medical facts be kept to a minimum should not be construed to mean that we feel patients and families should be kept in the dark regarding medical information. On the contrary, we feel that the more open the physician can be with medical information, the more family members will feel that they are participating in the care of their child, lessening their anxiety and feelings of helplessness. We caution that medical information be shared at a pace that allows the family to assimilate the news offered. Too much and too detailed information given too quickly can be overwhelming for troubled families; then anxiety mounts rather than diminishes.

SUPPORTING THE FAMILY

Had we extended the story of Eddie Nichols, his cystic fibrosis, and his family into subsequent interviews, the category of providing support would have been illustrated. As time went on, Eddie and his parents required considerable support from medical staff, first with accepting the diagnosis and subsequently with all sorts of issues, particularly the use of medical equipment and the almost overwhelming feelings of isolation that each parent disclosed during a subsequent hospitalization of Eddie. These issues were discussed in succeeding family interviews with a pediatrician. We have used inpatient family interviews in many similar situations, during times when families have specifically requested help in coping with their child's medical difficulties.

PREPARING FOR SURGERY

The need for adequate preparation of a child who is to be hospitalized is well recognized. The subject has received considerable attention (2,3,4,5,6). Such preparation is usually initiated before a child's hospitalization and is extremely valuable. One aspect of preparation for the hospital is often handled after admission: the preparation of a child for surgery. This subject also has had extensive consideration in pediatric literature (7,8,9,10,11,12).

Enlightened understanding of the psychosocial needs of children has diminished the frequency with which damaging statements are made to a child concerning an upcoming operation. It is rare now, we are happy to report, that a child is prepared for a tonsillectomy by being told that she will be going to a nice place where she can eat lots of ice cream. And parents no longer bring their children to our pediatric ward telling them only, "Mommy and Daddy are going to take you on a trip to San Francisco where we will take you to the zoo," leaving out the detail of surgery first for an undescended testicle. Although laughable, these were once commonplace occurrences.

Now, it is recognized that children require forthright preparation for anticipated surgery because children, just like everyone else, often cope better with the known than with the unknown. To deny that pain lies ahead contributes to a child's sense of betrayal and distrust. Anticipatory talk about what will take place can mobilize a child's anxiety in a useful manner, allowing the child to disclose worries and discharge some of them. It will also furnish an entree for the delivery of emotional support by those providing care. A sensitive, accurate, somewhat matter-of-fact prediction of what lies ahead, together with reassurance about the child's most pressing fears is required. For children under the age of 4 years, separation from the parents is an almost universal terror (13,14). Aside from any explanation of the surgery itself, a child this age needs particular reassurance that his parents will be with him or her as much as possible. Abandonment will not occur—before, during, or after the operation. For children this age and older, the fear of separation gradually becomes supplanted by one equally terrifying: the fear of mutilation and pain (15). A child struggling with this worry also requires honest reassurance in addition to an explanation of the operation. Depending on the circumstances, such reassurance may mean that the physician can say to the child that neither of these eventualities will occur. For other children, it may mean acknowledging that pain will happen but will be temporary, that medicine will be available to make the pain go away, that there will be no scar, or that the incision will heal without a trace. And if in fact disfigurement is to occur, that also must be anticipated and discussed with the child ahead of time.

Almost always lurking in the background with children, particularly between the ages of 3 and 7 years, is the notion that the surgery is a form of punishment for real or imagined misdeeds (16). Reassurance on this score is always needed. Wishing to place one's younger brother in the trash compactor and undergoing surgery for strabismus are *not* related, and children need to hear out loud that surgery is not punishment for their "evil" thoughts or acts.

Some children's apprehensions may be connected to family relationship issues of trust, abandonment, separation, and punishment. It makes sense then that the family should be involved in the child's preparation for the surgical event, and a family interview can be useful in helping family members prepare themselves and go over the preparation that they wish to carry out with their own child. Preparation of a child by the family seems in many ways a more appropriate maneuver than preparation by a stranger. However, for such family preparation to succeed, the family must be informed so as to do the job well. We have often used family interviews for the surgical preparation of children, helping family members decide what, when, and how they will tell their child about an upcoming operation. The Baxters were one such family.

THE BAXTER FAMILY

Michael Baxter was 5 years old. Four months ago he had undergone surgery on his left eye for a malignant growth of the orbit. The eye did not have to be removed. Neurosurgeons were cautiously optimistic that all tumor had been excised, but they could not be certain. Surgery was followed by 6 weeks of radiation therapy, during which time Michael was an outpatient. Until 2 days before this present admission, he had been doing well, gradually returning to normal routines including kindergarten. Suddenly, signs and symptoms of tumor growth reappeared: proptosis, discoloration, decreasing visual acuity, and some soft tissue swelling around the affected area. Michael was immediately hospitalized. Neurosurgical and ophthalmologic opinions agreed on both the problem and the treatment needed. Michael's tumor, a rhabdomyosarcoma, highly malignant and invasive, had spread throughout his left eye; the left orbit would have to be removed immediately. His parents were informed of this on a Wednesday; surgery was scheduled for Friday morning. Panic ensued. The family had less than 2 days to prepare their son for a horrific event, one that he had worried about several months before with the first surgery. At the time, he had been told removal of the eye would not be done. Now he was to have his worst fears confirmed. Mr. and Mrs. Baxter turned to the ward social worker, whom they knew well and whom Michael trusted, asking her for help in preparing their son. She then asked for assistance from one of us regarding the crisis.

The staff felt overwhelmed by this problem, and after discussion, they decided to handle the situation "by committee" in an interview led by a pediatrician from the Division of Behavioral and Developmental Pediatrics, with Michael's nurse, the social worker, and Mrs. and Mrs. Baxter in attendance. Michael would not be included in this initial family session.

The parents, in their mid-40s, arrived on time for the interview. Their other two children, both teenagers, were in school and did not attend. In retrospect they certainly could have participated and would have been welcome. The two parents and three staff members sat around a conference table. Mr. and Mrs. Baxter looked very upset. The mother was visibly agitated, doing most of the talking, and smoking; her hands trembled. Striving for control, she was barely able to stay in her seat. Her husband, more subdued, looked sad and frightened. He remained quiet for stretches throughout the session.

A few words should be said about the appearance of the staff as well. Not one of them looked eager for this interview to take place; all were feeling overwhelmed by the subject matter and very worried. It was their collective helplessness that had led to this interview format. No one wanted to tackle the subject alone; each wanted the other's support, and so all were attending. Like the parents, each staff member was experiencing turmoil over how in the world one tells a child that his eye is about to be removed.

Pediatrician: This is an awful business. Let's see, how can we get started?

Mother: I just don't know what to tell him. I just don't know.

Sensing that both parents were about ready to jump out of their skins with worry and fear, the pediatrician took advantage of his role as newcomer with this family, attempting to slow emotions down by asking the parents first for details of Michael's illness, the sequence of events leading up to the present crisis, and their understanding of Michael's condition. It also afforded an opportunity to find out about them, their coping styles, and their present array of feelings.

Mrs. Baxter took the lead in this family. She was articulate and had been the central coordinating figure for Michael and his illness. It was she who talked most often and most directly with the neurosurgery staff. She had explained Michael's first procedure to him and had sat by his bed during both hospitalizations. She continued to carry messages to their other children regarding Michael's progress and changing condition. And through it all, she continued to manage the household. She appeared to have basic good sense in helping their son deal with what had been a very difficult problem. The latest turn of events, however, seemed like just too much. She said she was nearing the end of her rope. Preparing their son for the removal of his eye was beyond her. She was lost.

Mr. Baxter, as mentioned, was generally quiet. He initiated little verbal activity, seeming to prefer that his wife remain in charge. He worked long hours in his own business and came straight to the hospital after work each day, not even stopping off at home first. He would remain for the evening with Michael, relieving his wife of her vigil. She would then go home to look after the rest of the family. The parents, during this hospitalization as during the first, were seeing very little of one another except to trade places. Mr. Baxter gave the impression of being quietly overwhelmed by an event that he could not fully comprehend. He was handling the situation by doing what he did best: working hard and staying out of the way.

Informing the Patient

As the interview progressed, the pediatrician asked how and what Michael was to be told.

Mother: I just think Michael has to know about his eye surgery before the operation. But how? How?

Pediatrician: What ways of telling him have come to your own mind as you've thought it through?

Mother: (laughing anxiously) Absolutely nothing comes. I haven't the least idea of how go to about it, and that's what we're asking your advice about. Any suggestions would be welcome. I just stop completely whenever I think about actually doing it. (pause) And Walt here doesn't think we should tell him anything.

Pediatrician: What *are* your thoughts about this business, Mr. Baxter?

Father: Well, I'm not sure, really.

Pediatrician: You have some doubts, it sounds like.

Father: My own thoughts about it, Doctor—if you want me to be very honest I feel we shouldn't tell the boy until after the operation. I think we ought to get him through this first of all and then take our time telling him about it. Now that's the way I see it, maybe you can change my mind. I dunno, but that's where I stand.

Pediatrician:	What would be your objection to telling him before the surgery?
Father:	I know he's worried, and I don't want him to worry more and get really upset before the operation. I guess that's it— I don't want to worry and upset him.
Nurse:	My concern, Mr. Baxter, is how will Michael react when he wakes up from the surgery and finds his left eye gone? I worry that *then* he will really be upset.
Father:	I hadn't thought of that really.
Nurse:	I've been able to be very honest with Michael ever since he first got sick. I don't want him to learn that he can't trust me to tell him the truth now.
Social Worker:	He's been so worried off and on about losing the eye. And until now we've always been able to reassure him that they were not going to remove it. He trusts what we've all said— you, his parents, and us, the staff. I feel that not telling him something would be a betrayal.
Father:	You're right. And yet . . . I don't want to upset him.
Social Worker:	I can understand your concern. Trouble is, I see no way for him to *not* be upset. This whole subject is very upsetting, very . . . for all of us as well. If we explain things ahead of time, you're right . . . he is going to be upset
Nurse:	And if we wait until after the operation he will feel upset and betrayed.
Father:	Yeah.
Mother:	Oh, Walt. We must tell him. I feel that strongly—as strongly as I've ever felt anything. But I don't know how . . . or what.
Father:	(after a silence) I do agree with you, Marge. He has to know something. I don't think I can do it, though.

The pediatrician was pleased with how this interview was developing. The magnitude of the event had drawn everyone into the conversation. It was not so much an "interview" as it was a mutual sharing of feelings by all the participants. Staff and family were each listening to the other. He also began to feel some relief. The active participation by both nurse and social worker meant that he could count on others to help during the course of this very difficult interview.

Pediatrician: So then who will be doing the telling?

Mother: (with a touch of resignation in her voice) I will.

Pediatrician: That's a big job for just one person. How did that fall to you alone?

Mother: (not looking at her husband) I most often get the tough jobs with the kids. That's just the way it seems to work in our family.

Pediatrician: Do you want it to be that way?

Mother: (after a long pause) Yes, I think I do . . . for this, I must.

Pediatrician: It's very important for you that you be the one to prepare Michael.

Mother: Extremely. I've handled things so far. I'm not going to back down now.

Pediatrician: And how is that for you, Mr. Baxter?

Father: OK . . . I think. I don't believe I could do it myself. That would be too hard.

Pediatrician: Do you want to be there when your wife speaks to him?

Father: Yes, I will be there. I'm not sure that I will say anything, but I will be there.

Pediatrician: And is that acceptable for you, Mrs. Baxter?

Mother: Yeah, that's how I imagined it would go.

Pediatrician: That's what you imagined. What is unclear is, do you want it that way or another way?

Mother: Well, when you get right down to it, I don't want it *any* way. But if Michael is to be told, then I want to be the one to do it.

Pediatrician: OK. I respect your courage.

Mother: (says nothing; her eyes fill with tears)

Pediatrician: What will you say?

| Mother: | Oh, oh . . . oh, as I was saying, I just don't have any ideas. I'm lost. |

Role Playing

The interview had now resolved if, when, and by whom Michael was to be told. Now the business of *what* he was to hear loomed large. Not proceeding into that territory, having now armed Mrs. Baxter with courage but no words, would be cruel indeed. Because the group in the interview had already demonstrated their intent to support one another, the pediatrician decided to capitalize on this spirit of mutual assistance when he heard Mrs. Baxter say next:

| Mother: | Actually I do know what I would tell him at first. That I can do, even though it means telling him about his eye. It's what comes after . . . |

| Pediatrician: | Do it right now. Something as important as this deserves a dry run or two. Tell me, as though you were talking to Michael himself about the operation. |

Mrs. Baxter protested that she felt silly "in front of all these people"; then she quickly settled into serious thought, planning the words she would use with her son.

| Mother: | I would say to him that . . . |

| Pediatrician: | I will be Michael. Say it to me directly. |

| Mother: | Michael . . . you know you have gotten very sick again. The doctors have decided that you must have another operation. Remember we said that you might have to have a second operation? Well, you do. But this time it is more serious . . . they are going to have to take out your eye . . . (She breaks off, visibly shaken. So is everyone else in the room.) |

| Pediatrician: | What is it? |

| Mother: | (brief sob) I can get that far every time. I've already done it in my head many times. It's what follows that I can't handle. I don't know what to do with all the questions I'm sure he will have. I don't even know what they will be. But the thought of his questions frightens me. |

| Pediatrician: | Perhaps the group here can give you some help with that. You've done a beautiful job so far. Rest for a minute, Mrs. |

Baxter, while I talk to the others. (turning to the other participants) All right. For just a few minutes I would like each of you to put yourself in Michael's shoes. That means you are 5 years old, that you know that you have had one operation on your eye, and that for some reason your mom says you are going to have another, but this time the doctor is going to have to remove your eye. Each of you think of one question that comes to mind. You may make it the most frightening question you can imagine. (turning back to mother) Mrs. Baxter, it seems to me what you need most right now is some practice in fielding the questions you dread hearing from Michael. So I am going to have each person here in turn face you—as Michael—and he or she will ask a question Michael might ask. Just respond with whatever comes to mind. Should you get stuck, one of us may have an idea to help you. One important thing to keep in mind: for the kinds of questions you will hear, there are most likely no single, correct answers. Everyone in the room would probably respond differently to the same question. It is mostly a matter of style. For the moment, just rely on your own very good style with your own son. You will be all right . . . Are you ready?

Mother: (indicates yes)

Asking family members to rehearse in the face of catastrophic expectations can be a useful device. The interviewer's strategy had several purposes. Mrs. Baxter was blocked by the thought of approaching the unapproachable and being asked the unanswerable. By using the supportive, safe environment of the present interview situation, he could allow her to practice, moving her through her self-imposed impasse. He also hoped, by encouraging her to experience and survive very difficult questions from simulated Michaels, to put her in touch with her resources for handling the actual event, rather than allowing her to persist with a focus on her inability. If necessary, he was also prepared to reverse roles in a second simulation, having Mrs. Baxter take the role of her son. Then she, as Michael, could ask someone else in the room, playing Mrs. Baxter, those terrible questions that she herself dreaded to hear. Having her first play herself was important to organize her thinking and to underscore her strengths. Having her play Michael would allow her to verbalize the questions that she herself most feared and then hear responses from others to those awesome queries.

The nurse volunteered to begin and, as Michael, faced Mrs. Baxter.

Nurse:	Mommy, is it going to hurt?
Mother:	During the operation? No, you will be sound asleep and it will not hurt. When you wake up afterward and come back to your room, I will be right there with you. It may hurt then: you may be sore.
Nurse:	Will I be sore a lot?
Mother:	I don't know, Michael. I hope not. The nurses and I can help by giving you medicine to make the pain go away. And I will stay right there with you.
Pediatrician:	(to mother) How is it going for you so far?
Mother:	This one I can handle, I believe. I did before when he had the first operation.
Pediatrician:	Good. You're doing great as far as I'm concerned. If you feel comfortable with that one, let's move on to another question. How about you, Mr. Baxter? Be Michael for a moment and ask your question.
Father:	(turning to his wife after some thought) What will it feel like, Mom?
Mother:	How do you mean, Michael?
Father:	When they do the operation.
Mother:	You still worried about hurting?
Father:	Yeah.
Mother:	Michael, tell me what you remember about the first operation.
Father:	It didn't hurt. I don't remember much. I was asleep, you said.
Mother:	That's right. This one will be like that too . . . are you scared?
Father:	(indicates yes)
Mother:	(stepping out of role) I think at this point I would just hold him and comfort him. Not talk, necessarily.
Social Worker:	Great. That's just what he would need at that point. I would hold him, too.

Pediatrician:	(turning to social worker) What would be your question, Mary, if you were Michael?
Social Worker:	What will I look like, Mom?
Mother:	Ohhhhhh, now that's getting into something really tough.
Pediatrician:	Do it. Answer your son (communicating his faith in her ability to take the next step).
Mother:	When you come back from the operation, you will have a bandage over your eye. Underneath your eye will look closed, that's all.
Social Worker:	Is it going to look all cut?
Mother:	No, Michael. The doctor says not. (again coming out of role) I know what he will ask next, and I think this is the one I've been dreading.
Pediatrician:	Say it.
Mother:	Michael will want to know if there is going to be a big hole in his face. (She breaks down. Aside from that there is silence.)
Pediatrician:	(after moments of silence and after Mrs. Baxter composes herself) Answer him.
Mother:	Well, no, Michael. There isn't going to be a big hole. Everything will look all right on your face except that your eye will look closed. No, honey, there isn't going to be a big hole. Have you been worried about that? (leaving her role) That's how I understand it—that the surgery is not going to be disfiguring. They are not planning to take out any bone or change the shape of his face?

Because she seemed to be asking for reassurance, the nurse spoke up and agreed that this was her understanding as well, that Michael's face would not be changed. The mother's own fear of this possibility had made answering the question so difficult for her. She was relieved to have now asked the question and been reassured that her fear was ungrounded. She also expressed her somewhat greater comfort in now approaching Michael about the subject. The pediatrician continued:

Pediatrician:	I have one further question as Michael.

Mother:	Yes?
Pediatrician:	Mom, after the operation, am I going to be able to see?
Mother:	Yes, of course, honey. People can see with one eye just about as well as with two eyes. You will be able to see . . . (leaving her role) and then I would love him again.

The interviewer brought the role playing to a close, with the goal accomplished. Mrs. Baxter had a sense of what to do and how. She seemed very capable. He then asked each person around the table to share a way in which he or she had been touched by the mother's approaches to her child. Everyone in turn, including Mr. Baxter, could acknowledge feeling moved by her caring and impressed by her savvy and courage in the various encounters. The comments themselves provided a touching moment in the session. Discussion was then held as to how mother wanted to arrange telling her son. Did she, for example, want anyone there besides her husband? How could the staff assist? She decided that, if Mr. Baxter were agreeable, she wanted the preparation talk to be a private time, involving just the three family members. Her husband agreed, and the interview concluded.

Later that afternoon Michael was told of his upcoming surgery, as planned. The parents reported to the social worker that things went reasonably well. They felt able to be open and direct in their own comments. Michael cried; they all cried together. Both parents said that the practice session had been very helpful in preparing them for the job that had to be done.

Tragically, Michael's surgery, although itself successful, was unable to save his life. He died less than 1 year later with extensive metastases.

References

1. Leveton A. Personal communication. March 1971.
2. Gofman H, Schade G, Buckman W. The child's emotional response to hospitalization. Am J Dis Child 1957;93:157.
3. Mason E. The hospitalized child—his emotional needs. N Engl J Med 1965;272:405.
4. Plank E. Working with children in hospitals. Cleveland: Case Western Reserve University Press, 1962.
5. Spitz R. Hospitalism. Psychoanal Study Child 1945;1:53.
6. Melamed BG, Ridley-Johnson R. Psychological preparation of families for hospitalization. Dev Behav Ped 1988;9:96.
7. Adams M, Berman D. The hospital through a child's eyes. Children 1965;12:102.
8. Bergmann T, Freud A. Children in the hospital. New York: International Universities Press, 1966.

9. Davenport J, Werry J. The effect of general anesthesia, surgery, and hospitalization upon the behavior of children. Am J Orthopsychiatry 1970;40:806.

10. Kenny T. The hospitalized child. Pediatr Clin North Am 1975;22:583.

11. Mattson A. Long-term physical illness and psychosocial adaptation. Pediatrics 1972;50:801.

12. Prugh D, Staub E, Sands H, et al. Study of the emotional reactions of children and families to hospitalization and illness. Am J Orthopsychiatry 1953;23:70.

13. Bowlby J. Grief and mourning in infancy and early childhood. Psychoanal Study Child 1960;15:9.

14. Bowlby J. Attachment and loss. New York: Basic Books, 1969:1.

15. Kenny, 583.

16. Wolff S. Children under stress. London: Alan Lane Penguin Books, 1969.

c h a p t e r **9**

Psychosomatic Conditions

THE ORTIZ FAMILY

Alice Ortiz, 15 years old, trailed after her parents. Her father, the first into the office, was a picture of crisp efficiency with a manner that said, "Let's get down to business." He was short, trim, and wore a three-piece suit; everything was well ordered—hair, moustache, white shirt, solid tie, handkerchief, dark socks, and black shoes. His somber face matched the outfit. Under his arm he carried a copy of *The New York Times* and a book. His wife, two steps behind him, acted as if she wanted to be invisible. She avoided Dr. Silver's eyes as he greeted her, extending her hand beyond her bulky coat sleeve only after she saw his outstretched; her coat was bundled around her so that only a portion of her head was visible above the collar. She moved to a chair quickly, two available seats away from her husband and motioned for her daughter, bringing up the rear, to join her on that side of the room. Alice complied, in many ways duplicating the entrance of her mother. She too was wrapped in a heavy coat. Even so, the pediatrician could see she was a beautiful young woman. Although Alice loosened her coat as she sat, her mother did not. All three family members looked anxious as the session began.

A fourth family member was not present. Alice's 19-year-old sister was away at college. The parents, both born in Guatemala, had come to the United States as young adults and met and married in this country. Mr. Ortiz had a responsible office position with a shipping company on the San Francisco waterfront. Mrs. Ortiz worked as a laboratory technician in a medical office complex. Alice's asthma had brought the family in. Previously, the pediatrician was told by the referring physician (Alice's allergist) that this was one of the few families in which he felt emotional factors were significant contributors to the symptoms; he himself had witnessed attacks triggered by the father's heavy-handed way with his daughter.

Because this was a teaching hour, a pediatric resident was present, observing her first family interview on the first day of her behavioral pediatrics rotation. Dr. Silver glanced over and winced; the trainee looked as uncomfortable as the family. The resident would be another responsibility and in fairness could not be expected yet to assist in the work of the interview. But she did look interested as well as anxious. And Dr. Silver generally enjoyed introducing family interviews to pediatric trainees by immersing them in an interview on the first day of training. It was seldom experienced as a boring or neutral experience and often served as "the hook" for capturing their attention and enthusiasm for the weeks to come.

Following introductions and a few words about taping the session, Dr. Silver opened the session by asking each family member what he or she understood about the meeting.

Pediatrician:	How about you, Alice?
Alice:	Well, it's about my asthma. Dr. Williams, my allergist, said we should come.
Pediatrician:	I see. For what purpose?
Alice:	I don't know. I think he thinks there may be psychological things about my asthma, as well as physical.
Pediatrician:	And what do you think?
Alice:	I'm not sure really. I'm wondering if we're going to be talking about medical stuff or . . . (glancing at her father) something else.
Pediatrician:	So you're feeling confused as to whether today's session is going to be a discussion of medical issues or psychological ones?
Alice:	Yes.
Pediatrician:	OK. I'll come back to that in a minute. Let me first move to your dad. Mr. Ortiz, what do you understand about this meeting today?
Father:	My wife asked me to come, Doctor. I really don't know—I assume that you are an allergy specialist, and you are going to help Alice with her asthma. Will you be giving her allergy tests, that sort of thing?
Pediatrician:	Oh, then you have been thinking that I am an allergist?
Father:	Yes.

Pediatrician:	I think I need to explain. I am not an allergist. I am a pediatrician, and I often work with children who are having some particular medical problem—like asthma, for instance. My special focus with them, however, is on the emotional or behavioral parts of that medical problem. And I prefer to work with the whole family, rather than just with the child alone. Alice mentioned a minute ago that Dr. Williams thinks there may be emotional or psychological issues connected with Alice's asthma attacks.
Father:	Yes . . . ?
Pediatrician:	Tell me how Dr. Williams explained that to you.
Father:	He didn't.
Pediatrician:	Oh, then you also must be feeling somewhat confused as to what this meeting is all about, especially since I have now just told you that I am not an allergist.
Father:	I certainly am.
Pediatrician:	Maybe we need to talk about terms . . . "psychological things as well as physical" . . . I wonder what Dr. Williams could have meant there? Anybody in the family have any ideas?
Father:	(very definitely) No
Mother:	I think what he is referring to . . .
Pediatrician:	Good, Mrs. Ortiz. I was beginning to worry that I hadn't yet gotten over to you . . .
Mother:	I think he means that Alice can get an attack just from getting upset.
Pediatrician:	And have you noticed that?
Mother:	Yes, often.
Pediatrician:	Tell Alice specifically what you have noticed.

The mother, still looking frightened, shared with Alice that attacks would often occur when the girl became stressed, anxious, or upset. Alice half-heartedly agreed and then countered that there were just so many things to which she was allergic. Her father entered at this point, listing off all her allergens and a description of his own recently surfaced allergies and the prolonged diagnostic evaluation in which he was currently involved.

It was not a particularly heartening beginning as family interviews go. The father thought Dr. Silver was an allergist; Alice, the identified patient, was showing reluctance in broaching psychological issues; her mother, though tentatively suggesting the presence of psychological factors, was looking scared to death. No one had visibly relaxed since the start of the hour, including the resident. Even the interviewer was not comfortable. He decided to retreat to territory that would feel more comfortable for the family and for the resident so that he could organize his thoughts and regroup. He asked Alice for a history of her medical condition. The interview settled into a discussion of the frequency of attacks, medications used, hospital visits, and duration of attacks. Alice and her parents talked freely, and the anxious pall seemed to lift. Even the resident uncrossed her folded arms. While Mr. Ortiz and Dr. Silver were discussing something about the use of albuterol, the interviewer glanced at Alice and noticed that she was close to tears. He said nothing, completing his conversation with her father, but felt a sense of relief; content would give way to process after all. He had no intention of discussing bronchodilators for the rest of the session. Using Alice's tears would allow him to venture a shift toward feelings and family relationships.

Pediatrician:	Alice, I'm wondering what you're feeling inside right now as we've been discussing all of this.
Alice:	(very quietly) I don't know.
Pediatrician:	I ask that for a specific reason. Just a few moments ago, I noticed that you were very upset, close to tears.
Alice:	Just a cold, I guess (blowing her nose).
Pediatrician:	Somehow, it seemed more than that.
Alice:	(Silent for a long time, she begins to sob quietly.)

Dr. Silver glanced over at the resident. She has crossed her arms again. Mr. Ortiz was sitting ramrod straight, unchanged. Mrs. Ortiz had started sobbing in rhythm with her daughter. Something important was happening; the interviewer chose to remain silent and let the situation unfold. Shortly Mrs. Ortiz rose from her chair, crying openly now and apologizing for her tears, "Oh Doctor, I am sorry . . . so sorry. Excuse me please." She headed for the door. The pediatrician rose, put one hand on her arm and the other on the doorknob, and gently asked her to stay. "Oh, I just shouldn't be crying," said the mother. The interviewer reassured her that in this room, it was all right to cry. Guiding her back, he asked her to talk about her tears. She indicated that she could not bear it when her daughter was upset—darting a look at her husband that he did not return—that when Alice got upset, she did too. The pediatrician acknowledged that the two of them must be very close and asked if she knew the origin of Alice's present tears.

Mother:	No, I don't understand.
Pediatrician:	Would you ask her now—ask her what her tears are about, see if she will put her tears into words?
Mother:	What's wrong, darling?
Alice:	Just . . . scared, I guess.
Mother:	Scared about what?
Alice:	(She shakes her head indicating that she does not know. A long silence follows.)
Pediatrician:	I bet you have a few ideas, though.
Alice:	(nods her head yes)
Pediatrician:	But it's very hard to talk about?
Alice:	(vigorously) Yes.
Pediatrician:	I can see that. I have some ideas too about what's happening on your insides. So don't talk—I'll share my ideas, and you can just let me know whether what I say fits or not. You can just nod yes or no.
Alice:	(nods in agreement)
Pediatrician:	If I'm Alice, I am feeling scared because this whole situation is frightening. Here I am with my family sitting in front of two strange doctors. I don't know them. It's hard to talk about important and private things with strangers. That's one reason I am feeling scared. Does that fit?
Alice:	Yes.
Pediatrician:	And there's more?
Alice:	Yes.
Pediatrician:	Another reason, if I'm Alice, for feeling scared is I'm worried

that people won't understand what I'm feeling or trying to say.

Alice: (again nods that he is correct)

Pediatrician: Those were my ideas. I wonder if you have some others of your own.

After a long pause, she indicates that she does. There is now a longer silence. Then, squaring her shoulders while continuing to look at her hands, she continues.

Alice: (almost a whisper) I cannot talk with my father.

Pediatrician: (allowing another silence) You sound very sad as you say that.

Alice: Very.

Pediatrician: Tell me, is there a part of you that would like to be able to talk to your father, a part of you that would like for the two of you to be closer?

Alice: (nods agreement)

Pediatrician: Could you tell him that directly, right now?

Alice looked at her father and did just that. He was listening. And the pediatrician was thinking so far, so good. They had successfully made a transition from medications to feelings.

Alice said that she wanted very much to be closer to her father, but that communication never seemed to work well between them. He seemed angry and dissatisfied with her. Because it was so hard to tell from Mr. Ortiz's unchanged facial expression what impact these comments had on him, the pediatrician ventured:

Pediatrician: Mr. Ortiz, you are obviously listening very hard. What do you see in your daughter's face right at this moment?

Father: Anguish. I see anguish.

Pediatrician: And what does that do to *your* insides?

Father: I don't know what you mean.

Pediatrician: What are you feeling?

After some searching, Mr. Ortiz acknowledged that his daughter's feelings triggered feelings of helplessness. He just didn't know what to do. He then began to defend his customary behavior with her, saying that it was not his intention to create distance, but that he was so worried about her asthma that her attacks often threw him into a panic. He displayed his worry by questioning her relentlessly about her behavior before the attack. He would probe for anything that might give a clue as to how she allowed an offending allergen into her system. She would have to list for him the food she had eaten, the places she had been, and her activities. Usually he would explode with an "AHHHHH, so that was it! How many times have I told you . . . " He would then severely scold her for being irresponsible for her own condition. Alice would be intimidated into tears. They would end the interchange in mutual bitterness and alienation. In an effort to support the father's good intentions, Dr. Silver pointed out that it seemed to be feelings of helplessness and concern for Alice's health that prompted Mr. Ortiz to be so upset with her. Both father *and* daughter nodded agreement.

The interviewer asked them if they were interested in learning to communicate in other ways and work at drawing closer together. Both said yes, and Mrs. Ortiz also signified her willingness to participate in additional sessions. Plans were made and the session terminated. From a tentative beginning, the interview had progressed well, Dr. Silver concluded afterward as he and the resident discussed the session. The resident was impressed and asked if the interviewer had in some way planted the family to demonstrate the effectiveness of a family approach. Dr. Silver took that as a compliment. Because the resident now seemed willing to enter the fray, she and Dr. Silver made plans for how they might jointly share interviewing responsibilities when the family returned in 1 week.

The family never returned. They canceled their next two interviews, then indicated that they did not wish to continue at all.

SOME OVERSIGHTS IN THIS FAMILY INTERVIEW

What happened? The resident and the interviewer both felt so positive about the initial meeting and sensed that the family had felt likewise. Yet their willingness to pursue the communication of feelings in subsequent sessions had obviously been misread. Why? What had happened that the interviewers seemed to win the battle only to lose the war?

The reader may have answers to these questions. In retrospect, we too developed some explanations for the family's disappearance after just one session. Our answers stem from three possible omissions or oversights by the interviewers: failure to achieve the necessary goals of an initial family interview, inattention to ethnic issues, and insufficient respect for the elegant defenses found in families with a psychosomatic member.

Failure to Achieve Goals for an Initial Family Interview

Achievement of goals has already been discussed in chapter 5. Briefly reviewed, interviewer aims are as follows:

1. To establish that the interviewer will be in charge of the session
2. To develop a beginning formulation of the problem and a tentative treatment plan
3. To make the interview a touching experience for every family member
4. To ensure the family's return

During the Ortiz family interview, there was never much doubt that the interviewer was in charge, so the first goal was met. The second goal was achieved by formulating the problem (i.e., the expression of feelings was blocked) and beginning a tentative treatment plan (i.e., "unblocking" the family's expression of feeling with one another). However, the failure of goal number four (ensuring the family's return) was probably related to a simultaneous failure of goal number three, making the interview a touching experience for every family member. In retrospect, Alice had been touched in the interview; her feelings were heard, acknowledged, and discussed. However, little attention was given to Mrs. Ortiz, and it was unclear whether or not the brief interchange around her own tears was sufficient acknowledgment of her distress. More time and care should have been spent with her in the hour. Considerable time and care were spent with Mr. Ortiz, eliciting and acknowledging his feelings in direct attempts to "touch" him. From the interviewer's vantage point, contact seemed to take place. In retrospect, Mr. Ortiz was not touched deeply enough because it was he who refused to return or to allow the family's participation in subsequent sessions. Or so said Mrs. Ortiz who actually made the call to cancel. Repeated attempts to talk directly to Mr. Ortiz were unsuccessful.

We believe that Mr. Ortiz would have been touched more deeply if the interviewer paid more attention to the father's feelings of discomfort surrounding the family interviewing process itself. This should have been done well before asking the father to expose his vulnerable feelings regarding his daughter and her illness.

This notion of attending to the comfort of interviewees, particularly in psychosomatic situations, is not just our idea. Susan McDaniel, Thomas Campbell, and David Seaburn discuss somatic fixation and how an interviewer can handle it in *Family Oriented Primary Care* (1). Briefly, somatic fixation is that process in which patient, family, and often a physician focus exclusively and inappropriately on the somatic aspects of a complex problem. This process frustrates the expansion of either the diagnosis or the treatment into more comprehensive, useful directions.

In these situations, these three authors urge a caregiver to develop a relationship with the patient that is collaborative. The interviewer achieves this by returning often to the patient's and family's strengths and areas of competence and eliciting their suggestions for diagnosis and treatment. Forming this collaborative relationship eases the anxiety of the group, making them feel comfortable and more in control. Additional work by Dr. Silver to form such a relationship might have been useful with Mr. Ortiz.

The idea is expanded further in another work dealing with psychosomatic problems:

Emotional postures can either open or close possibilities for therapeutic dialogue. All mammals, including humans, show two broad groups of emotional postures. Emotional postures of tranquility are the different configurations of a bodily readiness to care for oneself or another . . . (as seen in) reflecting, composing, listening, musing, affirming, understanding, trusting, loving. . . . Emotional postures of mobilization however are different configurations of a bodily readiness either to defend or to prey on . . . (during) scorning, shaming, blaming, criticizing, justifying, walling off, ignoring. (2)

These authors, influenced by the narrative therapy ideas of Michael White and David Epston, seek to create an environment that favors dialogue, not monologue, with patients, encouraging family members to adopt postures of tranquility rather than those of mobilization (3). The clinician's job is to "enter the interaction with an emotional posture of respect and acceptance if he or she assumes first that building a relationship is more important than gathering information and, second, that the patient may hold a valid understanding of the problem in which there is indeed wisdom in self-disclosing only with caution" (4). In retrospect, every member of the Ortiz family demonstrated postures of mobilization to Dr. Silver, and few postures of tranquility were displayed. Greater attention to building a relationship with this frightened family was needed.

Inattention to Ethnic Issues

Issues of ethnicity are integral parts of any therapeutic encounter. Historically, this fact often has been overlooked as a generation of family interviewers embraced clinical interventions based mostly on white, middle-class norms. The reader is certainly aware by now that the approaches outlined in this book are squarely rooted in that tradition, reflecting both the authors' backgrounds and the patient populations often served.

In our own work, we have attempted to amend this bias for our trainees by referring to the writings of Minuchin, which emphasize both ethnicity and economic status as important determining factors in family problems. As early as 1967, Minuchin was interested in poor families, coauthoring *Families of the Slums* (5). In a 1993 book he states, "I have returned to my early work with poor families" (6). Minuchin, himself from Argentina, has been keenly interested in ethnic variables as well. Describing Latino families, he might well have had the Ortiz family in mind when he wrote: "Hierarchies may be extremely clear, with roles explicitly organized around generation and gender. Women may be expected to be submissive, and men expected to protect their women. A mother may be expected to be self-sacrificing and devoted primarily to the children" (7).

Mr. Ortiz communicated on several levels the importance he placed on being a responsible individual and being regarded as head of his family. His attire, manner, and interaction with his wife and daughter emphasized this fact. The parents' Guatemalan roots very likely supported this clear role definition for both parents. Dr. Silver seemed to overlook this important issue and entered too quickly into the family's private business over which Mr. Ortiz was guardian and protector. It may well have been that the interviewer's well-intentioned intrusion was felt as just that—an intrusion and an implication that father was not managing his family well. The interviewer's goal of taking charge of the interview may have clashed with this father's sense of paternal leadership and control. Were this the case, the father's decision, when safely out of the interview, not to return for future sessions is understandable. The importance of considering ethnic variables in family interviewing has been well reviewed by other authors as well (8).

Insufficient Respect for Family Defenses Surrounding Psychosomatic Symptoms

In our experience, psychosomatic symptoms in a family member are often the feelings of that person expressed in disguise. As one of our staff has noted:

> *It is a useful generalization to consider that it suits the body's economy to discharge feelings of all kinds. If the expression of feelings is forbidden by family rules of behavior, those feelings will still press for release although by indirect means. I generally expect to find the most "psychosomatic" difficulty in those families that are most intent on teaching their children to suppress the expression of feelings. The parent's motive is usually based on his own dread of some feeling of helplessness. For example, "If I let my child cry, I won't know what to do to stop her." Or, "If my child loses his temper, I will not be able to stand up under her anger." Since there is nothing that can be done directly to prevent someone from having an emotion (short of drugs, psycho-surgery, etc.) families that are fearful of being overwhelmed by other people's feelings generally work to discourage expressing feelings. Certain body organs seem far more immediately involved in the discharge of feelings that are not being handled directly. As you might expect, the more vulnerable organs are those which are in dynamic equilibrium between the organism and the environment, e.g., the nervous system, the gastro-intestinal tract, and the respiratory tract. Breathing seems an especially sensitive interface between the self and the outside world. In fact, the German word "angst" from which "anxiety" derives, means a narrowness and refers to the feeling of restricted respiration and tightness that accompanies anxiety. (9)*

It is interesting how often metaphor and simile come to mind when working with a psychosomatic symptom. We believe that it is more than coincidence that an individual with a tension headache will generally describe his pain in terms such as, "I feel like I'm going to explode" or "I'm going to blow my top," and that these statements are widely accepted metaphors for the expression of anger as well. In this and other examples, there is an uncanny, almost poetic connection between a given psychosomatic symptom and the language used to describe a particular feeling. As James Griffith and Melissa Griffith have said, "The splitting of language and silencing of the body seem to be the soil in which somatic symptoms grow" (10). We have worked with families repeatedly in which someone had:

Headaches (expressed as ready to "blow my top")

Chest pains (and felt "sick at heart" with something he needed to "get off my chest")

Constipation (and felt "tied up in knots")

Vomiting (and could not "stomach" something in the environment)

Dysphagia (and experienced something in the family that was "hard to swallow")

Asthma (and felt "choked up," "breathlessly excited," or both)

Enuresis (and felt "pissed off ")

These individuals, finding direct methods for the communication of feelings blocked, sent their message in code, thwarting the family proscription against revealing feelings. Thus, psychosomatic symptoms and the indirect expression of feelings seem inextricably linked. We like Griffith and Griffith's view of a somatized symptom as "the public performance of an unspeakable dilemma" (11). These ideas are not far removed from some of the early writings of Breuer and Freud, who postulated connections between the symbolic expression of unacceptable feelings and somatic symptoms (12).

Because an individual develops, at least in part, psychosomatic symptoms to symbolize and express emotions that are considered unacceptable in that person's family environment, a rapid entry into this area by the interviewer may be intrusive and too unsettling. This may have been the case with the Ortiz family. Challenging family members so quickly and so directly to transcend their accustomed style of avoidance and denial may have frightened them off. Looking back, an alternative would have been to go slower, proceeding at a pace better matched to the level of the family's defenses, allowing them more time to feel safe in the interviewer's hands.

This discomfort with the direct expression of feelings is one important characteristic of a family with chronic and entrenched psychosomatic symptoms. Once again, we refer to Minuchin, particularly his book titled, *Psychosomatic Families: Anorexia Nervosa in Context* (13). This book presents the orientation and approaches of Minuchin and his coworkers at the Philadelphia Guidance Clinic to psychosomatic families. It is a model we have continued to use up to the present time with families. Although this model has not fit all psychosomatic families in our own work, it has certainly provided a useful structure upon which to begin with these families.

A Conceptual Model of the Psychosomatogenic Family

For several years, Minuchin and his colleagues were engaged in a study of patients with one of three psychosomatic conditions: anorexia nervosa, "brittle" diabetes mellitus, or intractable asthma (the last two disorders were judged to be psychosomatic if the symptoms were produced or exacerbated by emotional stress). They found certain characteristics that were consistent across the families and nonspecific with respect to the type of symptom. This fact supports the observation that "there is no evidence for the view that specific family constellations create specific family illnesses. What is more likely is that stresses associated with living with a dysfunctional family trigger the physiologically vulnerable organ or system with subsequent ill health" (14). The group in Philadelphia proposed a type of family whose organization predisposed or supported somatic symptoms as an expression of emotional distress. This group also felt that the somatic symptom bearer was not merely the recipient or expresser of emotional stress in the family but, in a dysfunctional way, also a reliever of stress. They developed these observations into a conceptual model of the psychosomatogenic family. In their view, the development of psychosomatic illness in a child was related to three factors: a characteristic mode of family functioning, involvement of the child in parental conflict, and physiological vulnerability.

A Characteristic Mode of Family Functioning

The repetitive transactional pattern of a psychosomatogenic family is characterized by enmeshment, overprotectiveness, rigidity, and lack of conflict resolution. With enmeshment, the family members are overinvolved with one another and overresponsive. Interpersonal boundaries are diffuse, with the family members intruding on each other's thoughts, feelings, and communications. Subsystem boundaries are also diffuse, which results in a confusion of roles. An individual's autonomy is severely restricted by the family system. Chapter 5 described Laura French, a patient with anorexia nervosa, who was asked to construct a family sculpture. The patient put together a small, tight, family circle and inserted herself in the middle. The interviewer then demonstrated that they could not take a step without everyone falling. Their enmeshment was unmistakeable.

Members of an overprotective family have a high degree of concern for each other's welfare. Protective responses are constantly elicited and supplied. When there is a sick child, for example, the entire family becomes involved. Parental conflicts are often submerged in the process, and the child in turn feels responsible for protecting the family, as illustrated by the Ortiz family. Father's heavy-handedness stemmed from his desire to (over)protect his daughter from her condition. And some of Alice's reluctance to open up in the session could well have been her own desire to protect the family (even the father she feared) from the prying of the interviewers. Rigidly organized families often present themselves as not needing or wanting any change in the family. Preferred transactional patterns are inflexibly maintained. Rigidity is a frustrating characteristic for interviewers to face because a family is almost always asking for help with a particular child *and* indicating, "But don't ask us to change anything." This pattern is often at the root of a family's resistance to change and certainly influenced the Ortiz family, as shown by their canceled appointment. They preferred their accustomed transactional patterns to those suggested by the interviewer. Again, a slower pace by the interviewer might have challenged the family's rigidity less directly and encouraged them to return.

Finally, the lack of conflict resolution in a family reflects a low tolerance for conflict. Some families handle this by denying the existence of any conflict. In other families, one member is a confronter, but another is an avoider. In some families, all the members bicker equally; however, they manage to avoid any real confrontation that leads to change. In each case, conflicting issues are not negotiated or resolved. The psychosomatically ill child plays a vital part in the family's avoidance of conflict by presenting a focus for concern. This family system reinforces symptoms in the child as a way to preserve its pattern of conflict avoidance. Difficulties with conflict resolution were prominent in the Ortiz family through Alice's reluctance to speak up to her father in the face of his angry overreaction to her wheezing.

Child Involvement in Parental Conflict

Minuchin and others have felt that the previous characteristics alone are not enough to explain the cause and maintenance of a child's symptom from a family systems point of view. They have suggested an additional key element: a child's ongoing involvement in parental conflict, which acts to detour, avoid, or suppress that conflict and to support the child's symptom.

The symptomatic child may be involved in parental conflict in particular ways. For example, parents who cannot deal with each other directly might unite in protective concern over their sick child. Another case might involve a marital conflict that is transformed into a parental conflict over the patient and care. Still other children might be recruited into taking sides by the parents or may intrude as mediators with them. In many families that we have seen with an anorectic child, we have been struck with the family's insistence on portraying the perfect marriage and family, only to find that when the child's symptom of not eating diminishes, profound marital dysfunction bubbles up to the surface.

Physiological Vulnerability

Some type of physical predisposition in a child, though not enough by itself, is a necessary fact for the appearance of a psychosomatic syndrome. For example, a person does not develop diabetes mellitus without some abnormality in the Islets of Langerhans. However, not all individuals with diabetes develop psychosomatically induced episodes of acidosis; other features of the psychosomatogenic family must be present for these attacks to be triggered. The same premise is true of asthma. A physiological hypersensitivity to specific allergens underlies asthmatic symptoms—even those attacks precipitated by emotional stress.

To conclude our retrospective guesses with the Ortiz family, certainly some interviewing mistakes occurred, and the work could hardly be considered successful. In part, we included a review of our work with this family for that reason. We find that interviews that go badly are frustrating but are not rare. Even with clear principles in mind, we sometimes feel like bumblers in our work. Interviewing families is difficult, complex work. Exposing our failures along with our successes communicates our expectation that both will occur, whether one is a novice or a seasoned interviewer.

SCHOOL PHOBIA

In no situation have we encountered psychosomatic symptoms more regularly than in the group of conditions collectively referred to as school phobia or school avoidance. There are several excellent reviews of this syndrome (15,16,17). School phobia is defined as a "partial or total inability to go to school that results from an irrational dread of some aspect of the school situation" (18). The definition more to our liking is "poor school attendance, based on unwarranted fear of school and/or inappropriate anxiety about leaving home" (19). This syndrome is different from truancy, in which the child does not usually return home and his parents are not usually aware that he is not in school. On the contrary, in situations of school phobia, the parents are usually painfully aware of the child's nonattendance. We will summarize a consistent picture that has emerged for us in working with certain families of children who refuse to attend school by invoking a psychosomatic complaint (e.g., abdominal pain, headaches, nausea). We recognize that not all cases of school avoidance are psychological in nature and a reflection of family imbalance. The physician must rule out other causes, such as a brain tumor or a physically threatening situation in the classroom or playground involving a teacher or classmates. Having excluded such cases, the majority of school avoidance referrals will remain unexplained.

The Family Configuration

Figure 9.1 illustrates a sociogram for the family of a child who freely attends school. Mother and father are shown to enjoy some degree of closeness, relatively closer to one another than either is to the child. The child is at a reasonable distance from his parents, between them and school; both parents and school are fairly accessible.

Almost without exception, we have found a different pattern for the family of a child with psychosomatic symptoms who is refusing to attend school. In Figure 9.2, the father and mother are not close; their distance may be psychological or literal. In either case, the parents are somewhat alienated. Usually the father has assumed a peripheral position in the family. In addition, the school is often positioned differently. Some factor at

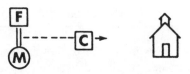

Figure 9.1. Family sociogram fostering regular school attendance.

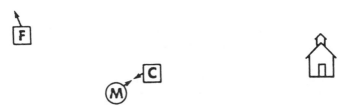

Figure 9.2. Family sociogram predisposing to school avoidance.

school has rendered it a less inviting environment for the child; hence, it is perceived as less accessible and uncomfortable. There may be peer pressures, academic stresses, or the child may have some conflict with teachers or curriculum. The result is that the school seems distant and threatening.

It may take no more than an upper respiratory infection or a bout of diarrhea to transform the preceding situation into one in which the mother and child become glued together at home. Each is frightened for his or her own survival should they be apart, and each is concerned about the survival of the other if separated. The mother, unconnected to her husband, is alone. The child, unconnected to his life at school, is alone. They latch onto one another with a vengeance, striving to assuage their own feelings and those of the other simultaneously. At this point, a physician may be consulted. Resolution of the crisis requires not only attention to the physical symptom, but a return of the family to a configuration at least approaching that of the first diagram. Disengagement of the central duo (i.e., mother and child) necessitates that the physician find another connection for each person. Ideally, the mother needs to reconnect with the father. The child needs help with a rapid return to a school that understands the situation. This process requires work with the child, the school, and the family, as the following story demonstrates.

THE NAKAMURA FAMILY

Fourteen-year-old Nathan Nakamura and his mother were first seen in our general pediatric clinic on November 26. They were both concerned about Nathan's headaches, nasal congestion, skin rash, and "poor" vision. An accompanying note from Nathan's counselor at Franklin Middle School indicated that the school was also concerned. Nathan had missed 20 days in the last month and a-half of school. A new patient workup with appropriate laboratory studies was done by the pediatric resident. She concluded that the patient had slightly decreased visual acuity, a skin rash suggestive of mild psoriasis (which was later confirmed), school phobia, and obesity. Plans were made for refraction in the eye clinic as well as an offer to help in Nathan's steady return to school through family counseling. Nathan and his mother were not interested in the latter, preferring to have him get glasses first to "see what difference that makes." The resident wisely let the family know that the family counseling door would be open for their return if they wished.

On November 28, Mrs. Nakamura called. She had reconsidered and asked for an appointment. The pediatrician with whom they spoke said he would be happy to work with them and stressed he would need to see the entire family.

Mother: Well, now, I don't know about that, Doctor. My husband is awfully busy. I thought perhaps that you could see Nathan by himself. Actually, with my heart condition I shouldn't be making so many trips myself. I had planned for my sister to bring him in.

The pediatrician inquired about her heart condition; it did not sound serious enough to prevent her participation in the visit. Thus, he repeated that he needed to see the whole family. Even though Mr. Nakamura was busy, his presence would be essential for the first visit. She agreed to discuss the situation with her husband and to call back the next day regarding confirmation.

Dr. Drew, the pediatrician, did not hear from Mrs. Nakamura for the next 6 days and attempted to contact the family himself. No one answered. The next day, December 5, was their scheduled appointment. They did not call or show up. Dr. Drew returned the chart to medical records, deciding he would push no further and that he would probably not hear from the Nakamuras again. He was wrong.

On January 7, Mrs. Nakamura called, apologetic. Two days before their scheduled appointment in December, Nathan had voluntarily returned to school, protesting that he would continue regular attendance if his mother would promise that they "did not have to go see that doctor as a family." She agreed. Three days after the missed appointment, Nathan resumed his customary refusal to get up and go to school. Dr. Drew made a new appointment for January 10, again for the whole family.

January 10 arrived; the Nakamura family did not. However, the pediatrician did receive a call early that morning. Once again Nathan had voluntarily returned to school because of the threat of an impending family interview.

Mother: I just don't know what to do. He promises that he is going

	to go from now on. And I certainly want to give him every chance. I really think he means business this time and that we've got this problem licked. What do you think? Should we cancel today's visit? He seems so willing now.
Pediatrician:	(with some duplicity) It certainly sounds to me that you've taken care of this problem yourself. That's terrific. Keep up the good work. Why don't we do it this way . . . I doubt that I am going to need to see you, things are coming along so well. I do have one more opening on January 17 that I will hold open for you, just in case, although it doesn't sound as though you will need to come. I will need you to call me on the 16th to let me know whether you will be using the time or not.
Mother:	That would be fine. I want to show Nathan that I have every confidence in him at this point, doing it on his own.
Pediatrician:	Absolutely. Good luck. You can let me know on the 16th. It will probably be the last appointment time I can hold open for you.
Mother:	Thank you so much, Doctor. I will be calling you.

On January 16, Mrs. Nakamura called, leaving a message that the family would be coming in the next day.

Finally, after almost 2 months, the pediatrician met Nathan and his mother and father. It was an interesting meeting indeed. The mother, less than 5 feet tall, alternated between apologizing for being 5 minutes late and scowling at Nathan, who caused their tardiness by insisting on buying a candy bar in the lobby. As for her husband, she did not even look at him. The mother and Nathan engaged in a mild struggle at the door, with Mrs. Nakamura literally pushing Nathan into the office. Nathan, a head taller than his mother, easily resisted her efforts. When clear of her, he petulantly entered the office and slammed himself into a chair, not the one his mother indicated for him. Mr. Nakamura, trailing behind, appeared proper and very uninvolved in the struggle between his wife and Nathan. He and the pediatrician shook hands and exchanged pleasantries. His blank smile raised the interviewer's worst fears, and Mrs. Nakamura confirmed them: "Oh yes, Doctor, this is my husband, Mr. Nakamura. You will have to excuse him. He doesn't speak English, only Japanese."

She must have seen the pediatrician's face fall because she hastened to reassure that *she* would be happy to translate whatever was necessary. Above all, the pediatrician was not interested in her giving his words (and who knows what else) to Mr. Nakamura in a way that Dr. Drew could not possibly check out! Three pediatric resident trainees were joining him that day for the interview. One winked at him, a second covered his mouth with his hand, and the third offered to find the Japanese translator generally available to the clinic. Dr. Drew knew that individual was not in the building and decided to conduct the session on his own.

It was not strictly true that Mr. Nakamura did not speak English. He said "yes" and "oh" a lot. It was not clear whether he understood his own words, but obviously he did not understand what the pediatrician was saying. This lack of communication coupled with the interviewer's suspicion that Mrs. Nakamura was adding her own flourish to translations made this a particularly memorable interview in Dr. Drew's experience. Even with the language barriers, the residents and Dr. Drew eventually were able to get an understanding of the family's repeating sequence around the issue of school avoidance. These were the events on a typical school morning:

1. Mrs. Nakamura would wake at 6 AM and gently rouse Nathan. Nathan kept no alarm clock in his room.
2. Mrs. Nakamura would then proceed downstairs to begin elaborate breakfast preparations. "Nathan likes hot muffins for breakfast." A breakfast bed tray was prepared.
3. At about 6:20, she would release the family dog into Nathan's room. The dog would lick Nathan's face, waking him a second time.
4. By 6:25 both the dog and Nathan would be asleep in bed.
5. Mr. Nakamura, having gotten up at about 6:15, would finish dressing, have a quick breakfast alone, and be out the door by 7:00 for his long day at the bank in Japantown.
6. Nathan would complain of a headache and not feeling well.
7. Mrs. Nakamura would feel his forehead and then plead that he try to go to school anyway.
8. They would argue.
9. Mrs. Nakamura would give up and return to the kitchen for her own breakfast, leaving the breakfast tray with Nathan.
10. Nathan and the dog would eat from the breakfast tray in bed.
11. Mrs. Nakamura would notice by about 7:20, after her husband's departure, that the time was getting short. Charging up the stairs, frustrated that Nathan was not moving, she would begin screaming.
12. Nathan would handle this in several ways. He might lock his door, hide under the bed, or run past his mother down to the basement, where he locked himself in a closet until 10:30.
13. Mrs. Nakamura, upset with these maneuvers and her numerous trips up and

down the stairs, would remember her heart and go to her bedroom for quinidine and a rest.

14. By midmorning, Nathan and his mother would be playing Scrabble both promising aloud that tomorrow things would go better.

15. Mr. Nakamura would arrive home at 6:30 PM to find his wife and son had spent another day together. By 7:30, he was at his desk with a briefcase of office work.

Although the pediatrician and the residents knew that Mr. Nakamura spoke no English, they did not know until later that Nathan spoke very little Japanese. At home then, mother and father spoke Japanese together while Nathan and his mother conversed in English. Nathan and his father did not and could not speak together. However, that did not stop them from shouting at one another—the father in Japanese and Nathan in English. The mother felt that she often had to be the intermediary between her demanding husband and her sensitive son. The father criticized her perpetual giving-in and acknowledged that some of his early leave-taking for work was to avoid the morning drama.

Mother: What my husband doesn't understand is how helpful Nathan is around the house. Yes, I would rather he were in school also, but he's been such a help to me this past fall. My condition has been acting up, and he's such a good child at helping me with heavy things around the house. My husband is too busy to take care of some of these things at home—I understand that. You'd think he would be grateful for Nathan's help. But . . . what's that? (Responding to a comment from her husband. The two had a lively exchange for a few moments. This caused Nathan to shake his head in disgust, at which mother chided him for his lack of respect. She then turned to the pediatrician.)

Mother: My husband wanted you to know that one reason he especially wants Nathan in school is that he doesn't want him to be at home where he could be on the street. We don't really like him to be out at all unless one of us is with him. But what my husband doesn't understand is that when Nathan stays home from school, he doesn't leave the house. He and I are home all the time together.

Nathan: (Complains that he never had any time to himself in the house, that neither parent seemed willing to leave him alone or to trust him.)

Mother:	Well, Nathan, when you're ready to show us that you are responsible, then we'll believe it, not before.
Nathan:	(scowling) See what I mean? They'll never change.
Mother:	And what about you, Nathan? What about you?

This family may begin to sound familiar. They are a verbatim copy of a family sequence described by Haley and summarized in chapter 3: the family with a "two-generation problem," one that includes an overintense parent–child dyad, which alternately includes and excludes the other parent. Such was the Nakamura family system. The mother and Nathan were seriously over involved, while the father was drifting in and out of their relationship, mostly out. Thus, the family also illustrated the typical configuration that we have come to associate often with school phobia as shown in Figure 9.3.

Minuchin's conceptual model for a psychosomatogenic family is also well illustrated by the Nakamuras. *Enmeshment,* particularly between the mother and son, was a prominent feature, as demonstrated by both parents' reluctance to have Nathan away from them on his own. They had few social contacts outside the immediate family and prided themselves on being a "close-knit family, except for my husband's long working hours, which of course are necessary." To the pediatrician, the phrase "close-knit" in this case suggested a form of bondage in which all were trapped. It was paradoxical that this family could visualize themselves as very close, yet have no common language. *Overprotection,* particularly by Mrs. Nakamura

Figure 9.3. Family sociogram seen in school phobia, as shown by the Nakamura family.

toward Nathan, was clearly evident. Such solicitude was in the reverse direction as well because Nathan's staying at home enabled him to keep a watchful eye over his mother and her heart. *Rigidity* was illustrated by the family's insistence on the same sequence of behavior over and over again. The outline of a typical school morning did not occur just once; it had happened regularly and in the same way for approximately 30 school mornings. The family's *difficulty with conflict resolution* was present in all of their behavior with one another. Resolution never took place; a lack of resolution seemed to meet some need.

▶ The family's sequence, structure, system, and configuration was clear. The question was how to proceed and help them alter their pattern. Dr. Drew felt he would have to include the school in any treatment considerations and told the family this. Both parents were delighted that he was willing to contact school. Nathan resented the intrusion, declaring that he would not go back to school now, no matter what. They ended the session by making a return appointment in 1 week, during which time the pediatrician would consult with the school and make plans for continuing work with the family.

A few weeks before, Dr. Drew had worked successfully with a suburban high school, helping one student with school phobia return to full-time attendance. The school staff had been well informed and effective in their efforts to support his work with the child and family. He approached this situation similarly, assuming that the school would be easily incorporated into therapeutic efforts; however, he had not worked with an urban San Francisco public school before. Just finding the appropriate (and last remaining for the entire school) counselor required four phone calls. The counselor reluctantly agreed to help. Dr. Drew explained that he anticipated difficulty, and a simple insistence on Nathan's return would not be successful. He would be working with the family to get Nathan out the front door in the morning. In the event of refusal, would Mr. Davis, the counselor, be willing to arrange for someone from the school to drive to the Nakamura's home and take Nathan to school. (The school guidance counselor in well-to-do Hillsborough had not blinked at this request several weeks ago, agreeing easily.) The counselor balked, citing legal constraints and lack of available personnel. The pediatrician, with pleading, ultimately had Mr. Davis agree to use his own car to drop by Nathan's home if necessary. Dr. Drew closed by letting him know that he was drawing up a written protocol for the family to follow. Each family member and Mr. Davis would be given a copy.

Satisfied that a plan involving the school was now in place, Dr. Drew made up several copies of the following plan:

Family task (to begin January 25):

1. Nathan is to return full-time to school immediately.
2. For now, Mrs. Nakamura is to wake Nathan at 6 AM by saying, "You must get up *now* for school"; "I expect you to get up and go to school"; or "I have confidence in your ability to get yourself there." There is to be no further discussion by Mrs. Nakamura: no punishments, no recriminations, no promises, no threats. This aspect is to be enforced by Mr. Nakamura.
3. If Nathan should choose not to attend school, Mrs. Nakamura is to notify Dr. Drew and Mr. Davis, who has for now kindly agreed to come to the house and take Nathan to school as needed.

The task was designed with certain goals in mind. First, the interviewer wished to communicate to everyone that an *immediate* return to school was planned. He also wanted everyone to be involved in the process and designed a plan giving each family member something to do. Nathan was to get to school; the mother was to wake him, and the father was to monitor the mother's approaches. The pediatrician did not expect the mother to say the precise lines listed; however; he wanted to focus on her approach to Nathan and stress that she should not allow herself to be drawn into extended dialogue with him. Because the pediatrician expected that the return would be a stormy process, probably often sabotaged by the family, he hoped that writing the task down would enable him and the residents to see at what point and with whom things were not working. That issue could then be addressed in family sessions.

On January 24, the task was presented to the family and discussed. To ensure that all family members understood, the residents and Dr. Drew encouraged the family to role-play a situation in which they carried the plan to completion. To the surprise of the interviewers, the family actually complied and demonstrated their understanding of the task. Nathan was, true to type, sullen and noncooperative; Mr. Nakamura expressed surprise and delight that the solution could be so simple, in Japanese of course. Mrs. Nakamura said repeatedly, "We'll do whatever you say, Doctor." Although Dr. Drew did not suggest they would fail with the task, a prediction of failure could have been a useful strategy. Predicting difficulty sometimes stimulates a family to prove the predictor wrong and complete a designated task successfully.

The next morning, the first for the plan, Mrs. Nakamura called. Nathan had not yet gotten out of bed, and it was 8:30 AM. The pediatrician asked for a brief report of what had happened. Mr. Nakamura had not supervised his wife's approaches to Nathan but had gone to work as usual. The mother and Nathan had screamed at one another.

Mother:	What do I do now, Doctor?
Pediatrician:	Do you have your task sheet available?
Mother:	Well . . . yes. I call Mr. Davis?
Pediatrician:	Right. You know what to do next. Thanks for letting me know.

Hanging up, the pediatrician felt uncomfortable. He called the school and learned that Mr. Davis was out sick. The house of cards was tumbling fast. Neither Mr. nor Mrs. Nakamura could be counted on, nor could Mr. Davis, it appeared. Dr. Drew asked to talk with one of Mr. Davis' coworkers or anyone else who might be able to help. He was eventually connected to the principal.

Principal:	Look, I don't know what this is all about. Mr. Davis was way out of line when he agreed to come out to the student's house. We don't have enough personnel for that sort of thing. And it's against school policy. No, we couldn't possibly send someone else out. You're the doctor—why don't you go over to his house? That would probably have much more meaning anyhow. Do you know how many kids we have here?

Defeated and confused, Dr. Drew decided to do nothing other than to call the mother back. She hastened to tell him that Mr. Davis was ill, and no one at school seemed to know what to do. He thanked her for the update and agreed the task would have to be shelved until Mr. Davis returned to work.

By the next day, the principal must have reconsidered. Mrs. Nakamura reported that Mr. Davis was still out, but the school had sent out a psychology intern who was doing field placement at the school. The intern had pleaded with Nathan through the locked bathroom door, but Nathan did not budge. The intern positioned herself in front of the door and stayed there for an hour doing needlepoint, leaving when she ran out of yarn and when it became clear that Nathan would not emerge.

On January 29, the family arrived for their scheduled family interview at the clinic. However, Mr. Nakamura was not with them. According to the mother, "He just can't keep taking time off from work. He won't be able to come anymore until after tax time is over." By now, any semblance of the pediatrician's being in charge was gone. He announced that the task should be scrapped, and the remainder of the hour was spent working with Nathan and his mother on their bitter feelings. Dr. Drew was weighing whether or not he was willing to continue without the father's presence. By the close of the session, however, he had decided to go on with the two of them.

The mother and son were scheduled to return on February 3. However, 1 hour before their appointment, Mrs. Nakamura called. She was frantic, and Nathan was screaming in the background.

Mother: Doctor, I can't get Nathan to come in for our appointment today. He just refuses. Couldn't we consider putting him in the hospital, please? I'm not sure how much more of this I can stand.

Nathan: (Howls in the background and swears at his mother. He is so loud that the pediatrician cannot hear words, just noise.)

Pediatrician: Mrs. Nakamura, I . . .

Mother: What's that? I can't hear you, Nathan is so upset. A psychiatric hospital, maybe?

Pediatrician: (surprising himself that he is angrily raising his voice) I will not talk to you under these conditions. Get him quiet. I cannot even hear you.

Mother: What?

Pediatrician: Unless I can hear you, I am going to hang up.

Mrs. Nakamura left the phone. The pediatrician heard angry, raised voices in the background, with the mother louder than the son. Then Nathan was quiet. The mother returned to the phone, and the pediatrician congratulated her on her ability to do what was necessary. She then asked if she could come in alone; Nathan would not agree to continuing sessions.

Pediatrician: I couldn't possibly do that, Mrs. Nakamura. I am unwilling to work with the family unless you both come.

Mother: Well, how do I get him there, Doctor?

Pediatrician: That will be up to you. However in order for me to continue working with the family, you must both be here. I can see you on February 7 at 4 PM. I will expect you then.

On February 7, the mother and son arrived, with the son smiling for the first time in the pediatrician's memory. Although the mother was successful in getting Nathan to the session, she could not get him to attend school. A few minutes into the interview, this remarkable exchange took place:

Mother:	Nathan, I don't know why I have to keep picking up your room. You should be able to do that. I've told you over and over again that your room is your responsibility and that I'm not going to pick up after you again.
Nathan:	Yeah, well, you don't mean it. We both know that. You give in too easily on everything.
Mother:	I just can't stand it looking like a pigsty.
Pediatrician:	Hold it, everyone. Nathan, say that again.
Nathan:	What?
Pediatrician:	What you just told your mother
Nathan:	Well, it's true. You give in too easily . . . on everything.
Mother:	If that isn't gratitude . . .
Pediatrician:	(interrupting) Nathan, is there a part of you that would like your mother to say "no" more often?
Nathan:	(after a period of thought) Yes.
Pediatrician:	Tell her that now.
Nathan:	(pause) Mom, I would like you to say "no" more often to me.
Pediatrician:	Say it again.
Nathan:	Mom, I *would* like you to say no more often to me.
Pediatrician:	Mrs. Nakamura, were you aware he felt this way?
Mother:	I'm floored. I don't believe it.
Pediatrician:	Are you serious, Nathan?
Nathan:	Yes, I am.
Pediatrician:	Then you're going to have to convince your mother. She doesn't believe you.

Nathan proceeded to tell his mother that he was uncomfortable with her giving in, that she did not stand up for herself at all with him, that it was almost like there were no rules in the house, and that somehow that was not right. The pediatricians exchanged glances. After all the turmoil and false starts with this family, they finally were approaching the substantive issues between this mother and her son.

The mother heard his request that she set stronger limits and acknowledged that such a shift would be very difficult for her for two reasons. First, Nathan was her only child, and saying no to him had always been difficult. Second, she had spent her early years during World War II in one of the Japanese relocation camps on the West coast. She remembered it as a bitter and difficult experience full of privation. Her father had died within 1 year of internment; financially, the family had had great difficulty. She resolved then that no child of hers would ever want as she had at Manzanar; her child would have everything asked for and more. With time, this resolve came to be construed as a determination to avoid the word "no" with Nathan. She glimpsed through her son's words the high price both she and he had paid for her resolution.

When the hour concluded, they both expressed for the first time a willingness to continue in future sessions. Mrs. Nakamura also shared a letter she had received from the school. It was an order for Nathan and his family to appear in court the next day for a truancy hearing. Obviously, the school had decided on its own course of action. Dr. Drew asked the family to keep him posted.

At the following session, the pediatrician learned that Nathan and his parents did report to juvenile hall in San Francisco for the hearing. It had been a preliminary event, during which the parents, child, school counselor, and the authorities met to discuss future plans. Nathan was shown the room he would occupy in juvenile hall if he was declared truant, which would occur if he missed one more day of school. Official court procedures were explained to the family. The counselor then offered to drop Nathan off at school for the remainder of the day. He went without a sound.

However, the next morning Nathan resisted going to school. There was a different sequence this day. The father rose first and told both his wife and his son that he would not leave the house until Nathan was headed for school and he was going to drive Nathan there himself. When Nathan challenged his father, he was cuffed for his protest. Nathan then got himself up, dressed, fed, and out the door into his father's waiting car.

There were no more school absences. In fact, in a few months time, when a citywide teachers' strike caused pupil attendance in San Francisco to drop to less than half normal, Nathan did not miss a day. Later, he was given an award for being one of the few pupils who had not been absent during the strike.

Clearly, a substantial shift had occurred. Why? In our view, several factors were responsible for the gratifying change in this family's intransigence.

Certainly the mother showing some strength (e.g., getting Nathan to the pediatrician's office), together with Nathan's request for more limits and the mother's insight into the origins of her own behavior were hopeful signs. However, we believe those facts could not account for such a dramatic reversal, particularly in father's behavior, which was crucial to resolving the crisis. The physicians, using the psychosomatogenic model described earlier, were aware of this fact when they unsuccessfully attempted to involve him in the beginning family work (i.e., finding a role for him in the written family protocol). The school provided the needed push for Mr. Nakamura, stimulating him into an active and responsible parenting role by setting up a clear consequence: juvenile hall for his son and possible public shame for the family. With that impetus, the father swung into action, and Nathan swung into school. The combination of some beginning, subtle shifts within the family system followed closely by a stern stance from the public institution involved, destabilized the family enough to move them toward change and more adaptive function.

Everyone in the family, including Nathan, expressed relief that the dilemma of school avoidance had resolved. Both mother and son asked to continue family counseling to pursue changing their relationship at home. Mr. Nakamura kept himself unavailable for future sessions. Because it seemed unlikely that the mother and father would make any significant changes in their marital relationship, the pediatricians focused on helping the mother establish a wider circle of social relationships in her community so that she could tolerate letting go of Nathan, allowing him to pursue his own adolescent growth, without herself feeling stranded and isolated. They encouraged her to get a part-time job, which she did. Nathan became interested in some after-school activities and began to spend less time at home, which was acceptable to his mother and father because he was in a supervised program and not just out on the streets.

The crisis with this family covered 3 months, beginning with their first visit to the pediatric clinic in November for a medical evaluation and ending with Nathan's steady return to school in early February. During that period, a total of five family interviews took place, two with the entire family and three with mother and son. Subsequent work with the family after the crisis continued for 3 more months, with the mother and son attending weekly sessions. The principal issue was their ability to tolerate separation from one another. Subsequent follow-up with the family (i.e., notes to

Dr. Drew once a year) extended over 8 years. There were no recurrences. When Mrs. Nakamura last sent a note to Dr. Drew, she was employed full time, Nathan was a college graduate, and Mr. Nakamura was very busy at the bank.

In psychosomatic conditions, just as in common behavioral problems, it is less the specific complaint that matters and more the family system. This system is what the interviewer needs to detect and alter. Children with psychosomatic complaints are common in pediatric practice. Youngsters with recurrent abdominal pain, chronic headaches, ulcerative colitis, tics, and encopresis are a few of these patients. In our practice, a successful outcome with these children depends on an alteration of the family system, communication pattern, structure, and repetitive sequences of behavior.

References

1. McDaniel S, Campbell T, Seaburn D. Family-oriented primary care: a manual for medical providers. New York: Springer-Verlag, 1990.
2. Griffith J, Griffith M. The body speaks: therapeutic dialogues for mind–body problems. New York: Basic Books, 1994:66–67.
3. White M, Epston D. Narrative means to therapeutic ends. New York: Norton, 1990.
4. Griffith, Griffith, 90.
5. Minuchin S, Montalvo B, Guerney B, et al. Families of the slums: an exploration of their structure and treatment. New York: Basic Books, 1967.
6. Minuchin S, Nichols M. Family healing. New York: The Free Press, 1993.
7. Minuchin S, Lee W-Y, Simon G. Mastering family therapy: journeys of growth and transformation. New York: John Wiley & Sons, 1996.
8. McGoldrick M, Pearce J, Giordano J, eds. Ethnicity and family therapy. New York: Guilford Press, 1982.
9. Leveton A. Personal communication, 1972.
10. Griffith, Griffith, 42.
11. Griffith, Griffith, 65.
12. Breuer J, Freud S, Strachey J (ed and translator). Studies in hysteria. New York: Basic Books, 1957.
13. Minuchin S, Rosman B, Baker L. Psychosomatic families: anorexia nervosa in context. Cambridge, MA: Harvard University Press, 1978.
14. Lask B, Fosson A. Childhood illness: the psychosomatic approach. New York: John Wiley & Sons, 1989.
15. Eisenberg L. School phobia: a study in the communication of anxiety. Am J Psychiatry 1958;114:712.
16. Nader P, Bullock D, Coldwell B. School phobia. Pediatr Clin North Am 1975;22:605.

17. Schmitt B. School phobia—the great imitator—a pediatrician's viewpoint. Pediatrics 1971;48:433.
18. Johnson A, et al. School phobia. Am J Orthopsychiatry 1941;11:702.
19. Schmitt, 433.

chapter 10

Neurodevelopmental Disorders

Our original edition of this book stated that the term *developmental disorders* was often incorrectly used as a euphemism for mental retardation and that its proper use should include a broader range of physical, mental, or psychological development problems. If a restricted, limited view of the term was incorrect then, it is even more so now. Developmental disorders, termed *neurodevelopmental disorders* now, have become increasingly researched and play an important role in the behavioral, learning, and performance problems of children referred to us. Clinicians are awash in a sea of children with assorted letters for diagnoses: SLD (specific learning disability), NLD (nonverbal learning disability), PDD (pervasive developmental disorder), AD (autistic disorder), HFA (high function autism), AS (Asperger's Syndrome), ADHD (attention deficit hyperactivity disorder), OCD (obsessive-compulsive disorder), TS (Tourette's syndrome), and others. Some of these terms are officially recognized and listed in the DSM-IV, but some are not. Many neurodevelopmental disorders seem to have shared differences in nervous system physiology and function, including alterations in available levels of certain brain neurotransmitters. Altered levels of these neurochemicals have been shown to influence brain function, producing, it is hypothesized, many of the clinical signs and symptoms found in children with these diagnoses.

Several of these disorders were once believed to be psychological rather than developmental and were treated by exhaustive psychological intervention (i.e., years of individual psychotherapy, residential treatment, or both). Children with autism, Asperger's Syndrome, obsessive-compulsive disorder, and Tourette's syndrome were particularly targeted for such intensive treatment approaches. Parents could be drained financially by the treatments and sometimes made to feel responsible for the diagnosis. To make things worse, the psychotherapeutic treatment was often unsuccessful, with treatment failure attributed to the resistance of the parent (usually the mother) or parents. More than a generation of parents was led through an appalling sequence of blame and guilt as they struggled to help their children. This trend of blaming parents unfortunately persisted until the late 1970s, when rapid advances in the field of psychopharmacology introduced specific medications designed to affect neurotransmitter metabolism, often with striking clinical success. Psychodynamic theories, which had ruled both cause and treatment of these disorders for almost 50 years, fell like straws in the wind, and an era of drug treatment was ushered in and remains today.

For some clinicians, this era seems a troubling one of overdiagnosis and overtreatment, as unreasoned as the worst excesses of previous psychodynamic therapies. Other clinicians have been impressed by the rapid symptomatic improvement often shown with medication in obsessive-compulsive disorder, attention deficit disorder (ADD), and Tourette's syndrome. However, even clinicians who have embraced the new psychopharmacology recognize that autistic spectrum disorders have not shown dramatic medication responses. Though recognized as disorders with neurodevelopmental origins and no longer tyrannized by such psychological notions as "the icebox mother" as cause, autistic spectrum disorders have been affected only marginally by the array of medications currently used for some of the other conditions. Autistic disorders stand as reminders that single-pronged treatments of any kind for complex issues can be appealing but usually disappointing.

As the pendulum has swung, in effect de-psychologizing many of these disorders, children with certain diagnostic labels now visit psychiatrists less, arriving instead in alarming numbers at the pediatrician's office. Autistic spectrum disorders, obsessive-compulsive disorder, and Tourette's syndrome are among those in this group for which pediatricians must now provide diagnosis and ongoing care. This group of children join two other groups already at the pediatrician's office: children with specific learning disabilities, considered appropriate for pediatricians for more than 30 years, and children with attention deficit disorder. Collectively, these groups have come to be known as "the new morbidity" in pediatrics, vying with infectious disease to become the center pin of clinical pediatric practice (1).

The category of developmental disorders includes not only these more recent entries, but also a huge population of children with physical disorders, mental disorders, or both. One may include under this heading deviations in physical development (e.g., short stature, precocious puberty, rickets, various congenital anomalies) and deviations in the central nervous system, such as delayed language development, clumsy child syndrome, deafness, blindness, and meningomyelocele. What about family intervention in these cases?

In cases described in earlier chapters, we suggest that a clinician's working knowledge of family issues surrounding a pediatric patient is important. Such knowledge becomes vital also in caring for children with developmental difficulties because the family is the main developmental context for these children. Much is expected of families whose children have significant developmental needs. These families must learn to assist, support, and adapt to children whose needs are extraordinary and often not well understood. By working with the families of such patients, clinicians may assist them and facilitate good care. The following case reports illustrate our work with families dealing with four common developmental conditions: specific learning disability, developmental retardation, a disorder with genetic implications, and attention deficit disorder.

SPECIFIC LEARNING DISABILITY (SLD)

Parents are frequently told these days that their child "is not learning as he should." Depending on the local custom and resources, what may follow is a recommendation that the child see the special educational staff in public school or be referred to an individual or agency outside the school for diagnostic evaluation. Frequently, the family consults the child's pediatrician, who then takes on the role of informed resource. As the informed resource, the pediatrician is expected to understand children's learning difficulties, know about diagnostic and treatment resources, and lead the family through a complex chain of professional educators, consultants, diagnostic tests, and legal advocacy maneuvers designed to establish the appropriate educational path for the youngster. An informed resource's involvement may range from referring a family to the appropriate professionals to oversee this process to participating in a multidisciplinary diagnostic team devoted to working with children experiencing school failure.

Some of our previous publications summarize our work in this area, including the evaluation process that we recommend for a child referred with the chief complaint of "school learning difficulty" (2,3,4,5). Lagging academic progress is not just a problem for the child but often for the family. A diagnostic family interview is useful for evaluating firsthand the impact of a child's school failure on the family. The interview also enables the examiner to assess the impact of the family's behavior on the child and his learning. The information gathered in such an interview helps with the diagnosis and treatment plan, which often needs to be medical, educational, *and* psychological in nature, as demonstrated by the Rivera family. Information provided through one diagnostic family interview supplied the missing pieces necessary to complete the puzzle and plan appropriate intervention with 8-year-old Alex and his learning difficulties.

THE RIVERA FAMILY

Mr. Rivera, on the phone with the pediatrician, explained a conversation with his son's first grade teacher at St. Edmond's Parochial School. "The teacher says that maybe Alex should go to a different school. The nerve of that woman—and to deliver that sort of news on the phone. . . . We just don't know what to do. This is Alex's second year in first grade there, and he hasn't been doing too well . . . but they certainly haven't suggested 'til now that he didn't belong there. She said something about a lot of tests being given, that Alex did very poorly on . . . we want Alex to have a complete evaluation somewhere else. Maybe my wife and I should meet with the principal. What do you think?"

The pediatrician agreed that a diagnostic evaluation was necessary. Because this case involved a parochial school that was then unable to provide comprehensive diagnostic assessments for learning difficulties, the evaluation would be done outside the school system. When the pediatrician offered herself as coordinator for this private assessment, Mr. Rivera agreed. Written teacher observations were gathered from Alex's school, followed by a history and physical examination. Neurological, psychological, and educational evaluations were also performed by consultants whom the pediatrician used in such cases.

The studies showed that Alex was above average in intelligence with a specific learning disability of neurodevelopmental origin. Alex's specific learning disabilities were limited to the area of visual perception. Spatial relationships and visual sequencing were problematic. Fine-motor coordination for paper and pencil work was another area of educational liability. Although he would require remediation and tutoring with a learning specialist, Alex could remain in a mainstream school environment and, with the right educational intervention, be expected to do well.

This information, although known by the pediatrician, had not yet been shared with Alex or the family. Dr. Han requested a diagnostic family interview with Alex, his parents, and his older brother, Rudy, age 10 years, before sharing findings and a treatment plan.

The session began in an unorthodox way. As the pediatrician greeted the family at her door, Mr. Rivera turned to his family:

Father:	Now I would like all of you to have a seat and wait for just a few minutes. I have some things I want to discuss with the doctor privately before we all meet together.
Mother:	Of course, dear . . .
Pediatrician:	Well . . .
Father:	Go on. It will be just a few minutes.

Without hesitating, everyone in the family retreated to the waiting room. Mr. Rivera maneuvered himself and Dr. Han into the office and pulled the door closed. The pediatrician found time to wonder what in the world was going on, and that was about all. Mr. Rivera continued, saying, "I thought there were some things that I ought to tell you ahead of time. We don't need to discuss them with the rest—it would just upset them, but it will help round out the picture."

In so short a time, the interviewer had stumbled into strategic trouble if she hoped to maintain control of the family interview (now already begun) and allow each person to have his or her own voice. She was having her interview participants chosen for her, and she was about to have the topics for discussion assigned—those discussible and those not to be shared. Further, the interviewer was being drawn into an alliance with one family member. By simply hearing Mr. Rivera's remarks, whether or not she agreed to honor his request for confidentiality, the pediatrician was jeopardizing her relationship with other family members, who were probably wondering, "What are they talking about . . . what are we being left out of . . . what are they saying about us . . . why can't we be in on it . . . who's really in charge around here—the doctor or my father (husband)?"

Frequently, we have found that an interviewer will be asked "for a few words alone before the rest of the family comes in." However, these private conversations can alienate excluded family members, may hamper their establishment of trust in the interviewer, and often immobilize the interviewer now saddled with secret information. Such requests may be attempts to prejudice the interviewer, confirm that one family member is "the patient," or limit discussion (e.g., "Please don't bring up my husband's drinking; he can't handle that in front of the children"). Often the individual requesting the time alone suggests by his or her manner that the request is for the disclosure of important information—and it often is. The interviewer's curiosity is aroused. And to deny the request may offend this very important person, the most controlling influence in the family. How to respond is a critical dilemma for the interviewer.

There are ways to exit this compromising position. First, the interviewer can use the request to initiate discussion in the family interview. In the Rivera case, this would require split-second reflexes on Dr. Han's part. She might have replied, "Mr. Rivera, it is important for me to meet with all the family. Come into my office—everyone—and maybe you and the family can discuss the purpose of your wanting to meet alone with me. They look very surprised by what you just said. You can talk about it together, and I'll just listen." Another method is to refuse the request with no explanation: "Mr. Rivera, I prefer that we all meet together initially." Still another way to handle this request is by disclosing the dilemma: "That puts me in a bind, Mr. Rivera. I am, of course, interested in what you have to tell me. Yet, I worry that I will then be placed in a compromising position with the rest of the family. That being the case, I prefer not to meet with you alone."

None of these strategies were used by Dr. Han. When she and Mr. Rivera were alone in the office, she began:

Pediatrician:	Before you begin, Mr. Rivera, let me set some ground rules. I am most willing to hear what you have to say. I am not willing to learn secrets from you that I then cannot openly discuss with the rest of the family should I think that important to do. Therefore, whatever we talk about, I reserve the final say as to whether it gets discussed with the rest of the family. You need to know this *before* you tell me anything. Do you understand?
Father:	Well, of course, Doctor.
Pediatrician:	That may mean that there are things you had planned to tell me that now you will not want to share. And those things you will have to keep to yourself. That is your decision.

In this way, the interviewer left an out for herself and would not hear confidences she might subsequently have to pretend she had not learned. This strategy had one error: the message was delivered only to Mr. Rivera; the rest of the family did not immediately hear that secret disclosures would be off limits. Their anxiety and mistrust would remain unrelieved. Mr. Rivera continued:

Father:	I don't quite know the purpose of this—what do you call it?—family conference that we are going to have. But I thought you ought to know that both my wife and Rudy, my older boy, are under a great deal of stress. Perhaps Ann explained the other day. I don't know, did she? No, well she has been having some serious physical problems—kidney problems with two major surgeries in the last 5 years and terrible complications with each one. She just isn't strong, and her nerves can't take too much. Now she and I don't always see eye to eye on this school problem with Alex. Since her own problems began, she's just so . . . isolated and withdrawn . . . I can't really convince her of the seriousness of his problem. Now all this has of course been getting to me too, and I have begun therapy with a psychiatrist—I felt that you should know that. My wife, who probably needs therapy more than any of us, won't have anything to do with it; I have asked her and asked her, but no. Rudy of course is a terribly sensitive child. He knows instantly when things are tense around the house, and they are tense most of the time right now. I don't think he can stand too much more . . . he gets so upset himself. Doesn't let on to anyone, but I can tell. I can always tell. He begins to look very worried, and he develops these stomach aches and diarrhea. My wife doesn't realize how sensitive he is. I'm sure she doesn't realize what pressure she is putting on him, but . . .

The father was controlling, using all the tactics previously predicted: striving to establish an alliance with the pediatrician; suggesting that he was the healthy parent, with his wife a patient, ominously near the breaking point but stubbornly refusing professional help. He was also suggesting that the interviewer stay away from stressful topics.

Pediatrician:	Mr. Rivera, I can appreciate your concerns as both husband and parent. It is clear that you want the best for both your wife and your children. What you are telling me is very important. I would, however, prefer that it be dis-

	cussed with the whole family here. I am uncomfortable at our talking in here and their sitting, worrying and wondering out there. I am going to have them join us.
Father:	Of course. We are very open as a family—I told my wife that I was going to have this chat with you ahead of time; she was in agreement. We can and do discuss everything together.
Pediatrician:	(the contradiction of father's last statement is not lost on her) Good.

The pediatrician asked the rest of the family into her office, greeting each member. Their seating arrangement was interesting. The mother sat alone, as did Alex. The father and Rudy were in a cluster with Mr. Rivera arranging his older son's chair, taking his coat, and asking him if his stomach was feeling better. The father seemed to have his eyes on everyone, always taking measure of his family and how each was doing moment to moment. Of the whole family, however, Rudy received the most observation.

Dr. Han explained, in an effort to recoup with those who had been kept waiting, that she preferred that all discussions should involve the whole family without secrets. She had stopped Mr. Rivera, she said, in his private sharing of concerns, feeling that other family members had a right to hear about his worries. They were obviously a family that cared and would want to be aware of one another's concerns. She then introduced the session itself.

Pediatrician:	Before getting to those issues, let me explain what this family session is all about. As part of Alex's evaluation for his learning difficulties, I want to meet with the whole family. Generally in families, particularly in close families such as yours, when something is going on with one member, all the others are affected by that in some way, perhaps differently for each one. I would like to know more about that from each of you. How you each get messages across to one another is something else I am interested in . . . all different kinds of messages, especially those that have to do with feelings—feelings of happiness, pleasure, sadness, worry, pain, and so forth. I'd like to learn more about your ways of doing that in this family.
Father:	We share our feelings openly with one another, have always felt that was very important. Isn't that right, Ann?

Mother:	Yes.
Pediatrician:	Let me start this way. Rudy, I'm sitting closest to you. I'll ask you first: How can you tell if your father, for instance, has had a good or bad day?
Father:	Come on, Rudy, you know the answer to that one I . . .
Pediatrician:	Wait, Mr. Rivera. Let Rudy answer.
Rudy:	Well, with my Daddy . . . well, if he's had a bad day, you sure don't have to guess.
Alex:	Yeah, right. Right.
Pediatrician:	What do you mean?
Rudy:	He yells. (Both boys agree.)
Father:	Now let's be fair, boys.
Rudy:	You do. Ask Mom.
Father:	Well now, mother's not feeling well. We mustn't upset her right now. Are you all right, Ann?
Mother:	It's all right, Sam. I'll be OK . . . sometimes, I do have to admit, your voice gets a bit loud. But you boys usually deserve it at those times, I might add. Your father works hard. The last thing he needs to hear is the two of you fighting. It's the last thing any of us needs to hear. I certainly don't, particularly on those days when I'm not even well enough to be up. Now Rudy's pretty good about that, but Alex . . .
Alex:	Geez, what do I do?
Mother:	I don't know what it is, but somehow all I have to do is be in bed and you seem to pick a fight with Rudy, Alex. It never fails.

Dr. Han had planned to make the rounds of every family member, asking how each was able to determine the moods and feelings of others. However, with just one question, they were off and running, providing a direct glimpse into their family communication system and structure. The father's need to control, illustrated in his private preamble to the interview, continued with his attempt to take over and answer the interviewer's question to Rudy. The boys seemed able to join with each other in alliance, at least in their common view of their father's yelling. The mother walked a perilous line, defending her boys and simultaneously agreeing with her husband. Blame was coming to rest on Alex as a provocateur, insensitive to his mother's condition and his father's fatigue. Family roles began to emerge: father, the long-suffering controller who was not to be crossed; mother, the sick intermediary, doing a balancing act between children and husband; Alex, the troublemaker; and Rudy, the sensitive, good child.

At this point, an interviewer must decide whether to hold on to a plan or allow the session to develop its own life, now heavily influenced by the family's own communication pattern and style. The interviewer, choosing to use predetermined plans, beginning with Rudy, might stay with him, exploring if and how he could tell when his mother had had a good or bad day. This would be followed by similar comments from Rudy regarding his brother, Alex. The interviewer could then ask Alex to disclose his method for sensing the feelings and mood of each other family member. Finally, the parents would be asked the same question. This method would begin to catalogue the family's expression of feelings and clarify the impact of these feelings on individual family members.

Following such a structure ensures that all family members will be given an opportunity to speak. Order and organization within the interview will certainly be upheld. However, that order may slip into rigidity causing the interview to become a lifeless exercise in "talking about," rather than "experiencing." An interviewer must strive for balance here, selecting a direction that is stylistically comfortable and tolerated well by the family, yet accomplishes the job at hand.

Dr. Han allowed the interview to develop on its own, abandoning a neat list of questions and order, because the family was now exposing its family system. Seeing that Alex was in the process of being scapegoated into a "problem," she turned to him:

Pediatrician: What are you feeling right now, Alex?

Alex: (looking sad) I don't know. I always get blamed. Always.

Father: For some reason, most of the time Ann and Alex just don't hit it off anymore. I don't know why that is. Well, I do know—they're so much alike, that's why. Stubborn as mules. If they would just listen to one another more. It really is upsetting, especially for Rudy. He's so sensitive.

	I can tell right now, for instance, that he's getting uncomfortable with this whole topic. Isn't that right, Rudy? I can tell.
Rudy:	Well . . .
Mother:	Just let him be, Sam.
Father:	Let him be . . . For what, to develop an ulcer? I don't think you ever understand how much this boy takes in and how it affects him . . . Do you have a bathroom, Doctor?
Pediatrician:	(somewhat taken aback, points to the door)
Father:	There now, see Rudy, don't worry. The bathroom is right there when you need it. Just relax. Here, let me rub your stomach, son. That helps. (Rudy, in grooming for the role of invalid, vulnerable child, allowed his father to massage his belly.) Your mother and brother just forget sometimes, Rudy. That's all. They don't mean anything by it.

What no one noticed was that, actually neither the mother nor Alex had done anything to upset or antagonize Rudy. They had not even spoken to one another or to Rudy during this interchange. Father had simply chided them for not getting along in general. The mother, now intimidated by the father's blaming, joined the solicitous ministrations to her older son.

| Mother: | Here, son, come over here with mother. I didn't mean to upset you. I'm just thoughtless sometimes. I'm not feeling well today either. |

Rudy pushed his chair over closer to his mother; she gave him a quick hug. Alex sat by himself looking penitent. He received no invitations for caring or rubbing. Responding to this observation of Alex's isolation, the pediatrician now shifted the interview in a direction that might more directly approach the important issue of positive validation of the children by their parents.

| Pediatrician: | Alex, can you think of some ways in which your parents are proud of you? What do you do that makes your mother or father proud? |
| Alex: | (silence) |

Pediatrician: How can you tell when your father, for instance, is proud or pleased with you?

Alex: (silence again) I don't know.

Father: (painful silence, noticed by everyone) Well, when you do your chores . . . of course, I wish you would do them more often without my having to remind you.

The father's validation was obscured by a simultaneous complaint regarding the boy's failure to follow through. Dr. Han tried again.

Pediatrician: I see. Think of something else, some aspect of Alex about which you feel proud and regarding which you don't need to add a negative comment.

Father: Let's see . . .

Mother: (unable to tolerate the awkward silence) Alex is very good about taking care of Jake. That's his dog, and we never have to worry on that score. Alex does a beautiful job there.

Father: That's right. He and Rudy both take care of their animals without any hassle.

Mother: Sometimes, with Alex, it's almost too much with that dog. Jake comes first and that's all there is to it. The rest of us just have to wait if Jake need something. I notice that especially when I'm sick in bed and need him . . . he spends so much time with the dog. He doesn't seem to realize how much I'm depending on him these days.

Now it was the mother's turn to discredit her own recognition of Alex's responsible behavior. Validation of Alex's emerging capabilities and worth was not done easily by either parent. The parents did validate Rudy, although in an injurious manner. Too often it was validation of Rudy's vulnerability. Such validation could be as crippling as no validation, training Rudy to become, as mentioned, an invalid.

This line of questioning around what in a child's behavior causes parents to feel proud has produced telling responses in our experience. Very often one or both parents will be genuinely stumped by the question, indicating that frankly they had never considered the matter. Hearing themselves acknowledge a disregard for the importance of validating their child is sometimes shocking to them. Worse yet we have interviewed parents who were not shocked by their disregard, nor did they see the need to support and affirm their kids.

If Alex was not receiving support for his behavior at home, what about school? He certainly could not be gaining much validation in that environment because persistent school learning difficulties had prompted this referral in the first place. This unhappy fact was underscored when Dr. Han turned to Alex and asked him to mention a few aspects of himself about which he knew his parents were proud. Alex fumbled with a few words, became silent, then said, sadly:

Alex:	There's nothing that I do that pleases them. Nothing.
Parents:	(looked chagrined and uncomfortable)
Pediatrician:	(to Mr. and Mrs. Rivera) What are you experiencing right now?
Father:	Well . . . er . . . I'm just realizing that Alex is right. I feel terrible. I never thought about it before . . . and yet . . . thinking about it now, I suppose that actually there is no one area of Alex's life in which he feels successful.
Mother:	He certainly doesn't at home with us. We're always complaining about what he doesn't do, the things he forgets. (turning to Alex) Is that true, son . . . does it seem like mostly criticism that you get from your father and me?
Alex:	(quietly) Yes.
Mother:	Oh . . . I'm so sorry.

Fortunately, neither parent rushed in to discredit him at this point. It was a useful moment for producing the desired impact, helping the mother and father see their son's predicament.

Dr. Han now shifted the interview again, this time focusing more directly on Alex's learning difficulties and the family's understanding and coping in the face of his continuing failure. Rudy, with all A's requiring a minimum of effort, tended to look down his nose at his brother, calling him stupid, according to Alex.

Father:	Come on, Alex—Rudy is very careful of other people's feelings. I'm sure he would never do something like that.
Alex:	He just doesn't do it when you're around.

Dr. Han tended to agree with Alex, noting that Rudy did not attempt to defend himself on this point. It seemed just more evidence that in this family one child was seen as always good, and the other was, if not always bad, then at least usually wrong.

As the father had attempted to explain before the interview, Mr. and Mrs. Rivera did not agree on Alex's learning difficulty nor on how to work with him. The father saw Alex's reading failure as a serious problem, stemming from poor study habits and mediocre schools and requiring scrupulous attention on the part of both parents. He saw the need for frequent teacher conferences, close supervision of homework, and a strict schedule of study in the home. Mrs. Rivera felt that Alex could really do his work if he would just apply himself. She wanted her husband to leave him to his own devices regarding school, so that he could learn for himself what was required. The father predicted certain disaster with such an approach, fearing that Alex would drop out before he finished middle school if they allowed him to handle "the problem" himself. With such discrepant views, it is not surprising that homework sessions became a battleground, often involving everyone in the family except Jake. Fighting between Mr. and Mrs. Rivera could be particularly intense, resulting in strained silences for days. Mrs. Rivera would often take to her bed during such times.

The parents were asked for information regarding their own upbringing and particularly their experiences in school. The father was raised by immigrant parents from Central America, who, contrary to the cliche of the American dream, did not successfully climb the ladder to a better life. They insisted that their children succeed where they had failed, however, and from an early age, Mr. Rivera was given direction, structure, and exhortations to study hard and do well. He did succeed, and he felt that his survival then and now depended on the diligence taught him by his struggling parents. He wanted the same for his own children. Mrs. Rivera had been a lackluster student; her parents had felt that education was not essential for a girl and had not pushed her. She wandered through her school years, never failing but never excelling either. Educational plans beyond high school were interrupted first by her marriage and then by her chronically failing health. Two such very different family-of-origin styles were proving difficult for the Riveras to integrate as they now attempted to find a common path with their boys.

As a final phase in this diagnostic interview, Dr. Han asked each family member to cite one aspect of family behavior that he or she would like to change. Alex volunteered first.

Alex: That's easy. I'd like my dad to stop smoking.

We have often heard this comment voiced by children regarding one or both parents. It can be simply a child's criticism of a parent's "bad habit." But it is often reflecting something else—a message of caring from child to parent, a signal that the child has burdened himself or herself with worry about the safety and health of a parent.

Pediatrician:	Alex, I am touched by your comment. It tells me that you worry about your dad's health.
Alex:	Well, sure.
Pediatrician:	Why?
Alex:	What do you mean, how come?
Pediatrician:	I mean, how come you worry about his health?
Alex:	Oh . . . you know.
Pediatrician:	I think I do. But I'd like you to tell him out loud.
Father:	Oh, he doesn't like the smoke in the house, I know.
Pediatrician:	Wait a minute. I think there's more to it than that. Is there?
Alex:	Well . . . yeah.
Pediatrician:	What?
Alex:	(embarrassed and looking at father) I care what happens to you.
Father:	(genuinely touched) I know you do, son.
Pediatrician:	(after a silence) How about you, Rudy? What would you like to change in this family?
Rudy:	What I would like to change is . . . when Mom and Daddy won't talk in front us, only after we're in bed.
Mother:	What's the problem with that, Rudy?
Rudy:	You always say that business . . . "Let's not talk about this in front of the children," and then I hear you at night hollering—since my room is so close. I feel like you're talking about me . . . especially when you're fighting in there.
Mother:	Oh Rudy! (concerned that her son is troubled)
Rudy:	That's true. Sometimes I feel like *I'm* to blame for your fighting.

Father:	There, you see. I tell you, this boy is aware, Ann; you need to be more careful.
Mother:	Sam, we both need to be more careful.
Father:	I am careful. I am careful.
Mother:	Our fighting is no good, no good at all. (Again there was a long pause.)
Pediatrician:	What would you like to change in the family, Mrs. Rivera?
Mother:	Some of my own actions and reactions . . . I would like to be more open with my feelings. I think Sam . . . er, Alex and I would get along better if I was able to do that better. Sometimes when I'm short with him—and I know I am much of the time . . . it's not that I'm angry with him. Maybe I'm not feeling well or I'm not happy with myself about how I just handled him or something. But he only sees that I'm mad. I wish I could find other ways to express myself.
Pediatrician:	Had you ever thought of some family counseling for just that purpose? (Dr. Han noted Mr. Rivera squirming in his chair.)
Mother:	Actually, I had been considering it recently . . .
Father:	But do you think you're well enough? You know I've started therapy myself, and it takes a tremendous amount of energy, I'm finding out.

The interviewer was remembering the father's earlier complaint that the mother would not participate in psychotherapy, although "I have asked her and asked her." Now, the father was the unwilling one, a curious stance for one who had tried so hard to involve his wife in treatment. This topic appeared loaded, and Alex's evaluation had not yet proceeded to the treatment recommendation stage. Dr. Han chose not to pursue this subject any further right now.

| Pediatrician: | Perhaps we can talk more about all that at another time, when we meet to go over the results of Alex's evaluation. Mr. Rivera, you haven't had an opportunity to answer my last question: what would you like to change in the family? |
| Father: | I would like all of us to express our feelings openly and to be a happier family. |

The pediatrician would have been more encouraged by Mr. Rivera's words if the father had not, when the interview concluded a few minutes later, sidled up to her and said softly:

Father:	Doctor, perhaps just before our meeting next time, I could have a few words with you first. The last point . . . there are some . . .
Pediatrician:	No, I won't be doing that next time, Mr. Rivera. I will need to see you all together. I, too, share your concern that the family learn to express feelings openly; consequently, I insist that we all meet together so that such an open sharing can occur. I think our next meeting is scheduled for Wednesday, am I right? Fine, I'll see you then.

Before this interview, the pediatrician knew that Alex Rivera had a specific learning disability with particular problems in the area of visual-motor function. She now had a family context in which to place Alex and his learning difficulties. She had learned several things:

1. Alex's father was a man who worked to control situations, people, and events. He was adroit at using predictions of doom ("Let him be? . . . for what, to develop an ulcer?"), secrets ("Perhaps just before our meeting next time, I could have a few words with you first"), blame ("If they would just listen to one another more"), generalities ("Of course, Doctor, we are very open as a family"), and pseudosolicitude ("So you think you're well enough, Ann? You know I've started therapy myself and it takes a tremendous amount of energy . . . ").

2. Alex's mother was a woman who retreated into and made a career of her "condition." She controlled others, her own illness being the tool used for this purpose ("I notice that especially when I m sick in bed and need him . . . he spends so much time with that dog. He doesn't seem to realize how much I'm depending on him these days.").

3. The family was polarizing the two boys into one good child and one bad child ("Now Rudy's pretty good about that, but Alex . . . ").

4. In addition, Rudy was being programmed to view himself as vulnerable and sensitive. He was being encouraged by his father to develop illness as a retreat and as a control manipulation ("There now, see, Rudy, don't worry. The bathroom is right there when you need it.").

5. Neither boy was receiving any consistent, clear validation of self-worth or growth toward independence ("Well, when you do your chores . . . of course I wish you would do them more often without my having to remind you.").

6. In fact, communication at several levels in the family was dysfunctional, particularly regarding the expression of feelings ("Maybe I'm not feeling well, or I'm not happy with myself about how I just handled him or something. But he only sees that I'm mad.").

7. There were strong indications of marital imbalance ("I would like to be more open with my feelings. I think Sam . . . er, Alex and I would get along better if I was able to do that better.").

8. At least one of the boys, Rudy, was feeling responsible for his parents' marital stress ("Sometimes I feel like I'm to blame for your fighting.").

9. Finally, no one in the family appeared to have an appropriate understanding of the dimensions of Alex's learning difficulties. His parents in particular showed widely discrepant styles for approaching and managing Alex with his neurodevelopmental disability ("Now she and I don't always see eye to eye on the school problem with Alex.").

The Process of Treatment Recommendations

Is the collection of this information necessary in such cases? One might argue that the boy had a mild neurodevelopmental condition and that appropriate special educational assistance would take care of the problem. Such intervention would help Alex develop better fine-motor coordination and improve his written language skills. But how should his parents be involved in his subsequent learning to facilitate his success rather than obstruct it? In what ways were Alex's difficulties on the school front interacting with his relational difficulties at home? Could the parents learn to provide Alex with appropriate validation of self-worth and competence at home while he slowly improved at school? Answers to such questions are important in planning therapeutic interventions with Alex and others like him. These answers may be obtained by close attention to family structure, communication patterns, and sequences of behavior. A family interview offers the opportunity to observe those aspects of family interaction. For us, such sessions have become an integral part of the diagnostic evaluation of any child with a suspected neurodevelopmental difficulty. Family influences are usually a part of the problem and a component of the solution in such patients.

Dr. Han considered how she might address these important family issues in the next interview, during which she would offer her treatment recommendations for Alex's learning problem. The parents would require specific information regarding the nature of his learning disability, and helping them understand that his persistent school failure was not caused by a lack of motivation, poor study habits, or faulty parenting would be the first step in enlisting their support. Beyond clarifying diagnostic information and suggesting learning assistance, it seemed appropriate to recommend ongoing family counseling because family stresses were numerous and fairly serious. Alleviating these stresses would require effort on the family's part, a willingness to continue family work for considerably more than just a couple of sessions. The family would need some understanding of its own dysfunctional style and the impact of such a style on each family member. Helping a family accept a recommendation for ongoing counseling is difficult and is frequently, as in this case, a primary pediatric caregiver's responsibility.

When considering ongoing family counseling, a clinician must take into account the complexities of a particular family's problems, which will dictate the type of counseling and time frame to be recommended. If the family's difficulties are mild or so chronic that nothing has changed in years, the interviewer may take additional sessions to discuss the areas of family difficulty. Such a leisurely pace allows the interviewer to build a trusting relationship with the family that helps the acceptance of a suggested referral. A leisurely pace is seldom possible these days for several reasons:

Family problems often are acute and serious, calling for rapid intervention.

Managed health care does not tolerate a leisurely pace.

Clinicians, even when able to avoid the watchful eye of an HMO, are generally pressed for time and unable to offer several visits toward effecting a referral.

However, disregard for these aspects of pacing can lead to failed follow-through on a family's part. A family in distress is frightened, angry, and confused. Such a group may well be put off by their clinician saying, "The tests are all negative. Marlene's stomach aches are functional. I recommend psychotherapy. I usually send patients with such problems to Dr. Baird. Here is her address and phone number. Give her a call."

No interviewer should settle for this quick approach, no matter how pushed for time. The task will always take longer because it is a complex transaction. When making a referral for counseling, the clinician must consider the "psychological mindedness" of the family members, their relative openness versus their resistance, and their readiness to acknowledge not only their distress but the need to do something about it. Getting a feel for the family's level of defensiveness is essential for planning how to help move them further.

The clinician must also be thinking of the specific resource being recommended. Obviously, if the interviewer feels that he or she can handle the task, then the referral process can be relatively simple. The completed evaluation and already established relationship can work to his or her advantage, so that the family feels that a transition from assessment to treatment with the same individual is the logical next step. However, a referral to someone else may require the interviewer to help the family with its discomfort at having to start over with someone new.

A successful referral depends on all four variables: the time constraints imposed by the family's presenting problem, the time available to the clinician to effect a referral, the family's level of readiness to accept the recommendation, and the features of the actual resource being recommended. We have all experienced clinical situations in which one or several of the variables has been problematic, leading to an unsuccessful referral. Although those times are inevitable, we have found them to be the exception, not the rule. Even accounting for substantial variation in these factors, a general rule is that families tend not to accept a referral for therapy if they do not feel that they and their situation are well understood by the referring clinician. Thus, a family interview in which this understanding is conveyed can be the determining factor in facilitating a successful referral.

The Riveras did accept the pediatrician's referral for ongoing family therapy. Three more 30-minute sessions were held with the family before a specific recommendation for ongoing family work was made. The family problems did not warrant immediate action (variable number 1). Dr. Han had the time to offer follow-up visits (variable number 2). And although it appeared that the family possessed some readiness to consider therapy, they were resistant to the idea of ongoing family sessions (variable number 3). Thus, additional sessions were spent highlighting the areas of family conflict. The family seemed most comfortable with parent–child issues, and discussions were limited to this area. Marital difficulties, which were obvious to Dr. Han, were not brought up for discussion in these sessions.

At a point in the last session when both parents agreed that communication was often ineffective with their boys, particularly Alex, Dr. Han said:

Pediatrician: Is this something that you would like to change?

Father: Oh my, would we ever, Doctor. I'm sure my wife would agree (still speaking for his wife).

Mother: (nods assent)

Pediatrician: Then I am wondering how you would feel about the possibility of ongoing family sessions, specifically geared toward improving your communication with the children and theirs with you?

Mother: Would it help?

Pediatrician: You have some doubts, it sounds like.

Mother: Well . . .

Pediatrician: I hear your doubtfulness. And it is also clear the current situation is not working very well.

Father: You can say that again. Ann and Alex, if they could . . .

Pediatrician: (hurrying to silence Mr. Rivera in his blaming of other family members) I would want you to be involved as well, Mr. Rivera. You are an extremely important part of the family, and I do not feel that any sort of counseling would be successful without your very important perspective on the family.

Father: I see. And the boys? You mean they would come too?

Pediatrician: Absolutely. Especially since it is communication between you, the parents, and your children that you want to change. Of course, you and your wife sometimes might have some things that you would like to discuss privately, in which case the children could stay home for that session, but that could be arranged as the situation arose.

Mother: Would we come to see you, Doctor?

Pediatrician: I would like very much to continue seeing you. However, I can also arrange for you to see a counselor closer to home, if you wish. I am aware of some excellent resources in your area.

Father: Oh no, I think coming here makes the most sense. You know us now. (The mother and the two children agreed.)

The referral was accepted. There remained some particulars of the recommendation to be discussed. Dr. Han told the family that she would want to see them weekly for 1 hour each visit. She wanted the family to know that the work on communication was going to require several months of work, that they could evaluate the duration of counseling more clearly as the work got underway. The family agreed. The referral was successful because Dr. Han attended to all four of the variables.

In fairness to the reader skeptical of such good results, we should state that the Rivera family did participate in sessions as long as the pediatrician focused only on parent–child issues. When Dr. Han began to address marital difficulties more directly in the ninth family interview, the family abruptly terminated sessions because "this is getting too expensive." Until this point, there had been no mention of financial constraints. We suspect that Dr. Han had presumed on her relationship with the family and unwittingly entered an area in which she was not welcome. Here, just as during the initial period of referral, proper timing is essential. But, as the Rivera family illustrated, sometimes the proper timing can be evaluated only in retrospect.

Some comments about other aspects of Dr. Han's style and technique with this family are indicated. In her initial interview, she made very few direct interventions to alter family function. The omission was intentional. The Rivera family had not come to her initially asking for changes in their interaction with one another. They understood they were participating in a diagnostic effort to clarify the characteristics of their son's learning difficulties. Dr. Han recognized and honored their perspective in this initial setting, so she collected family data but did not try to create changes in their system. Our trainees have reported difficulties restraining themselves here sometimes. Recognizing dysfunctional behavior, particularly after learning some early strategies for altering that behavior, compels some to "wade in and straighten this mess out." But such a move is too often experienced by the family as offensive and intrusive. In initial diagnostic interviews of this type, caution regarding fancy intervention footwork is recommended.

The diagnostic family interview with the Riveras demonstrates that important family stresses are almost always present around a child with a neurodevelopmental learning disability. The initial interview is also a good example of a "sloppy" session, typical in our experience. By sloppy we mean that topics sometimes tumbled over one another, issues were not necessarily followed to any conclusion, and sometimes the interviewer seemed to have little form or structure to her questions. Family interviews are like that, particularly those held for the purpose of gathering specific diagnostic information.

DEVELOPMENTAL RETARDATION

In addition to being used to formulate a diagnostic picture, family interviews can also be used to share the results of neurodevelopmental diagnostic studies. However, it is one thing to explain to a family that their child has some difficulty with eye–hand coordination and quite another to share with a family that their child is mentally retarded. Can family interviews serve this purpose? We believe so.

Delivering this news to parents amounts to declaring a chronic condition of the most devastating variety. Such an interview needs to be structured closely around the guidelines presented in chapter 7 for the delivery of bad diagnostic news. The clinician must:

1. Respect the event, furnishing the time, energy, and support that a family will need
2. Keep medical facts to a minimum
3. Pay careful attention to the feelings of individual family members
4. Withstand the family's silence and grief
5. Resist the temptation to run
6. Share the diagnosis quickly

How to accomplish this last rule can be troubling when faced with the grim reality of telling parents that their child is retarded. How does one go about such a formidable task? Even with adequate attention to all the other rules, how is one to share this diagnosis—and how to do it quickly? Excerpts from work with the family of Maria Gates illustrate some of the methods of family interviewing in such a case, when the job entails helping a family hear for the first time the diagnosis of developmental retardation in one of their children.

THE GATES FAMILY

Mrs. Gates had originally brought her daughter to the pediatrician for a hearing test and a checkup. Maria, at age 3 1/2 years, was developing language slowly, so slowly that the mother was worried that there was something wrong with her child's hearing or her tongue ("Could she be tongue tied, Doctor?"). Mr. Gates had chided his wife for being overanxious; he believed Maria's hearing was normal. He had noticed how much she liked to sit and rock to the music of television commercials. She was certainly hearing the music. And her speech was coming along; she was making more sounds all the time. Although her speech was often not understandable, pronunciation would improve with time, he maintained. Maybe his wife should go back to her part-time job, he suggested. Being home with Maria just made her too watchful. However, Mrs. Gates could not shake the idea that something was not right. It was this concern that prompted the visit to the pediatrician.

After obtaining a history and spending some time with Maria, the physician shared Mrs. Gates' concern. The child had very little expressive speech beyond some unintelligible single syllables. Her large motor skills were lagging; she still took stairs one at a time, would not attempt riding a tricycle, could not button, nor was she successful in putting on any of her clothes. Toilet training had not been successful. She *did* seem able to hear, but Maria was evidencing serious developmental delays across a wide range of abilities. The physician suggested a formal diagnostic evaluation to give a clearer picture of Maria's developmental progress. This evaluation would include a hearing test and an evaluation of her language development and measures of muscle coordination, thinking abilities, and general development. Mrs. Gates readily accepted the suggestion of this evaluation, adding:

Mother: But my husband will think it's all a waste.

Pediatrician: I'm glad you mentioned him. Because that reminds me, I will certainly want to discuss the testing with you *both*. So I would like to arrange an appointment when you and Mr. Gates can come. In fact, you have two other children, right? George . . . ah yes, that's right. He's 7 years old? And Tracy is 2? I would like them to come also. I will want to go over the evaluation with the whole family.

Mother: Well, I don't know about my husband . . .

Pediatrician: He must come. It is essential. Would you like me to call him?

Mother: Oh . . . no. I'll . . . talk to him and see.

Pediatrician: Good. If you do find you want me to speak to him, give me a call. As Maria's father, he is a very important person to include in this process.

   This was one situation, and there are such times, when the physician's positive expectations regarding father's participation were insufficient. Mr. Gates refused, saying he was either unavailable, sick, held up at work, or out of town. The evaluation dragged on, incomplete, the physician felt, without this family interview. As a compromise, rather than losing father altogether, the physician offered to combine the diagnostic family interview and summary discussion of evaluation results into one interview. Mr. Gates reluctantly agreed to come in with his wife and all three children.
   The pediatrician did not have good news to share with the family. Maria had had a severely traumatic, hypoxic birth. Complete physical, neurological, laboratory, psychological, and developmental evaluations had yielded no more specific explanation for the fact that Maria was developmentally retarded. At 3 and one half years, she was functioning in almost all categories of development as an early 2-year-old child. Motor skills, language development, and social development were all at this level. Formal measures of intelligence placed her IQ in the low 60s, consistent with the child's behavior and demonstrated developmental pattern. The family could hardly be expected to receive this diagnosis with equanimity: mild mental retardation, cause unknown; perhaps pervasive developmental disorder.
   After greetings and introductions, the interview began.

Pediatrician: I am glad the whole family was able to come today. I wanted to talk with all of you about Maria's development—your concerns and the various tests that she has had. Mr. Gates, your wife has already shared her questions and worries about Maria. I would like your view on the situation as well. How do you see Maria's development?

During this overture to Mr. Gates, the interviewer noted Maria solidly nestled in her mother's lap, sucking two fingers, whimpering at times. Tracy, age 2 years, was curious and had wandered over to the toy shelf and was exploring. George, age 9 years, sat next to his father. The two males formed a unit on one side of the room, whereas the mother and Maria formed another on the opposite side. Tracy drifted back and forth between the two groups. Of the five individuals, only Tracy appeared to be enjoying herself.

Pediatrician: (interrupting Mr. Gates before he responds) Hold it just a minute. Mrs. Gates, see if you can interest Maria in joining Tracy with some of toys over there.

Mother: Oh that's all right. I think she's a little tired this morning. You'd probably rather stay here, eh, Maria? (holding Maria more tightly)

Maria's response was nonverbal. She buried her face in her mother's shoulder and did not budge. They looked glued together. The pediatrician had not missed Mrs. Gates' coded message to her daughter: "Do not leave my lap, Maria." That one interchange between mother and daughter verified that there were issues on more than one level with this family. Many of Maria's difficulties were developmental in nature, stemming from some neurological malfunction of her own brain. She was also reluctant to separate from her mother. Deciding whether this difficulty was a reflection of developmental delay only or represented different issues was needless. Because her mother was directly encouraging the child's reluctance to separate, the problem was interactional, as well as developmental.

The pediatrician was about to learn that he had unwittingly played into father's hands.

Father: Actually, that's a large part of the problem right there. I tell my wife that Maria would be all right if she just wouldn't baby her. Why don't you just let her play with Tracy, hon?

Mother: She doesn't want to, do you, Maria? You never seem to understand, Rod, that she's uncomfortable in new situations. And it takes her a while to feel relaxed.

Serious developmental difficulties, then interactional problems between mother and child were now joined by marital dysfunction. The pediatrician realized he would have to organize the session in order to share the news for which this meeting had been called.

Pediatrician: That's an excellent point, Mrs. Gates. Of course she's uneasy in this situation so far. Why don't you move your chair closer to Tracy and the toys so that Maria will continue to feel comfortable near you as you ease her off your lap and onto the floor with her sister? (The mother complied and father continued.)

Father: You see my wife worries too much. She . . .

Pediatrician: And you, do you have any worries about Maria?

Father: Well, not like my wife, but sure. I wish she was talking more. I guess we all wish that.

Pediatrician: Tell me what you have noticed about her speech.

The father explained that he too was worried that Maria was developing speech slowly. He noticed the problem particularly because George had been very quick with language development, and Tracy was already using more words than Maria.

Pediatrician: You are a careful observer of your children. I've been notic-ing also here today that Tracy is talking much more than her older sister.

Father: That's right. And I tell my wife, if she wouldn't baby Maria, then Maria would have to begin to talk more.

Mother: (rolls her eyes and says nothing)

Pediatrician: Looks like you've heard that one before, Mrs. Gates.

Father: (embarrassed, laughs)

Mother: I sure have. I tell him if I baby her, it's because in many ways she seems like the baby of the family. He won't listen.

Pediatrician: It's a bone of contention between you two. (George, silent up to this point, nodded agreement vigorously.) That's a bother for you George?

George: They always fight on this one! (George's remark caused everyone to laugh. The pediatrician was grateful for his en-try.)

Pediatrician: Let me return, Mr. Gates, to your observations of your daughter's development. I hear clearly that you and your wife don't necessarily agree on the reasons behind Maria's slow speech development, but it sounds like you both agree that her speech development is slow.

Father:	Yes. I guess you would have to say that.
Pediatrician:	Now in what other ways have you worried that Maria was a little behind?
Father:	Well, I know that her teeth are slow in coming in, but I don't think that means anything. And they're beginning to come through now.
Pediatrician:	Uh huh. (silence)
Father:	My wife complains that she doesn't try to dress herself. But that's another one of those . . . if she wouldn't do it for her, maybe Maria would pick it up.
Pediatrician:	Have you tried that approach yourself with Maria?
Father:	Yes, I did. I tried to teach her about putting her pajamas on . . .
Mother:	Tell him what happened, Rod. It didn't work. He's too impatient. He gets mad, and she starts screaming.
Pediatrician:	Now you're back to that bone of contention . . .

Maria had slid off her mother's lap toward Tracy and the toys. The difference in the play activity of the two children was striking. Maria seemed confused by or uninterested in most objects, using them for the wrong purpose, handling them clumsily, putting many of them in her mouth. Tracy was appropriately using the toy telephones, drinking out of teacups, and managing a small train set. Maria watched, sometimes attempting the same activity, but her play lacked the creativity of Tracy's. Using this information, the interviewer brought the interview around to a discussion of the evaluation results.

Pediatrician:	Mrs. Gates, you've done an excellent job encouraging Maria to play with her sister. You were right—she needed to feel comfortable before moving away from you. Is that the way it often is?
Mother:	(with a sigh) Yeah. She really sticks close.
Pediatrician:	I need to talk about that a little more. However, as we are talking for the next few minutes, all of you keep your eyes on the two girls and their play, just pay attention to how they seem to be playing.

They agreed to watch as the pediatrician continued his discussion with Mrs. Gates regarding Maria's "sticking close."

Pediatrician:	Sticking close—that must sometimes be confining for you?
Mother:	(guarded) Well, yes.
Pediatrician:	When do you find time for yourself?

A trace of sadness flashed on the mother's face, and she acknowledged that Maria afforded her little time for her own needs. With the pediatrician's encouragement, she admitted not liking the situation, wishing that she could find more time both for herself and her husband. Mr. Gates was listening. The interviewer returned to his previous request of the family.

Pediatrician:	OK. Let's go back to Maria and Tracy. You folks are good observers. While they are playing, at what age level would you say each is operating? You first, Mr. Gates.
Father:	You mean Maria?
Pediatrician:	I mean each girl.
Father:	Well, I would say that Trace is playing much as I would expect for a 2-year-old; if anything, she's maybe a little ahead of her age. But probably 2 . . . 2 and a half, I would guess.
Pediatrician:	And Maria?
Father:	She's just about where Tracy is—maybe not even quite as far along, but well—they've been doing most of the same things there on the floor. So I would have to say Maria is about a 2-year level too.
Pediatrician:	Does that match at all with what you notice at home?
Father:	Yeah, the two of them copy one another all the time. Maria likes to play with her sister more than any of the older kids on the street.

The mother and George were asked for their appraisal of each child. They agreed with father that the two girls, both in the office and at home, acted more like twins than siblings, even with an 18-month spread in their ages.

The way had now been prepared for some discussion of the evaluation results.

Pediatrician:	You are all right on the button. The studies that we have done with Maria, and I want to go over them with you, show exactly the same thing. In almost all respects, Maria is per-

	forming and behaving at a 2-year developmental level, rather than her age level of 3 and one-half years. (There was silence. The mother looked up wearily.)
Mother:	I knew it. I knew something was wrong.
Father:	What does it mean?
Pediatrician:	Tell me what you understand about what I have just said.
Father:	Well, that is . . . you are saying that Maria is slow, that there's some problem with her development. But what do you mean by that? What kind of a problem and in what kind of development?
Pediatrician:	Slow down, Mr. Gates. For right now what I am saying is that our tests agree with your own observations. Maria is mostly at a 2-year-old level in her behavior and in her abilities.

The pediatrician presented specific examples of Maria's performance on developmental measures, demonstrating that in motor coordination, speech, language development, and social development, Maria was succeeding at the 2-year level and consistently failing on items beyond that. The parents listened, George was respectfully silent, and the girls continued to play on the floor.

For some families, it is enough at this stage to have heard that their child is significantly behind in development. The term *mental retardation* is not spoken aloud nor discussed with the physician. It is not necessary to assault families with the term out of a sense of honesty. If the family is loath to utter the phrase, particularly in the initial stages of hearing that their child is slow, their reticence should be respected. There will be abundant time for a discussion of terms. With other families, the physician's initial declaration forces the question.

Mother:	Does that mean that Maria is mentally retarded?
Pediatrician:	Tell me what you mean and understand by that term.
Mother:	I don't know, really. I guess mostly what I know is from TV, seeing a program on kids who look different and have . . . Down's?
Pediatrician:	No. I need you to hear me clearly. Maria does not have that condition. What else do you know about mental retardation?
Mother:	(stunned) I don't know.

Pediatrician:	How about you, Mr. Gates?
Father:	Mostly I think that it has to do with people who are vegetables, who can't learn, and who have to be in institutions.
Mother:	(nodding her head in agreement)
Pediatrician:	Do you see Maria as someone like that?
Father:	Absolutely not.
Pediatrician:	I agree. She is not. That is one reason I am uncomfortable with the term mental retardation. Parents so often have terrible . . . and wrong ideas about what the term means. Maria does not have Down's syndrome. She will learn, but it will be slow. And she is certainly not a vegetable. What I need you to understand is that she is developing slowly in a number of areas at the moment. Period. It looks to me as though you are all hearing me on that point. Right? (Even George nodded assent.)
Pediatrician:	OK, now take some time . . . and breaths. Tell me what you are each feeling now that you have heard the news.
Mother:	(tears in her eyes) I am not surprised . . .
Pediatrician:	But there is pain, just the same?
Mother:	(nods yes and quietly breaks down)
Pediatrician:	(pause) What about you, Mr. Gates?
Father:	It's just . . . one of those things, I guess.
Pediatrician:	How are you feeling inside?
Father:	She'll come along. I'm hoping.
Pediatrician:	This has been hard news for you to hear . . . and accept.
Father:	Yeah.
Pediatrician:	I can appreciate that (pause) . . . George?
George:	(tears run down as he notices those of his mother)

In a loving gesture George rose and put his arms around each of his parents in turn.

In chapter 7, we paraphrased six questions raised by families faced with the diagnosis of chronic illness in a child (6):

1. What's the matter?
2. What (who) caused it?
3. What can the physician do?
4. What can the parents do?
5. How long will the condition last?
6. Will the child be completely cured?

A diagnosis of mental retardation raises all of these questions. Essentially, only question number 1 was handled in the initial Gates interview. It was in no way resolved. Mr. Gates partly heard what the doctor had to say; however, his last comments indicated his denial and ambivalence at the news. He and his wife would need additional discussion sessions just to accept the fact that their daughter was actually lagging in her development.

Questions 2–6 were not even approached. With the Gates family, the remaining questions were threatening to break through into the open at any moment. Regarding who caused it, Mr. Gates had been holding his wife responsible for Maria's difficulty. That issue could become more prominent should the fact of Maria's hypoxic birth be raised as causative by either parent, and this information could easily intensify the notion of maternal blame. Succeeding interviews demonstrated that Mrs. Gates blamed herself as much as her husband did. Much of her solicitude toward Maria was offered to handle her own feelings of self-blame for having "caused the problem." Regarding what the physician could do, the parents wanted further tests to confirm the diagnosis. As to what they themselves could do, the parents wanted to be involved in a program of diet supplements, language stimulation, instructional play, or anything else that might accelerate their daughter's progress, as expressed in later interviews. They also had many questions about the future, such as prognosis, schooling, and their dreaded fear of institutionalization, reflecting concerns over how long will this condition last and will the child be cured.

Each of these questions required discussion and revisiting along with a willingness on the pediatrician's part to recognize that just because she had reassured them on two separate visits about, for example, the inappropriateness of institutionalization for Maria, the subject was not necessarily closed. Multiple follow up visits took place but were not frequent. The family saw the pediatrician for a talk session approximately every 2–3 months over 2 years. About 8 months after the initial session, the parents asked for help in locating a parents' support group for the families of retarded children. The fact that they could see themselves as being able to use such a group signaled to the pediatrician that this family had come a long way in accepting the reality of developmental delay in their daughter.

DISORDERS WITH GENETIC IMPLICATIONS

After the initial diagnosis of neurodevelopmental disorders, family members struggle to reckon with the condition. Shock and denial have been replaced by acknowledgment of the facts. Along with that acknowledgment may come a preoccupation with Steinhauer's second question: what or who caused it (7)? The question is often personalized: am I (are you, are we) responsible?

These queries can become troublesome foci for family rumination. Parents indict themselves and one another with a variety of issues, from medications taken during pregnancy, to dietary indiscretions, to smoking, to illness recent or long ago, to not wanting the baby in the first place. One of the most painful concerns for parents of a developmentally disabled child is the notion that they, the parents, have caused the child's condition because of "bad" genes, particularly when the condition is one actually associated with hereditary factors, such as genetic dysfunction. Parents of these children are routinely urged to seek genetic counseling as an integral part of proper medical care for the family, a process that may unwittingly increase their already heightened sense of shame and blame.

THE STRAND FAMILY

The prototype of a neurodevelopmental problem for which genetic counseling is sought is Down's syndrome, now recognized by most parents, even before they are told, as connected to genetic factors. How does a physician impart the information essential for appropriate genetic counseling to the parents of a baby with Down's syndrome in a way that does not intensify parental feelings of guilt? Dr. Burnett was facing such a task with the Strand family. The parents, a young couple in their late 20s, had asked for genetic counseling. Their only child, Sheila, now 5 months of age, had been suspected in the newborn period of having Down's syndrome, and chromosome studies had confirmed the clinical diagnosis. The parents were told this when Sheila was almost 1 month old. Shaken by the news initially, they seemed to cope reasonably well. They were now beginning to face, among other dilemmas, the question of having other children and the risks involved. Chromosome studies had characterized Sheila's problem as one of straightforward trisomy 21. The Strands, without chromosomal evidence of translocation, with a negative family history, and with maternal age under 35 years, stood approximately 1 chance in 100 of having another child born with the same condition. This information had not yet been shared with the family.

Dr. Burnett was anxious and studied beforehand to make sure that she had the right genetic information at hand. She found that this was a condition with statistical certainty. The clarity with which numbers had been established in Down's syndrome was reassuring, and she hoped the family would feel likewise.

Physician:	Mr. and Mrs. Strand, you asked to meet with me so that we might discuss some of the genetic factors in Sheila's situation. I think it might be useful if we were to back up and start from the beginning. What do you understand about what causes Down's syndrome?
Mother:	Just what you told us when we first talked with you, that there is something wrong with Sheila's—er—chromosomes. She got that from us somehow—we gave her too many or the wrong kind or something. But I felt perfectly fine all during the pregnancy. I don't understand it.
Father:	I worry about all those dental X-rays you had, Jean, before we even knew you were pregnant.
Mother:	He had me wear a shield, Harry. What do you think, Doctor? Could X-rays have damaged genes or whatever? I was only about 6 weeks pregnant at the time. Incidentally, you had . . .
Father:	The first 12 weeks of the pregnancy are the most impor-

tant—that much I know. And it's chromosomes that are the important things to consider; genes are different. Yes, I know I had some X-rays too about then, but not as many as you.

Physician: Let me explain a little about genes and chromosomes. It may help to clarify . . .

From her reading, Dr. Burnett had prepared a short description of the cause of Down's syndrome. She was eager to use it so that the parents would have a correct understanding of the origin and would stop blaming each other.

Physician: While the underlying causes of Down's syndrome are still unknown, an extra chromosome is always present. Chromosomes are very tiny structures that contain the hereditary factors—genes. Every cell in the body has a complete set of chromosomes. In a normal human, a complete set of chromosomes equals 23 pairs. In each of the 23 pairs, one chromosome comes from the mother and one comes from the father, to make a total of 46. In Down's syndrome, the baby has an extra chromosome in one of the pairs, making a total of 47 chromosomes. This extra chromosome is responsible for Down's syndrome and Sheila's condition.

Mother: The extra chromosome—it must come from the mother, am I right? I remember that you said before that mothers who are over 40 have a greater risk of having a baby with Down's. And you certainly never hear anything about it being dangerous for fathers over 40 to have babies. It's always older mothers . . .

Physician: Sometimes it is the mother. But the extra chromosome can come from either parent. Let me draw some diagrams for you. (She does that.) Now there are X and Y chromosomes, but for the time being we don't need to bother with the Y. That's the male sex chromosome and the female doesn't have any. The problem in Down's isn't on the Y chromosome anyway. It's on the twenty-first X chromosome. Now the egg from which the baby develops usually receives one chromosome of each pair from the mother and one from the father. Since each cell has 23 pairs, a baby receives 23 chromosomes from each parent. Therefore, a normal baby has a total of 46 chromosomes in every cell in the body, as does each parent. In the case of Down's, a mistake occurs. The egg from which the baby develops receives two chromosomes of the twenty-first pair from one of the parents and one chromosome 21 from the other parent, giving the baby an extra chromosome. Therefore, a baby with Down's syndrome has a total of 47 chromosomes in every cell in the body, not 46, the normal number.

Dr. Burnett felt it was going rather well. The parents had stopped talking to one another and appeared to be listening. She had been careful to use understandable English and still maintain medical correctness in the information delivered. So far, so good, she thought. Now on to the next, for she knew these parents were worried about having another affected baby. She wanted to give them statistics on that issue.

Physician: Do you have any questions about what I have said so far? (Neither parent spoke. They looked dazed.) Let me go on. I know that you are worried about having other children. Let me reassure you on that one. Only in rare cases is Down's inherited, and in yours it is not. In your situation, a woman younger than 35 has 1 chance in 100 of having another child with Down's. By age 45, as you remembered, the mother's chance of having an affected child is 1 in 50. But you're a long way from that. Now, although the chances are always in favor of having a normal child, no one can be certain. That's why amniocentesis is done—it's a chromosome examination of the baby inside the womb. With a needle some amniotic fluid is removed from around the baby. This fluid has cells shed by the fetus. They can be examined to find out whether or not the baby is affected. Amniocentesis can be performed safely at about 15 weeks of pregnancy. Depending on the diagnosis from that test, you would then have to decide whether or not to continue the pregnancy.

This time when she asked the parents if they had questions, Dr. Burnett did noticed that the father managed only an inquiry about medical costs of amniocentesis; the mother offered a polite thank you to the physician, and they left. They did not come back.

In subsequent talks with another physician, the Strands disclosed their great unease and turmoil as a result of that session. It was, they said, an interview they would never quite forget. We are not surprised. Dr. Burnett provided accurate information without ever hearing this couple. She unwittingly demonstrated a common error of health care providers in family interviewing work: focusing on content and information to the exclusion of process and behavior. In her desire to transmit correct facts, she had relegated the family's interactional behavior in her presence to background status, something to be circumvented in order to accomplish the business at hand. She had failed to notice that both parents were preoccupied with the question of genetic blame for their daughter's condition. The father had suggested that the mother was the carrier of defective genes, absolving himself of any contribution. His wife had been similarly concerned. Her pain was, if anything, more intense around the issue; she agreed with her husband's innuendoes, believing herself to be the contributor of the extra chromosome. Dr. Burnett never acknowledged this issue between them nor their pain surrounding it. The couple left the session with feelings of self-blame and other-blame intact, perhaps even intensified by the episode because the physician had talked about increased risks relating to advanced maternal age, a facet that Mrs. Strand had already used to conclude it is mothers, not fathers, who are to blame for Down's syndrome. The family had not been helped by this encounter.

As discussed in previous chapters, we advocate that interviewers pay equal attention to the necessary medical information and to the feelings, behavior, and process displayed by a family. Weighting an interview too heavily in either direction produces difficulties. A preoccupation with facts and risk ratios leads to the sort of difficulties experienced by the Strands. Too much emphasis on feelings and behavior with no information provided leads to inadequate medical care and a feeling by the family that they have had some kind of counseling, but the data they received was insufficient for planning their present or their future. The balancing between content and process in genetic counseling interviews is particularly delicate. Although the physician must observe the family's process, the information that is shared in genetic disorders is vital. A family must be taught about future risks in later pregnancies, the danger of later onset in currently well siblings, the risk for future generations of the family, and the advisability of sterilization. Because this content is so important and health care workers are often more comfortable giving information than discussing feelings, genetic counseling interviews are particularly vulnerable to becoming data discussions without regard for feelings, as the Strand family discovered.

Diagrams, such as those offered by Dr. Burnett, are often used in medicine. However, what a physician sees as clarity, the family may experience as informational overkill. All too often, it has been a painful experience for us to watch an earnest student physician tallying on paper the X's and Y's of a given condition, never realizing that the family has gotten lost. Too polite to hurt the young physician's feelings and perhaps too embarrassed to express their confusion, family members patiently wait for the physician to finish. The interviewer, as with Dr. Burnett, has no inkling that the information presented was useless.

Interviews for genetic counseling need not end this way. An interviewer can provide a family with information *and* a discussion of feelings. Had Dr. Burnett received some supervision along these lines before her encounter with the Strands, the following exchange might have occurred:

Physician:	Mr. and Mrs. Strand, you asked to meet with me so that we might discuss some of the genetic factors with Down's. I think it might be useful to back up and start from the beginning. Tell me what you understand about Down's syndrome.
Mother:	Just what you told us when we first talked with you, that there is something wrong with Sheila's—er—chromosomes. She got that from us somehow—we gave her too many or the wrong kind or something. But I felt perfectly fine all during the pregnancy. I don't understand it.
Father:	I worry about all those dental X-rays you had, Jean, before we even knew you were pregnant.
Physician:	I hear that a big problem for each of you right now is . . . what or *who* is responsible for this whole business.
Mother:	Well, of course—she's our child, after all. We had to cause it somehow.
Physician:	You're feeling very responsible.
Mother:	(nods yes)

Physician: That's a very heavy feeling to be carrying around. How do you bear it?

Mother: Sometimes I think I can't. (very sad)

Physician: I don't blame you. Mr. Strand, were you aware of this particular problem pressing down on your wife?

Father: She talks about it all the time. Sure.

Physician: How is it for you?

Father: Well, like I say, the only thing I can come up with are those dental X-rays at the beginning.

Physician: No, no. I wasn't explicit enough. What I meant was how is it for you to see your wife in so much distress, feeling that she is somehow at fault for Sheila's difficulty?

Father: (pause) . . . very hard.

Physician: How are you able to comfort her at those times?

Father: I'm not really. There's nothing I can say, it seems like.

Physician: And how does that make you feel?

Father: Pretty . . . helpless.

Physician: What an awful spot for each of you. One is feeling responsible, and the other is feeling helpless.

Both parents admitted the feelings labeled by the physician were correct. She had begun to direct them away from blaming or defending one another.

Physician: I think both of those feelings need more discussion. It is clear to me, Mrs. Strand, that you are not responsible for Sheila's condition. And it is equally clear to me, Mr. Strand, that you do not need to continue feeling helpless. Yet my saying that does not change things, I know.

Mother: (emphatic) Nope.

Physician:	From the sound of that, you will not easily allow blame to be lifted from your shoulders.
Mother:	(nods in agreement)
Physician:	As I say, it is an issue that needs talking about. However, I am also aware that you wanted to talk about some specifics of future pregnancies. And I do not want the time to get away from us. Would you prefer that we continue talking as we are about your feelings, or do you want to shift to your questions? We are going to need to talk about both your questions and your feelings.
Mother:	Well, I do want to know about having other babies.
Father:	Yeah, me too.
Physician:	OK. I'm not forgetting about your feelings, I want you to know. (pause) What specifically do you want to know about having babies?
Mother:	Well, should we even consider it or what? I certainly would never want to have this happen again.
Physician:	Let me say that only in rare cases is Down's inherited. And I can reassure you that in yours, it is not. The . . .

Dr. Burnett could now continue with an informational discourse regarding risks and safeguards in future pregnancies. A return to discussion of feelings might be achieved afterward as follows:

Physician:	If what I've told you about future pregnancies now seems understandable, I would like to return to that earlier issue— one of you feeling helpless and the other feeling responsible. Mrs. Strand, I would like you to tell your husband one way in which he might help you to feel even slightly less responsible. I say even slightly because—he can't take the feeling away. I know that, but how could he help?
Mother:	Well, he could stop talking about those damn X-rays for one thing.
Physician:	Tell him that directly . . . now.

There can be room for both information and interactional feeling issues in an interview of this sort. Such room, however, must be organized, developed, and encouraged by the interviewer.

ATTENTION DEFICIT HYPERACTIVITY DISORDER (ADHD OR ADD)

Nothing is more illustrative of the new morbidity in child health care than attention deficit disorder. Today, it seems unbelievable that the syndrome was not even mentioned in our original text of 1979. Deserved or not, attention deficit disorder has become the condition of this decade, offering something for everyone. Child development specialists, neurologists, psychiatrists, neurochemists, educators, behavioral therapists, pediatricians, pharmacologists, providers of adult medical care, parents, and even tabloid newspapers have embraced the condition, offering their own perspectives on diagnosis and treatment. We periodically receive an attention deficit disorder catalogue, a publication that describes itself as " . . . specializing in products for attention deficit/hyperactivity and related problems: books, videos, games, newsletters, feature article, training & assessment products, for teachers, parents, adults, teens, kids, and health care professionals." We are unaware of any other medical entity that has its own mail order catalogue!

Although we worry about the professional and public zeal in overdiagnosis and overtreatment, which often includes long-term use of medications, we are not nihilists. Attention deficit disorder does exist, can be very handicapping, and merits appropriate treatment (pharmacological, behavioral, and educational). We have been using diagnostic family interviews with the families of children referred for diagnosis of attention deficit disorder for more than 25 years, in much the same way that we have been using such interviews for comprehensive evaluation of children with other forms of school learning difficulties. In fact, the differential diagnosis of attention deficit disorder includes family stress and entrenched family relational difficulties (particularly between child and parent), both of which are appropriately assessed through a diagnostic family interview.

Today, managed care plans would prefer we use a diagnostic checklist in one abbreviated interview and, if results indicate, prescribe a stimulant, then send the patient and parents home. We object to this simplistic, inadequate plan and have been successful in resisting the imposition of such a model in our clinical practices. Checklists have disadvantages as definitive diagnostic instruments. Checklists are subjective, unilateral, are targeted toward outward manifestations (i.e., behaviors), and offer little regarding causal stressors and feelings states. Checklists are unscientific because they depend on the report of one of the participants in a two way interaction. Direct observation in a school visit or in the family setting offers more objective information. Thus, a family interview continues to be an important diagnostic *and* treatment tool in our work with inattentive children.

THE JOHNSON FAMILY

Sam Johnson, 14 years old at the time of treatment, was the only child of divorced parents. Sam was 6 years old when his parents divorced and behaviorally became such a handful that Mrs. Johnson felt unable to manage him. She relinquished both legal and physical custody. Sam came to live full time with his father, and they had been in this arrangement now for 8 years. The mother remarried, moved to another state, essentially dropping out of Sam's life by the time he was age 10 years. The father remained unattached, dividing his time between full-time work as an appliance repairman and his often-out-of-control son. At age 13 years, Sam was diagnosed as having attention deficit hyperactivity disorder by his primary care physician. The assessment, according to Mr. Johnson, had consisted of his completing the parent version of an attention deficit disorder scale and a brief physical examination for Sam. Treatment included four components: a prescription for Dexedrine, a telephone call back in one month, referral for Mr. Johnson to an attention deficit hyperactivity disorder parents' support group, and a return appointment for Sam in 6 months. Since Sam's initial diagnosis, his course on stimulant medication had been rocky with some positive effects noted in his selective attention and degree of distractibility. However, side effects of anorexia and rebound were troublesome, for which the dosage was adjusted to no avail. Then alternate medication was tried. Eight months after the first follow-up appointment, Sam had worked his way through Dexedrine and Cylert; he was now taking Ritalin tablets with inconsistent results. Impulsive behavior at home and at school was mushrooming out of control. Sam's physician was certain about the diagnosis but could not explain the troublesome course on medications that he usually found to be dramatically effective and quick. He suggested that Mr. Johnson and his son seek a second opinion with a behavioral pediatrician. It was then that our colleague, Dr. Lofland, received the call. The father, sounding desperate, asked to be seen immediately. When it was explained that there would be a 3-week delay before the first appointment, Mr. Johnson pleaded: "I don't think you understand, what's happening here, Dr. Lofland. I don't think anyone understands. That's why I'd like to tape what goes on at home. Please, could I send you a tape so you can get the full picture? Maybe it might even help to get us in there sooner. The medicine just isn't working." Although this was an unusual request, Dr. Lofland agreed, hoping he would ease this father's anxiety at having to wait three weeks. The pediatrician also asked for written observations from the teacher about Sam's learning and behavior in the classroom.

The information from school, along with a call to Sam's primary care physician, certainly seemed to support attention deficit disorder as a proper diagnosis. All the telltale signs were reported by both individuals. Even before seeing Sam, Dr. Lofland had obtained the criteria needed for a DSM-IV diagnosis of Attention Deficit Hyperactivity Disorder, Combined Type.

The next day, the tape arrived. It contained 45 minutes of chunks of dialogue between Sam and his father, recorded at different times. The following example is one 2-minute section, which Dr. Lofland found important and appalling.

Sam:	(sullen) Is my ball in your car?
Father:	No.
Sam:	WHERE is it then? Where's my BALL?
Father:	What do you mean?
Sam:	Where's my stupid ball?
Father:	Calm down. I don't know. I think it's outside, don't you remember? You wanted to leave it in my car, I said don't leave it in my car, because then I'd go off with it.
Sam:	Where? Where the [expletive] is it? I didn't LEAVE IT ANYWHERE!
Father:	Stop. Would you stop? Get in control for a minute.
Sam:	Well where is it then?
Father:	Well, will you please get in control so we can talk about this?
Sam:	NO!
Father:	Can I ask you a question? It's important.
Sam:	What?

Father:	Did you take the Ritalin?
Sam:	YES!
Father:	You didn't throw it away or anything?
Sam:	No.
Father:	OK . . . what caused you to . . .
Sam:	(unintelligible screaming)
Father:	Don't get mad, OK?
Sam:	Where's my basketball? I . . . . . (mumbles)
Father:	You what? . . . . You want me to help you find your basketball, right?
Sam:	Yeah.
Father:	I will help you find your basketball as soon as you help me pick up the mess.
Sam:	NO! FINE . . . I DON'T CARE.
Father:	Come on, son. OK, look, life is a reciprocal process.
Sam:	It's your loss. IT'S YOUR LOSS. I don't care.
Father:	Sam, it's not my loss. You know that, OK? I'm trying to help you; you try to help me . . . OK? Now all I'm asking you to do is turn the TV off for a second, come help me put this stuff . . .
Sam:	(quietly) If you find my ball, then I'll come.
Father:	If I find your ball, what? If I go find your basketball, then you'll come help me clean this stuff up?
Sam:	(mumble)
Father:	I'll go find your basketball, then come back in and we'll clean this up . . . ?

Father and son had unknowingly furnished Dr. Lofland with a compendium of the best of dysfunctional communication from Virginia Satir, along with the prototype for a family with boundary difficulties a la Salvador Minuchin, and a repeating sequence of family hierarchy/organization confusion to delight any Jay Haley student.

Both Sam and his father had adopted dysfunctional communication styles: messages sent and received tended to be unclear; meanings were not well checked out; neither individual was listening well to feedback from the other; and each found the different stance of the other somewhat threatening and a reason for challenging defensiveness.

Their boundary seemed enmeshed, overly diffuse; horizontal delineation between the two was blurry; they felt uncomfortably, unreasonably close somehow to Dr. Lofland's ear. From a vertical boundary standpoint, that of hierarchy, things were unbalanced between the generations. Sam, inappropriately, was in control, shaping the course of the episode with his escalating, demanding, oppositional stance. The following sequence repeated several times during other segments of the tape:

1. Sam demands.
2. Father begins to bargain ("I will help you find your basketball as soon as you help me pick up the mess.").
3. Sam refuses and demands louder.
4. Father in response weakens his bargaining stance ("All I'm asking you to do is . . . help me put this stuff . . . ").
5. Sam responds by setting his own terms ("If you find my ball, then I'll come.").
6. Father agrees to Sam's conditions ("I'll go find your basketball, then come back in and we'll clean this up . . . ?").
7. Sam remains in charge.

On the tape, their relationship was limited to a series of such deals arranged around the same sequence: Sam's outrageous behavior handled by the father with a willingness to bargain and ultimately cave in to the son's demands. Sam was by far the better bargainer, although the initiator of negotiations on the tape was always the father. He had negotiated himself into a position of pleading and powerlessness with his own son. Ritalin, no matter if delivered by intravenous drip, was not going to alter this sequence, Dr. Lofland concluded.

This preview of the family's interactional style allowed Dr. Lofland to design an intervention, which it should be stated, never included a formal family interview. Sam was seen alone for a neurodevelopmental evaluation to confirm the correctness of the diagnosis of attention deficit hyperactivity disorder. That done, Dr. Lofland asked to meet with Mr. Johnson individually. Further details of medical history were obtained and the tape segment above was played for the father. Mr. Johnson was embarrassed and shocked by what he heard and at the same time recognized it as a pervasive component in his relationship with his son.

He and Dr. Lofland agreed to a series of four appointments together without Sam. The appointments were used to help the father establish a firm interpersonal boundary between himself and Sam. For example, the father was coached to stop asking his son's permission through the repetitive use of the term, "OK. . .?" More importantly, Mr. Johnson was encouraged to take more arbitrary, fatherly stands with his son, without the sabotaging effects of negotiating. A system using immediate incentives of money ($1 per day) in exchange for Sam's compliance at home without abusive verbal behavior was drawn up in writing and implemented. No bargaining was permitted. As the father developed clarity in his approach and in his hierarchical position as father, the escalating episodes between them diminished dramatically.

Ten months after that series of visits, the Johnsons are still struggling and making progress with one another. Sam remains on Ritalin, which now seems to be an effective assist for his selective inattention, distractibility, and impulsivity. No medication changes are anticipated. Follow-up visits with Sam and his father have occurred about every 2 months, and the behavioral incentive system was dropped recently without negative consequences.

There may be critics that say this case, without the benefit of a traditional family interview, is inconsistent with the thrust of this book. We do not agree. The Johnson case is securely rooted in family systems principles, arising from the decision to review the family's interaction on audiotape and then intervene around a dysfunctional pattern of communication, structure, and sequence. Sam, Mr. Johnson, and Dr. Lofland allow us to illustrate a point we make with trainees: family intervention for a pediatric problem often has more to do with what is in the interviewer's mind than with who is actually in the room. In some cases, we believe that a family interview can occur with one person.

The Johnson case serves as a reminder that children with attention deficit hyperactivity disorder and their families are complicated systems indeed. When treating these children, a multimodal approach, which uses family, school, and medical components to develop a treatment plan, is best. Such children seldom are successfully managed solely by the administration of medications. Effective intervention also requires a respect for the complexity of human relationships and an understanding of those important repetitive behavior patterns that have reinforced, often for years, a family's ways.

References

1. Haggerty R J. Child health 2000: new pediatrics in the changing environment of children's needs in the 21st century. Pediatrics 1995;96:811.
2. Gofman H, Allmond B. Learning and language disorders in children: Part I, the preschool child. Curr Probl Pediatr 1971;1:10.
3. Gofman H, Allmond B. Learning and language disorders in children: Part II, the school-age child. Curr Probl Pediatr 1971;1:11.
4. Tanner JL. Learning problems: differences in learning styles to school failure. In: Rudolph AM. Rudolph's Pediatrics. 20th ed. New York: Appleton & Lange, 1996:118–121.
5. Tanner JL. Family effects on children's learning and school performance. In: Wender EH, ed. School dysfunction in children and youth: the role of the primary health care provider for children who struggle in school, Report of the 24th Ross roundtable on critical approaches to common pediatric problems. Columbus, Ohio: Ross Products Division, Abbott Laboratories, 1993:95–106.
6. Steinhauer P, Mushin D, Ray-Grant Q. Psychological aspects of chronic illness. Pediatr Clin North Am 1974;21:825.
7. Steinhauer, Mushin, Ray-Grant, 825.

chapter **11**

Issues with Adolescents in Family Interviews

CONFIDENTIALITY

THE CHIEU FAMILY

Dr. Roth had not seen Judith or her family for some time. He had worked with them in his behavioral pediatric practice 4 years ago when the family was coming apart. His role had been to watch over the marital separation, providing supportive counseling and as much damage control as possible, particularly for the children. At that time, Judith was age 11 years and her brothers were ages 7 years and 6 years. There were seven family meetings during 5 months. The father attended the first two meetings, then angrily refused to return, his new wife actively supporting his nonparticipation. Ms. Chieu and the three children continued, and after five family meetings, they were beginning to come to terms with their situation, learning that rebalancing the family would be a long, painful process. However, their managed care insurer declared that there had been enough therapy, and after a denied appeal, the sessions were discontinued.

Now Judith was 15 years old, and her mother called the pediatrician with several concerns: Judith was not sleeping well, her eating was idiosyncratic, she was now a vegan, and she was losing weight. Ms. Chieu added that Judith herself was worried and agreed to a visit with the pediatrician alone but was not willing to "go in for one of those family things." The mother agreed that a family meeting did not seem necessary, thinking that Judith just needed Dr. Roth to "check her out." Even Mr. Chieu, now divorced from his second wife, expressed worry and, when called by Dr. Roth, gave his permission for Judith to come in. The pediatrician agreed to a first appointment with Judith. When speaking with Judith to set the appointment, Dr. Roth mentioned, as he often did in preparation for interviewing an adolescent alone, that whatever they discussed would be kept between the two of them. She understood, she said. The mother, father, and Judith all stressed how well she was keeping up with school in spite of her symptoms: she was maintaining straight As in a difficult school.

The pediatrician was not prepared for this Judith. He remembered her as a sweet, compliant 11-year-old child in a plaid skirt and white blouse dressed for the parochial school. The teenager Judith entered with electric blue hair (what there was of it), multiple piercings, lots of black, a gaunt figure, and an attitude. She did not look well, and her story substantiated that she was not. Throughout the past academic year, a new experience in a high-pressured, San Francisco private high school, she had worked hard to keep her grades up. She felt inadequate to the work and not up to the performance of her peers in this new setting. She sought out others who felt the same, a group labeled at school as thrashers, many of whom were heavily into drugs. As the year progressed, Judith felt increasingly tense and exhausted; yet, she could not sleep. In fact, her sleep pattern was erratic, and sometimes she would go for days with no sleep. At other times, she could retreat into sleep for more than 24 hours. Her appetite was poor, and she was eating a lot of beans and peanut butter on her vegan diet. She had lost 14 pounds since beginning the diet 7 months ago. Her moodiness was striking, even to her. She could explode at a moment's notice about nothing and find herself in tears "for no reason." In spite of all of this, her grades were up, and she was on the honor roll.

Sleep deprivation, acute depression, incipient malnutrition—any of these seemed possible. Until, that is, reminding the pediatrician of his promise of confidentiality. Judith divulged that months ago she became terrified of not making the grade in this new school, disappointing her parents, incurring their anger, and wasting their tuition money. These terrors loomed so large that 6 weeks into her ninth-grade year, she began using methamphetamine; she was now "snorting crank" daily. The drug enabled her, she said, to concentrate, do her work, and stay on top of her academic game. She actually was not using it recreationally, but rather to study. Without it, she was convinced she would be flunking out, and she was equally convinced that her parents must never be told of this. Her mother would be destroyed, and her father's rage would be frightening and vengeful. (There was supporting evidence from the past that the father could become irrational and violent. Those qualities had contributed to both his divorces.)

Dr. Roth had wandered into difficult territory. This young woman was confiding in him and at the same time insisting that critical information not be shared with those responsible for her well-being. If he included the family now, he might lose Judith altogether, crushing any confidence she had placed in him. Also, her catastrophic fears regarding her mother's fragility and her father's wrath could be correct. If he did not include the family, Judith would probably continue to self-destruct, snorting chemicals up her nose; her parents would remain ignorant of the danger overwhelming their daughter. Those were ethical and moral issues, but there were others. What was the pediatrician's legal responsibility to this teen and to her parents?

The issue of confidentiality is one that distinguishes family interviewing with young children from family interviewing with adolescents. Confidence and privacy with young children in interviews is handled with some flexibility because parents often need specific information in order to help their children when they are very young. With adolescence, however, one expectation is that the teen is separating, becoming independent. That process is supported when an interviewer promises confidentiality in individual discussions with a teen. However, even when that promise is made, as Dr. Roth shows, some flexibility is needed to preserve confidence and credibility. For example, the pediatrician might have gained maneuvering room by saying, "Judith, in the course of our talk, I consider what we discuss is private, between you and me. You may, however, tell me something that I feel must be shared with your parents, like something that involves your physical safety. I will tell you that and we will discuss it first, before we decide how it should be shared with your folks." But Dr. Roth did not say this, and even if he had, Judith, hearing his words, might well have chosen to remain silent about her crank use. Uninformed about the real problem, the pediatrician would have proceeded with other diagnostic possibilities; he might even have considered the use of antidepressant medication, complicating Judith's situation even further.

Working to build trust with an adolescent is complex work, made more difficult, we are coming to believe, when the adolescent is split off initially (prematurely) into a private interview such as was done with Judith. In retrospect, we wonder what would have happened had Dr. Roth insisted on an introductory family interview first, to include at least the mother, the father, and Judith. We too have become trapped by the promise of privileged communication when we have sequestered ourselves alone with a teen. However, if a family interview is required before any individual meet-

ings, issues around confidentiality with a teen can become less troublesome, as the Jackson family demonstrates.

THE JACKSON FAMILY

Dr. Stuart knew Ruby Jackson slightly as a nurse at the local hospital. On the
telephone, she sounded desperate. Her 16-year-old son, Kevin, was driving her
crazy. Two recent episodes of coming home drunk had prompted her call.

Mother: I really wonder if he has a substance abuse problem; I mean
                     it. He wants to stay out all hours on the weekend. Party,
                     party—that's all he talks about. He gets frantic if he can't be
                     with his friends . . . calls me every name in the book if I de-
                     cide he's not going to go out on a Saturday night. I do think
                     he should spend some time with the rest of the family. He
                     says that's stupid . . . actually, he says I'm stupid. We've got
                     a real problem here.

The pediatrician inquired about the rest of the family. Besides mother and
Kevin (who was adopted), there were 6-year-old twins, Angie and Russell (who
were biological offspring). Mr. Jackson died 4 years ago. While working as a
roofer, he had been fatally injured in a freak ladder collapse at work.

Mother: I told Kevin he needed help. He just laughs. He might listen
                     to you, if you could see him and talk to him about his drink-
                     ing . . . and drugs. He might listen to a doctor. He tells me,
                     what do I know about life today . . . I'm from another cen-
                     tury is how he sees it. Can you see him?

Dr. Stuart's policy, unlike that of Dr. Roth, was to have an initial joint appointment when teenage issues were present. He informed Mrs. Jackson of this,
asking that she and her son be seen together. Because he sometimes regretted
not having other family members available to be included as needed, he added
that he would like the twins to come along. "They would be out in the waiting
room while the three of us are talking. But at some point, I may want them to
join us. I will begin with you and Kevin, however." Mrs. Jackson protested that
Kevin would not agree to a session with her, but the pediatrician held his ground
and stressed how important the joint meeting would be.

Pediatrician: Seeing you together first is the best way I know to hear what
                     each of you has to say—and in the presence of the other.
                     That is very important if I am to help you and Kevin take the
                     next step with this problem, whatever it is. I may at some

point want to meet with each of you alone. That actually gets
decided during the time I meet with you together.

He brought the call to a close, mother's protests notwithstanding. She took the
appointment offered.

On the scheduled day, they arrived. After settling the twins in the waiting
area, Mrs. Jackson and Kevin walked into the interview room. She walked; he
slunk, radiating contempt and a recognizable sweetish smell as he slammed down
into a chair and folded his arms. His clothes were baggy to excess with strategic rips and frays.

Mother: Please take your hat off.

Kevin: Why should I?

Mother: Kevin, you heard me.

Kevin: So what's that supposed to mean?

Mother: I don't know what's wrong with you anymore!

Dr. Stuart had done little more than say hello. He had already tallied up two
important observations: Kevin was using marijuana; the mother was powerless
with her 16-year-old son. Her chides and his defensive posturing continued over
the next 10 minutes, at which point the pediatrician was able to add a third item
to his list. Mrs. Jackson was complaining about the change in their relationship:

Mother: Honestly, I don't understand. We used to be so close.

Kevin: Don't give me that crap . . . (under his breath) we're not
               even related.

Mother: You are so hurtful. Why are you so hurtful? When you don't
               know what else to do, you drag that out.

The fact of Kevin's adoption was in the mix also. The interviewer faced a
choice: should he allow this embarrassment of riches to continue so that issues
tumbled helter-skelter into the interview? Or should he opt for some control
over the proceedings? He chose control, remembering that an initial
parent–adolescent interview is often a triage operation, done to get the diagnostic lay of the land quickly and then point a family in the direction of help,
wherever that might be. As the mother and son paused to refuel, he interrupted:

Pediatrician: Hold it everybody. Mrs. Jackson, what are you feeling now?

Mother: Like I don't even know my son anymore.

Pediatrician: And that leaves you feeling . . . ?

Mother:	Sad and scared.
Pediatrician:	Tell your son what frightens you.
Mother:	He won't listen.
Pediatrician:	He came here today. You thought he wouldn't do that. He's here now. Tell him.

Although Kevin was rolling his eyes, the pediatrician noted that he was in his chair, not about to bolt; nor was he verbally refusing to let the conversation continue. In fact, he was waiting for his mother to speak. Their attacking one another had been halted temporarily by the pediatrician's decision to focus on feelings of vulnerability lying quietly underneath the more obvious emotions of anger and irritation.

The mother disclosed her enormous fears for Kevin around the issue of alcohol and drug use. Aside from his several episodes of outright drunkenness, she mentioned his explosive irritability, sudden mood changes, precipitous decline in both school attendance and grades, his wanting to sleep for up to 18 hours after Saturday night parties, along with her discovery of marijuana paraphernalia in his backpack when she washed it. The pediatrician attempted to coach her through this part of the interview, so that what was emphasized was her fear, rather than her rage, frustration, and need to blame. However, Kevin still heard her comments as blaming. Dismissing her concerns as simply her own worry about what people would think of her as a parent, he turned to the pediatrician:

Kevin:	Will you tell this woman to get off my back! She thinks I'm just a pothead. Geez.
Pediatrician:	If that's not right, tell her so . . . now.
Kevin:	(sullen silence)
Mother:	See . . . you can't do that, because I am right. I am right, I know it.
Kevin:	Yeah, you know everything.

They were back at one another again with moves that seemed so practiced that the interviewer felt they could go on for hours. He allowed them to go on while he planned. His own internal triage had led him to place Kevin's use of substances in a priority position. If this were a teen in serious trouble with drugs, and the data suggesting that was mounting, then getting him off drugs would take precedence, even over the hurtful relationship. How could the interviewer determine

Kevin's level of drug use without sending him storming from the room? Should he ask to see Kevin alone? His decision was no. Relying on his observation that the teenager, although verbally mean-spirited, had not once denied alcohol and drug use (and therefore might be willing to admit to use), Dr. Stuart would push for more disclosure in this meeting.

Pediatrician: Kevin, it's time to level with your mother.

Kevin: About what?

Pediatrician: About what you've been putting in your body.

Kevin: It's none of her business. I knew I shouldn't have come here.

Once again, the pediatrician noted Kevin's lack of denial and, even more, his actions. Although verbally protesting being in the room, he made no attempt to leave. Kevin was illustrating how important it is to read the subtle behavior of teens. Limiting the interpretation of an adolescent's message to words alone is just that—limiting and often incorrect.

Mother: I do know what's been going on, Kevin. Why can't you ever tell the truth?

Pediatrician: (entering quickly) Mrs. Jackson, your son was about to level with you. Is that something you would like?

Mother: That's something I always want.

Pediatrician: Were you aware you are getting in the way of that by accusing him?

Mother: (sputter)

Pediatrician: Tell him instead: I need you to be truthful with me

Mother: I do, Kevin. Be honest.

Kevin: (fell silent, then exploded) F——! What IS the big problem here? There's nothing wrong with smoking pot—you and Dad did it, you told me that. Everyone I know does it. Big [expletive] deal. You are so lame. You don't even know what's goes on with kids now. I do. It is NOT a problem . . . I AM NOT THE [expletive] ALCOHOLIC IN THIS FAMILY!

Dr. Stuart allowed those words to hang in the air, silencing the mother who was about to speak. She was tearful. He maintained the silence. When the mother later spoke, it was to explain with emotion Kevin's thunderbolt. As a child she and her mother had been forced to flee, literally in the night, her father's irrational rage fueled by alcohol abuse. She never saw him again. And her own husband's death might have been alcohol related; no one was quite certain. It was known that he drank heavily. The subject was seldom discussed. She had come to the reasonable conclusion that men and alcohol were a horrifying combination. Seeing her son embark on this path had now thrown her into a panic of watchfulness, ever increasing rules, distrust, and nagging. Kevin, the pediatrician hypothesized, had responded with the clumsy self absorption of adolescence, portraying a teenager who needed watching and could not be trusted. His substance use was in part adolescent overreaction to his mother's over response to past events. Dr. Stuart also hypothesized that the degree of Kevin's use of alcohol and marijuana was substantial, probably more ominous and complex than a simple case of adolescent risk taking, experimentation, and defiance. The danger to him should not be minimized.

It was this conclusion that compelled him to urge Kevin's assessment at Thunder Road, an adolescent drug treatment facility in Oakland, California.

Pediatrician:	I am very concerned about what's going on. And frankly I don't feel that I can figure it out alone. I am going to ask you to make an appointment at Thunder Road for an assessment. The folks there are very good in determining, one, whether or not there is substance abuse and, two, what sort of treatment, if any, is indicated. That needs to happen right away—and before we go on with anything more here.
Kevin:	(now out of his chair) I TOLD YOU THIS WOULD BE A WASTE OF TIME! No way, no way, NO WAY!
Pediatrician:	(after Kevin quieted) That will be a decision the two of you will need to make. Mrs. Jackson?
Mother:	(sounding resolved) I have no choice. I will do it. (To Kevin with firmness) You will too.
Kevin:	(mumble, swearing)
Pediatrician:	Here's the number. I will call them also.

As before, Dr. Stuart based his moves on Kevin's behavior over his words. The youngster was still in the room. He *was* kicking at the rug with his foot and regarding all adults in the room with fury, but he was doing very little to frustrate the referral from proceeding . . . beyond shouting that he would never come back to this place, that the session and Dr. Stuart were a bunch of crap. Missing from Kevin's diatribe was any refusal to go to Thunder Road, a point not lost on Dr. Stuart. The interview concluded. Twelve days later, Thunder Road called to report that Kevin and his mother had made an appointment.

OTHER ISSUES

Confidentiality is just one of the variables to consider when holding to a family systems view in work with adolescents. There are other issues, all of which reflect basic differences between families (and therefore family interviews) with adolescents and those with younger children. The following issues, all of which were present in the Jackson family interview, should be considered when conducting family interviews with adolescents (1).

- **The stakes are higher.** An elementary school child may get suspended from school or tear up his or her room when angry. Teenagers take drugs, shoplift, get pregnant, run away—engaging in seriously dangerous activities that can have long-term consequences for their futures.
- **Different parenting skills are needed.** With a 6-year-old child, a parent can always pick her up and put her in her room. Parents of teenagers must use other skills of persuasion, reasoning, and verbal enforcement. During these years, lack of parental power is only exceeded by a similar lack of parental credibility in the teen's eye, which is not a winning combination for the limit setting that is still essential. Both Kevin and his mother were acutely aware of this dimension.
- **Others outside the family have increasing influence.** Younger children are most affected by their home and school environments, settings created by adults who are in charge. Teens, however, react to a wider circle of powerful friends who pull them in various directions. They are the other, usually stronger, voices that an adolescent hears. Kevin was listening to those voices with great interest.
- **Parents often underreact or overreact.** Recognizing their waning influence on a child, aware of the risks at stake, realizing that the time left to influence a child's life is running out can all intensify parents' reactions. Some parents, in a panic, overreact and over control their children—threatening, demanding, pushing for the child to be more responsible and stay away from trouble, or not to grow up at all. Other parents feel that it is too late to turn things around; they allow the child to have full rein over adults and their decisions. Such parents have essentially given up. Mrs. Jackson, by her own admission, had fallen into the former pattern of overreaction and attempts to over control.
- **Interviewers' reactions can be intense.** It is not only parents who are

sensitive to the risks and dynamics of adolescence; so too are health care providers and interviewers. When a family interviewer sees destructive family dynamics souring a child's life but faces parents who are too over-whelmed to change them, or when an interviewer wants the best for an adolescent but feels stifled by bureaucracy or limited resources, the in-terviewer too can feel that time is running out. He or she starts to believe that it is necessary to work hard and fast in order to avert disaster, or, like the parents and community, the interviewer may feel helpless and give up.

- **The adolescent has more opportunity to fill a surrogate role.** A child in elementary school can learn to copy and fill roles for those who are missing in the family. But filling in these roles becomes more powerful as the teen moves closer to adulthood. When occupied with taking on these roles, the adolescent sacrifices his or her own growth in the effort to emulate, for example, a missing parent. In the Jackson family, this variable was only conjecture after a single interview that contained no direct investigation of the issue. It is tempting to hypothesize that Kevin, the oldest male in the family now, was placing himself in his absent fa-ther's position around a shared symptom (i.e., substance use). Further interviews would be needed to confirm this hypothesis.

- **The adolescent can be more verbal.** Although they do not always com-ply, adolescents often have the capacity for complex verbal interchange. One of the main differences between a child interview and that of an adolescent is the ability of adolescents to do more talking. Not only is the adolescent's vocabulary and comprehension greater, but so is the ability to think abstractly. Right and wrong, for example, is not deter-mined by whether someone gets punished as it is in the mind of a 6-year-old child, but by a developing internal set of values, ethics, and morals that can be discussed.

Some adolescents become sullen grunters when interviewed. Robert Taibbi advises:

There are several ways of approaching a grunter. One of the best is to see him or her together with the whole or part of the family. This sidesteps the grueling one-on-one struggle. By your exploration of the entire family landscape, the adolescent sees that the focus isn't only on him or her, and anxiety goes down. Better yet, usually someone in the family will say some-

thing outrageous enough to ignite some response from the teen. All you have
to do is give him or her the space he or she needs to talk and be heard. (2)

Kevin was certainly not a grunter. To the contrary, he was, compared to
many teens in this setting, positively chatty. His verbal output was crude
and defensive. Beyond the rudeness, however, he delivered the winning line
in the interview—winning because it revealed what was hidden, true, and
painful in his family's life ("I AM NOT THE [expletive] ALCOHOLIC
IN THIS FAMILY"). He spilled the beans to the interviewer. We find that
children often do.

THE INITIAL INTERVIEW WITH ADOLESCENTS

Attendance

Because all of these variables can be examined directly by watching a family in action and because of fiascos of our own similar to that of Dr. Roth
surrounding confidentiality issues, we do begin work with teenagers by
first scheduling a family interview. Earlier in this book, we stated that we
see parents alone first to assess the appropriateness of using a family approach, and that remains the case for families with younger children.
However, in families with adolescents, we have shifted to meeting with
parent(s) and teenager(s) together initially. This sometimes improves our
credibility with adolescents because teenagers are not won over by the appearance of grownups ganging up on them in private meetings from which
they are excluded. Because interviewer standing can be tenuous to begin
with, it makes little sense to shoot oneself in the foot before even starting
with a teen.

Siblings may be included subsequently, depending on the circumstances. In the Jackson family's interview, it was Dr. Stuart's choice not to
use the twins because the pressing issue for him became facilitating Kevin's
referral for substance abuse evaluation. The children remained in the playroom and were never interviewed. In another interviewer's hands, they
might just as correctly have been included in this interview or in later sessions. Such a decision is most often the result of interviewer preference and
a judgment about who is needed to get the job done.

An interview with the adolescent alone may, and often does, come later.
Combinations of participants may also be used later (e.g., entire family,

parents alone, one parent and the teenager, children together without parents). As Taibbi says, " . . . you have to do a lot of juggling—between adolescents and parents, past and present, individual work and family work. . . . Unlike treatment of younger children, working with adolescents requires walking a fine line, carefully balancing the needs of the child with those of the family" (3). If the work becomes ongoing, extending beyond the initial family interview, the balancing gets even more complex. Too much siding with the teen (particularly by a young interviewer) results in parents who are offended and dismiss the interviewer as inexperienced about parenting. As mentioned, the teenager is often ready to disqualify the interviewer from the outset, merely because he or she is an adult. If an interviewer joins with the parents too vigorously, the adolescent may not be willing to attend or open up. One more reminder from Taibbi is good to keep in mind: "It's easy to feel like a bouncing ball if you're not careful, shuttling back and forth diplomatically between the generations like . . . Henry Kissinger. The way out of this is not to think in terms of being *between,* but *above,* your client isn't the adolescent or the parent, or even the adolescent and the parent, but the family system" (4).

Ron Taffel urges those working with adolescents to turn their attention to a teen's "second family," which he defines as the peer network, pop culture, school, and neighborhood ethos.

Family therapy has not kept pace with several decades of massive social upheaval. The world of an adolescent is now so powerfully defined by systemic forces other than home . . . that working with the family alone is rarely powerful enough to effect change in the life of a troubled teenager. . . . There is compelling evidence of the need to significantly redefine how family therapists work with adolescents and children. (5)

He frequently asks permission for specific friends to join in sessions with an adolescent, echoing a former generation of "network family therapists," who seemed to like crowd work in the 1970s (6). Taffel's approach sounds apt, particularly for those engaged in ongoing psychotherapy with teenagers, and we listen as he warns: "To do therapy in the old way—under the illusion that the family, regardless of its configuration, is still a self-contained unit—contributes to the centrifugal forces in our society that are already driving kids into a huge post-modern army of semi-homeless nomads" (7). His work sounds arduous and grueling, which may explain why we have not entered that arena yet. Also, note that he is discussing how *family therapists,* not necessarily *primary care pediatric providers,* work with adolescents. It is our belief that the latter, often able to use their relationship over years with teenagers and families, can provide effective intervention in work which is limited to the adolescent and immediate family and does not include the neighborhood.

Goals

The initial interview with a teen and parents together can often be a discrete, encapsulated piece of work, as the Jackson family interview illustrates. As a combination assessment and triage operation, the interview may yield a beginning diagnostic formulation, address medical issues involved, serve as springboard for a referral to someone or somewhere else, or provide an introduction for further interviews. Offering to help a family "take the next step" in the process or problem is a phrase we often use with trainees. This phrase suggests that the proposed interview will be limited in scope and leave the family in charge of itself. With this latitude, the clinician can either continue with the family if comfortable or jump ship after the session if he or she feels overwhelmed by the clinical picture emerging. Jumping ship is only acceptable, we stress, when a family has been directed to the appropriate resource. Dr. Stuart would have been irresponsible to uncover as he did a substance abuse problem needing formal assessment without also supplying a referral (i.e., Thunder Road).

Often the initial family interview is framed for the family as an opportunity to figure out the next step. Clinical situations with teenagers for which we have used this type of interview have included:

Attention deficit disorder within the family
Dual-career families with "no time"
Substance abuse
Alcohol or drug abuse in other family members
Running away
Delinquency, acting out
School failure
Truancy
Chronic illness (e.g., diabetes, epilepsy)
Depression

Issues surrounding adoption
Pregnancy
Parental separation, divorce
Blended families
Conflict over rules at home
Eating disorders
Obsessive compulsive disorder
Insomnia
Issues concerning the normative step of leaving home.

Interview Form and Style

The form of such an interview is no different from that illustrated by the Jacksons and that articulated in chapter 5. Opening stages are succeeded by a discussion of family concerns and an interactional portion during which the family is encouraged to show its system. The encounter is wrapped up with a planned ending by the interviewer. And interviewer goals are precisely those described in chapter 5 as well.

A comparison between the Jackson interview with earlier examples reveals some stylistic differences. With Kevin and his mother, the interviewer relinquished strict adherence to Satir's approaches (see chapter 2) surrounding communication within the family. There is often considerable urgency, as in this case, around the presenting problem with teens, coupled with a critically short period of time in which to connect with or lose the adolescent. Teenagers do not suffer fools gladly . . . or for long. There may not be time to develop a focus on "I" statements and other parameters of functional and dysfunctional communication. Communication patterns should not be overlooked in families with teenagers. And Dr. Stuart did attend to them at several points. For example:

Mother:	I do know what's been going on, Kevin. Why can't you ever tell the truth?
Pediatrician:	(entering quickly) Mrs. Jackson, your son was about to level with you. Is that something you would like?
Mother:	That's something I always want.

Pediatrician:	Were you aware you are getting in the way of that by accusing him?
Mother:	(sputter)
Pediatrician:	Tell him instead: I need you to be truthful with me.

However, such interventions were in the form of short bursts by Dr. Stuart. He deliberately let pass many other opportunities for shaping communication in a leisurely Satir styled approach. By doing this, he hoped to maintain his tenuous engagement with Kevin and to move the interview along quickly. If Satir's family communication theory was minimally called upon in this adolescent interview, Dr. Stuart liberally used structural approaches from Minuchin (see chapter 3), including joining and accommodation, restructuring techniques of actualizing family transactions, escalating stress, assigning tasks, and providing support and guidance. Attention to hierarchy and family sequences (per Haley, see chapter 3) was also used by Dr. Stuart.

Joining and accommodation (the methods used to create a therapeutic system and establish a position of leadership with the family) were illustrated when Dr. Stuart required a family interview and stuck to it, and when he highlighted mother's feelings of sadness and fear. *Restructuring techniques* were used often, including *actualizing family transactional patterns* (i.e., encouraging family members to talk directly to one another) when the pediatrician spoke to Kevin about smoking pot: "If that's not right, tell her so . . . now." He was clearly *escalating stress* when he offered this line: "Kevin, it's time to level with your mother." The recommendation for making an appointment at Thunder Road was an example of *assigning a task*. Support, education, and guidance were offered throughout the interview when Dr. Stuart voiced his concern about the seriousness of Kevin's substance use. He validated the importance of *hierarchy and parental boundaries* by refusing to cave in to Kevin's tirade against the drug assessment, turning instead to the mother for her input about the referral. His observation of a *repeating family sequence* was helpful in establishing his overall theme and direction with the family: by noting that Kevin's sullen petulance was met each time by the mother's helplessness (each reinforcing the other), the pediatrician focused on changing that sequence, positioning the mother as a parent taking charge of her family despite Kevin's intimidating style. The sequence did shift enough for the mother to declare about the Thunder Road referral: "I have no choice. I will do it." (And to Kevin with firmness), "You will too."

We do not claim that the work was ended here. It had barely begun. One brave stand on a mother's part is just that, no more. Families can return to accustomed sequences by the time they are out in the parking lot, and they often do. But even this small move turned out to be an assist for Kevin and his mother. Remember that the purpose of an initial interview with a teen and parent may be limited to helping them take their next step. For the Jacksons, this amounted to a diagnostic assessment for substance abuse, and it was a step that they took.

References

1. Taibbi R. Doing family therapy. New York: Guilford Press, 1996:120–122.
2. Taibbi, 148.
3. Taibbi, 129.
4. Taibbi, 130.
5. Taffel R. The second family. The family therapy networker 1996;20:36.
6. Speck R, Attneave C. Family network: retribalization and healing. New York: Pantheon Books, 1973.
7. Taffel, 36.

chapter 12

Shifts in the Traditional Family

DEFINING "FAMILY"

In the 1979 edition of this book, the families that were profiled reflected our experiences then, when families often came to us "intact" (i.e., two traditionally married parents with one, two, or three children all living together under the same roof). Exceptions were signaled by a chapter in the first edition entitled "The Single-Parent Family." With inclusion of that chapter, we had hoped to acknowledge the rapidly changing composition of typical American families. However, we were not prepared for the speed with which such changes were taking place, nor the magnitude of the upheaval. As soon as we put it on paper, the title was inadequate and naively limited because it seemed to suggest that families came in just two varieties: traditional and one-parent. This was not true then and certainly is not true now. As Dr. Ellen Perrin stated in 1996:

> *The traditional stereotype of a mother at home full time with primary responsibility for home and children and a father employed outside the home and with few primary responsibilities at home no longer serves us well. Over half of married mothers with children under 6 and 85% of single parents are employed outside of their home. Only 60% of the 65 million children in the United States currently are living with both biological parents, and more than 1 million children experience divorce each year. <u>Among the diverse patterns of family structure seen today are reconstituted and blended families, parents single—by choice or not, successive common-law relationships, homosexual parents, joint but separate care and custody, children with foster parents, and homeless families.</u> (1)*
> *[The emphasis is ours.]*

These developments have made a definition of the word *family* almost impossible, and we have steered clear of any attempt to do so until now. Our colleague Salvador Minuchin comments:

> *Most definitions of a family focus on the composition of a small group related by blood or commitment. But what wording could include all the possibilities? . . . Families in a kibbutz extend their boundaries to include the community. . . . With today's biotechnology, a family may include a couple's biological child, conceived of her ovum and his sperm but gestated in the body of a stranger. In a recent instance, a lesbian couple was brought to family court by the biological father of their child, a homosexual friend whom they had asked to donate sperm. When their daughter was two years old, the donor sued, seeking parental rights. The judge ruled that the daughter already had two parents and that it was in the best interests of the child not to upset her concept of a family. What then is a family? (2)*

In order to answer his own question, Minuchin invokes the importance of historical context on family development. Through the centuries, families have differed in different historical periods. This era is no exception, he points out: family arrangements taken for granted only a few years ago have grown increasingly irrelevant, and the organization of families is in great flux in Western culture. He expects, as do we, that the configuration of families will continue to change.

Citing the work of Arlene Skolnick, Minuchin lists three variables in particular that he believes will influence family organization in the United States (3). The first variable is *economic,* currently heralded by the large-scale movement of women into the workforce. Many women do not have the option of remaining at home anymore. The impact of women working outside the home, together with feminist ideas, is shifting the cultural ideal of marriage itself and the roles within marriage in a more egalitarian direction.

Minuchin lists a second important variable as *demographic.* Family size is decreasing, which is a response in part to the large economic burden of rearing children in today's world. At the same time, life expectancy is increasing. People now expect to grow old, and a couple plans on many years together alone, beyond their active parenting years during which they have raised fewer children.

A third factor, *psychological gentrification,* is associated particularly with the middle class, higher levels of education, and more leisure. Individuals in this group have become more interested in the emotional quality of relationships. "It is no longer enough for a husband and father to be a good provider. A woman cannot prove her wifely virtues by the contents of her pantry. A child can no longer be merely dutiful and obedient" (4). More is expected, and the rules and roles are shifting and expanding. Minuchin is careful to note that although reflective of middle class families, these observations stop short of accuracy for the lives of many other American families . . . the poor.

Minuchin does, however, synthesize a definition of family that transcends socioeconomic issues: "A family is a group of people, connected emotionally and/or by blood, who have lived together long enough to have developed patterns of interaction and stories that justify and explain these patterns of interaction" (5). This definition may be cumbersome, but we have not been able to improve it, and it has helped us sometimes to answer the question, "Just who (what) do you consider a family these days in your clinical work?"

In 1979, we wrote this then uncommon, but telling, illustration of how families were changing:

Pediatrician:	Now, George, when you come to the clinic tomorrow, we are going to be meeting with you and your family. Is your father going to be able to make it?
George:	Which father do you mean?
Pediatrician:	The one who is married to your mother.
George:	Do you mean my stepmother or my birth mother?
Pediatrician:	I'm not quite sure George. Which one are you living with?
George:	This week I'm staying with my aunt.
Pediatrician:	But your mother, the one who came with you this morning . . .
George:	That was my father's friend, Josie.
Pediatrician:	And is that your stepmother?

George:	She was, but she moved out. She brought me in today because my dad and Laurie went up to the Sierras for the weekend.
Pediatrician:	I don't understand—do you call your mother Laurie?
George:	No, my mother's name is Mom. Laurie . . . I haven't met her, she's going to be moving in with Dad . . . after Ron moves out.
Pediatrician:	Do I know Ron?
George:	I don't know. He's tall, has a moustache . . .
Pediatrician:	I guess not. Is he related to you?
George:	I'm not sure.

Invoking Minuchin's definition will not assist in this case. It's anybody's guess as to just who, properly, is George's family. The interchange is revealing; we no longer consider it uncommon.

We recall one family in which we asked a child's mother to invite the rest of her daughter's family for a diagnostic family interview on the pediatric ward. When they arrived, the group included: the 9-year-old patient, her mother and mother's second husband, their 22-month-old daughter, and two other children of the mother's first marriage, the patient's brothers. There were also: the patient's father and his second wife, their two children, and one child from the father's first marriage, again the patient's brother. This collection of 11 individuals made the interview even more confusing by their behavior in the room. The patient's mother and father, long divorced and now each remarried, chose to sit together; they obviously enjoyed a continuing close relationship. Their current spouses likewise gravitated to one another, seeming familiar. The patient spent the session sitting on their laps, disregarding both natural parents. The remaining children were a tangle; just calling an individual by the correct name loomed large for the interviewer.

Interviewing such a large group together may seem reckless. However, with this group it was exactly the essential lack of boundaries dramatically portrayed that was responsible for considerable stress in the hospitalized child. That feature formed the focus for change in this and three subsequent family interviews.

This family and that of George, illustrated in the previous dialogue, represent the end of the spectrum where there seem to be too many connected people. These patients are the product of our ever-changing views in the United States about marriage, divorce, separation, and family living arrangements. Many children are now accustomed to an array of adults and other children in their lives, with labels to keep everyone straight: mother, father, stepfather, stepmother, birth mother, brother, sister, stepbrother, stepsister, "aunt," friend, roommate, lover, or just "Ron."

SEXUAL PREFERENCE AND THE FAMILY

Sexual preference issues have also added complexity to one's understanding of family. We recently saw a 6-year-old girl, Renee, with attention deficit hyperactivity disorder (ADHD). She lived with her biological mother and the mother's new lesbian lover. The mother's former lesbian partner of 8 years now lived alone but considered herself a parent to our patient because she had lived with Renee and Renee's mother for many years. The child's biological father was gay and lived nearby with his lover. His previous partner had died of AIDS and was the biological brother of Renee's mother, thus Renee's biological uncle. Renee evidenced no difficulty around these roles and in fact considered it an advantage to have a total of so many parents in three separate households. The adults had organized themselves so that parenting responsibilities were acknowledged and divided among biological mother, her ex-lover, and Renee's biological father, each living in a separate place. It was that group of three plus Renee who attended family meetings. In this situation, who is in the family and who serves in what capacity has been determined by the family's own sorting out process over time. It may sound disorganized, but we can report that it seems to be working for all concerned. There is a growing body of literature on the subject of homosexual families (6,7,8).

THE BLENDED FAMILY

This family represents one form of a blended, reconstituted, or step family (i.e., a family in which at least one of the adults is a step-parent). Blended families are now familiar because 80% of divorced persons in our country remarry, and 60% of these individuals have children. Families in which there are children from a previous marriage are common these days, according to Visher and Visher (9).

We see many blended families in our own clinical practices. Interviews with these families do not necessarily require different approaches. We find ourselves using the ideas and strategies articulated in this text, continuing to depend on understanding a family's system, homeostatic pattern, communication, structure, and sequences of behavior. What is unique to step families (and somewhat predictable as our experience grows) is the list of concerns for which they seek help for children from a pediatric clinician. Often that list includes issues of trust and loyalty, space and boundary, and the assignment of roles and division of labor. Using our illustration from chapter 1 of the family as a mobile in dynamic equilibrium, a step family becomes two separate mobiles hanging from a single hook that are expected to balance harmoniously without jostling one another, tangling up lines, interfering with accustomed movement, or frustrating the delicate equilibrium. Children caught up in this process of family re-equilibration struggle with several issues, including dealing with loss, divided loyalties, figuring out where they belong, membership in two households, unreasonable expectations for themselves and others in the family, the continuing fantasy of natural parents reuniting, and persistent guilt over causing the divorce, an event that has led to the new, often unwanted blending. These topics surface in the process of routine medical care for such children.

Guidelines for Step Family Interviews

The pediatric caregiver may have an advantage, particularly if he or she has been providing medical care for some time to the family. Offering continuity and an established relationship may allow a caregiver to propose occasional family sessions to discuss the issues listed previously. We invite a caregiver positioned in this way and hearing these concerns voiced to offer a family interview with the blended family. In our experience, families rarely refuse. Because every member of the mobile has been feeling confused and frustrated, the chance to move forward out of chaos is often welcomed. When begun, the interview proceeds just as any other, with reliance on a family systems approach by the interviewer. We also incorporate specific content from the literature on step families to guide our own thinking in the work and to share in discussion with the family. Families are helped by knowing their issues have been studied, experienced, even sometimes resolved by others. The guidelines for step families set forth by Visher and Visher have become so useful to us and to our patients that we offer them here, excerpted from their first book, *Stepfamilies: A Guide to Working with Stepparents and Stepchildren:*

1. *It is difficult to have a new person move into another's "space," and it is difficult to be the "new" person joining a preexisting group. For these reasons it helps to cut down feelings involved with territory if families can start out in a new place.*

2. *Parent–child relationships have preceded the new couple relationships. Because of this, many parents feel that it is a betrayal of the parent–child bond to form a primary relationship with their new partner. A primary couple relationship, however, is crucial for the continuing existence of the stepfamily, and therefore is very important for the children as well as for the adults. A strong adult bond can protect the children from another family loss, and it also can provide the children with a positive model for their own eventual marriage. The adults often need to arrange time alone to help nourish this important couple relationship.*

3. *Forming new relationships within the stepfamily can be important, particularly when the children are young. Activities involving different subgroups can help such relationships grow.*

4. *Preserving original relationships is also important and can help children experience less loss at sharing a parent. So at times it is helpful for a parent and natural children to have some time together, in addition to stepfamily activities.*

5. *Caring relationships take time to evolve. The expectation of "instant love" can lead to many disappointments and difficulties.*

6. *Subsequent families are structurally and emotionally different from first families. Upset and sadness are experienced by the children and adults as they react to the loss of their nuclear family. Acceptance that a stepfamily is a new type of family is important.*

7. *Because children are part of two biological parents they nearly always have very strong pulls to both of these natural parents. These divided*

loyalties often make it difficult for children to relate comfortably to all the parental adults in their lives. Rejection of a stepparent may have nothing to do with the personal characteristics of the stepparent. In fact, warm and loving stepparents may cause especially severe loyalty conflicts for children. While it may be helpful to children for adults to acknowledge negative as well as positive feelings about ex-spouses, children may become caught in loyalty conflicts if specific critical remarks are made continuously about their other natural parent.

8. *Courteous relationships between ex-spouses are important, although they are very difficult to maintain. Although it may be strained, many ex-spouses are able to relate in regards to their children if the focus is kept on their mutual concern for the welfare of the children.*

9. *Children as well as adults in a stepfamily have a "family history." Suddenly these individuals come together and their sets of "givens" are questioned. Much is to be gained by coming together as a new unit to work out and develop new family patterns and traditions. Values do not shift easily. And different value systems are inevitable because of different backgrounds, etc. Having an appreciation for and an expectation of such difficulties can make for more flexibility in the stepfamily. Negotiations (using family negotiation sessions) are needed by such families.*

10. *Being a stepparent is an unclear and difficult task. The wicked stepmother myth contributes to this. Stepparenting is usually more successful if stepparents carve out a role for themselves that is different from and does not compete with the natural parents. While discipline is not usually accepted by stepchildren until a friendly relationship has been established (often up to 2 years), both adults do need to support each other's authority in the household. The natural parent may be the primary disciplinarian initially . . . at no time does it work out for either children or adults to let the children approach each adult separately and "divide and conquer."*

11. *Integrating a stepfamily that contains teenagers can be particularly difficult. Adolescents are moving away from their families in any type of family. In single parent families teenagers have often been "young adults" and with the remarriage of a parent they may find it extremely difficult to return to being in a "child" position again. Adolescents have more of a previous "family history" and so they ordinarily appre-*

ciate having considerable opportunity to be a part of any stepfamily negotiations, although they may withdraw from both natural parents and not wish to be part of many of the "family" activities.

12. *"Visiting" children usually feel strange and are outsiders in the neighborhood. It is helpful if they have some place in the household that is their own. If they are included in stepfamily chores and projects when they are with the stepfamily they tend to feel more connected. Bringing a friend with them and having some active adult participation in becoming integrated into the neighborhood can make a difference. Noncustodial parents often are concerned because they have so little time to transmit their values to visiting children. Since children tend to resist efforts by the adults to instill stepfamily ideals during each visit, it is comforting to parents and stepparents to learn that the examples of behavior simply observed in the household can affect choices made by the children later in life.*

13. *Sexuality is usually more apparent in stepfamilies because of the new couple relationship, and because children may suddenly be living with other children with whom they have not grown up. Also there are not the usual incest taboos operating. Sensitivity regarding sexual issues is important.*

14. *All families experience stressful times. Children tend to show little day-to-day appreciation for their parents, and at times they get angry and reject their natural parents. Because stepfamilies are families born of loss, the mixture of feelings can be even more intense than in intact families and therefore expectations that the stepfamily will live happily ever after are unrealistic. Having an understanding of this can result in less disappointment. (10)*

SINGLE-PARENT FAMILIES

For step families, the impact of societal changes in America has been to produce a striking increase in their dramatis personae and in the complexity of their family living arrangements. In other families, those same changes in society have yielded an opposite effect: a shrinking population within the household, often with a commensurate shrinking in resources and circumstance. Separation, divorce, and death can all divide families into fragments, sometimes leaving a group of just two, a parent and one child, to carry on the job of family life formerly shared by three or more individuals. Single parenting by choice, where there has never been two parents, is another configuration that has led to smaller rather than larger families. Rarely seen in our experience in the 1970s, this subset is fairly common among our patients today.

Theoretically, these families with fewer members should respond to our model of family interviewing as all others. The principles still apply whether dealing with an intact family, a blended family, or one in which only one parent is available. However, we do consider single-parent families more difficult to work with for several reasons. There is one less adult to contribute perspective regarding family behavior. Also, when one family member is absent, the temptation is great for someone in the family to speak for and about him or her, often distorting the facts. The interviewer may have no way to correct the distortions. "Talking about" behavior, if allowed to persist in these family interviews, can produce considerable mischief.

Families with one parent and one child present special problems. We refer to these families as "deadly duos." The typical situation is that of a mother living alone with her preteenage daughter. The two of them often coalesce in a grand manner, frustrating the interviewer's best efforts to introduce unwanted change into the family's existing pattern. Consider Paula, age 9 years, and her mother, Ms. Frazier. She and her mother have slept in the same bed since the parents' divorce several years ago.

Pediatrician:	I think we need to get back to the sleeping arrangements at home.
Mother:	That's not really a problem. Do you think so, honey?
Paula:	(shakes her head no)
Mother:	Actually, we help each other get to sleep. Sometimes my legs are aching so much, and no one can rub legs like Paula. She's magic! And her room is way down the hall, not very well heated, and there's a streetlight outside. It makes sleeping in that room very difficult. What don't you like about that room, Paula?
Paula:	The light—it shines in, right in my eyes. And the TV—that's in Momma's bedroom. We like to watch it in bed together . . . and snuggle when it's cold.

The arrangement sounds uncomfortably close, and what might help the interviewer would be the presence of another family member, for example a sister, to say, "I don't see why she gets to be in there, and you won't let me! She gets to do everything!" But there is no sibling. There is only mother and daughter, each committed to maintaining the status quo and easily able to form a tight alliance against intrusion by any interviewer hoping to change the setup. Undeniably, the pediatrician interviewer is running into trouble partly because she is imposing her judgment on the family, pinpointing a problem (i.e., sleeping together) where none exists in the family's eyes. Because it is a problem important only to her, the interviewer is bound to meet resistance from the family.

Even in situations not compromised by the pediatrician's beliefs, it is usually a simple matter for a family of just two to hold with a united front against incursions by the interviewer. This is harder for them to do if even just one additional family member is present. In a family of more than two, alliances are less fixed. There always seems to be someone who is for the moment "on the outside" of a two-person coalition—someone who is therefore able to provide the interviewer with some information, remark, or behavior that offers an entrance into the family system. We prefer to work with a family unit of three or more individuals. So much so that we have at times invited a grandparent or other relative to join a deadly duo in interviews.

Single-parent families are more difficult to interview for another reason. These families can be beset by profound real-life problems—economic, occupational, geographic. One grown-up has generally been asked to take on a job that traditionally and perhaps a few months earlier required the shared energies of two parents. The disruptions engendered by that fact alone can be staggering. A divorcing parent has often, in the course of becoming single, had many resources halved, while being asked to assume total responsibility for twice as much as previously required. Job, school, child care, finances, food, health issues—many of these stresses will depend on changes in the family's life circumstances for resolution, some perhaps beyond the family's ability to control or alter. This unyielding struggle over real-life issues can often force an interviewer to face his or her own limits in assisting such a family. The conclusion that "these single-parent families are hard" is reemphasized.

We are not saying that working with one-parent families should be avoided. Working with such families could not be avoided even if one wished; they are simply too numerous in our patient population. Although family intervention may be difficult and frustrating with these families, it can also be successful, as detailed in the following case.

THE "GLUED TOGETHER" FAMILY

We have often encountered single-parent families (e.g., Ms. Frazier and Paula) in which relationships appear to be stifling growth. Sometimes the closeness began as an appropriate drawing together following the event that precipitated the loss of the second parent, but then this closeness persisted. At other times, there never was a second parent, and the exaggerated closeness was present since the youngster's birth. Trouble was on the way as the mother (in our experience, it has been the mother) and child gradually became more and more interdependent, clinging to and preferring intensified contact with one another over relationships with age peers or those outside the household. The result has become a constricted, isolated family of two in which the child is not given opportunities to separate and grow toward independence, and the mother sees little need for expanding her own horizons into adult relationships.

THE GRIFFIN FAMILY

Ms. Griffin had no clear idea that togetherness was contributing to the difficulties she was having with her 9-year-old daughter, Anna. She knew only that she had an increasing problem getting her daughter to attend school. The pediatric resident, after giving Anna a clean bill of health, suggested that the two of them return to the office in 3 days for a longer conversation about the problem. Ms. Griffin agreed but hoped, she said, that the interview would not take too long; she had other things to do. This was the week before finals, and she was a full-time student. She would soon have her degree after years of struggling with work, single-parenting, and night classes. The pediatrician congratulated her on her soon-to-be-reached goal and said he would keep in mind that her time was short.

The interview began in an interesting way. The family was late. The car had broken down en route. Mother and Anna left it parked by the side of the street and came the rest of the way by bus. They looked tired, hurried, and exasperated. Anna was holding on to her mother's waist. Her mother scolded her, saying, "Don't do that, Anna. I'm hot. Stand up, stand up. Don't hang." Anna grumpily moved a few inches away. She did not return the pediatrician's hello and did not look at him.

Mother:	I'm so sorry, but could I use your bathroom? In all the business with the car, there just wasn't time . . .
Pediatrician:	Sure.
Mother:	(moving toward the door) Now wait right here, Anna. I'll be right back.

Anna shook her head no and moved right along with her mother. Ms. Griffin look exasperated and tried to peel Anna off to no avail. At the door, the mother conceded defeat: "Oh, all right. You can come in too, but I want to be able to be by myself once we're in there. Understand?" Anna's response was to engineer both of them inside and close the bathroom door. They emerged, together of course. The mother sat down; Anna joined her in the same chair, settling into her lap. The mother made no moves to discourage Anna, accepting the maneuver as though she were accustomed to it.

Ms. Griffin described her concerns about Anna. They were extensions of actions the pediatrician had already observed in the office. Anna whined about going to school in the morning and sometimes had stomach pains. Those usually disappeared by 9:30 after the mother had called in sick at work, resentfully deciding that she would have to stay home for the day. The usual day-care arrangement was not an option at this time because of increased fees. Anna balked in the same way when it came to sleeping alone at night. Ms. Griffin had handled that just as inconsistently, sometimes allowing Anna to sleep with her, sometimes joining Anna in the girl's bed, and sometimes refusing to give in to Anna's demands. The last action resulted in a sleepless night for both. Ms. Griffin, feeling that she had to reserve energy for classes and work, tended less and less to take any sort of stand.

Mother:	Anna, you're awfully heavy. Wouldn't you like to sit over there?
Anna:	No.
Mother:	Pleeeeease.
Anna:	No.
Mother:	All right for you (giving her a squeeze and to the pediatrician rolling her eyes up in exasperation).

Watching the two of them produced a tightness in the pediatrician's chest. It was this sensation that prompted him to act. Rising from his chair, he moved over and lifted Anna off her mother into a separate chair.

Pediatrician: Anna, I need you to sit there during our talk.

Anna: I don't like sitting here. I want to sit there (mother's lap).

Pediatrician: I need you to sit where you are.

Surprisingly, Anna made no effort to test the pediatrician's tone that carried no ambivalence or invitation to test. Not happy in her new spot, she nonetheless stayed put.

Pediatrician: How does that feel?

Mother: (sigh) Oh, much better. She's really a lapful at 9. I was hav-
                     ing trouble breathing.

Pediatrician: So was I, watching the two of you.

Mother: Anna tends to be somewhat shy around strangers.

Pediatrician: What about at home?

Mother: We're very close.

Pediatrician: What does that mean?

The mother described their life together. The incident with the bathroom in the pediatrician's office was not an isolated happening. Anna demanded the same at home. There was also the previously described problem with separate sleeping arrangements. And of course going to school was problematic now. Even study-ing had become a joint endeavor. When the mother did her studying at the kitchen table, Anna refused to be in another part of the apartment even if her own school work was finished. She would busy herself with some activity at the table. There was enough exasperation in the mother's voice that the interviewer decided to risk asking:

Pediatrician: Tell me, Ms. Griffin, when do you ever find time for your-
                     self—private time for you . . . alone?

Mother: To tell you the truth, I haven't had time to myself since
                     Anna's father cleared out 4 years ago. I don't really see that
                     I have much choice. I haven't had money for child care or
                     sitters . . . Sometimes I think to myself and this is embar-
                     rassing to say . . . Oh if I could only go to the bathroom
                     alone, what I wouldn't give for that!

Pediatrician:	Do you feel that you have a right to some privacy . . . for yourself?
Mother:	(looking taken aback) I've never considered much about my "rights" at all . . . in anything. I've been so busy for so long that I sort of assumed this is the way . . .
Pediatrician:	Is this the way you want it to be?
Mother:	Well . . . no, not exactly, but . . .
Pediatrician:	If you were to begin to arrange some time for you alone in your life, where would you start?
Mother:	I've never thought of it in terms like this.
Pediatrician:	It is very clear that you are a woman who puts a premium on responsible mothering, and . . .
Mother:	Well, of course. I want to do the best for Anna, and I'm worried about her.
Pediatrician:	OK—I would like you to tell her directly what your worries are.
Mother:	Oh, she knows.
Pediatrician:	I am sure you have discussed it before. Do it once more, this time, here.
Mother:	OK, Anna, are you listening to me? How can I say it? I'm worried about . . . your ego.
Anna:	(looks blankly at her mother, says nothing)
Pediatrician:	Find out if she understands.
Mother:	Do you know what I mean?
Anna:	No.

The mother explained that she feared that Anna lacked self-confidence and was so shy around others because she did not respect herself and her own abilities. She did not seem to have much faith in herself. Anna indicated she understood her mother's last words, so the pediatrician continued: "And how are you teaching Anna to have respect for herself?" The mother said with frustration that she did not know how to get that across; it seemed a difficult lesson for Anna to learn.

Pediatrician:	I wonder if you can teach her what you haven't learned for yourself?
Mother:	What do you mean?
Pediatrician:	Would you agree that you tend to put your own needs aside?
Mother:	Of course. Any mother ought . . .
Pediatrician:	(interrupting) Wait. If you are not demonstrating that you respect your own needs—for privacy and time alone, for instance . . .
Mother:	Yes?
Pediatrician:	. . . then Anna will not respect those needs in you, nor will she be learning any good models for developing the ability to see her own needs as important. Are you following me?
Mother:	Yes, I am.
Pediatrician:	You do put your own needs aside with Anna. That is clear . . . I often hear a resentful edge in your voice when you do so, at least here. Am I hearing correctly?
Mother:	(hesitating) . . . You're right. There is. I try . . . to do so much for her, and it never seems to be enough. There just isn't enough of me to go around.
Pediatrician:	Uh huh. Then perhaps in order for you to be able to give more freely to your daughter—especially a sense of strength in herself, you must first nourish and respect some of your own needs, so that you have something of that to offer . . . something beside resentment, so that Anna does not become for you simply one large insatiable demand.
Mother:	That's it! That is often the case, especially with work and school.
Pediatrician:	So back to my earlier question, if you were to insert some time for you, a time for you to be alone and meet some of your needs, where would you begin?
Mother:	(considerable pause) I think if I could have time to myself for studying in the evenings, that would help . . . now during finals.

With the pediatrician's help, Ms. Griffin planned the specific changes required to have evenings devoted to solitary studying uninterrupted by Anna. The mother would continue to work at the kitchen table. Anna would be required to stay out of the kitchen from 6:30 PM until her mother had finished studying. The mother said that until now she had not realized there was no place that was hers, rather than theirs, in their entire apartment. Even Anna had her own desk and alcove for privacy.

Mother:	What I'm saying is I guess I might like the kitchen to be my private space on weeknights from 6:30 until about 9.
Anna:	No . . . I can't study by myself at my desk.
Mother:	Well . . . would you rather be . . .
Pediatrician:	Hold it. Are you giving Anna the choice? Or is this one time you decide? Are you asking her or are you telling her?
Mother:	It's my decision, I guess.
Pediatrician:	You guess?
Mother:	Oh, dear.
Pediatrician:	If this time it is going to be your choice, then you need to tell her that directly . . . now.
Mother:	The doctor's right. I am going to do what is good for me, for once, Anna.
Anna:	(sulks)
Pediatrician:	So is this one way this whole thing could not work out for you—that you would continue to put your own needs aside and let Anna decide?
Mother:	It's almost automatic with me.
Pediatrician:	Right. Tell me some other ways in which the two of you could make the proposed change not work out.
Mother:	I'm sure Anna could insist on being in the kitchen, no matter what I want.
Pediatrician:	OK, and how could you handle that?
Mother:	If need be . . . I would just have to pick her up and carry her out of the room.

Pediatrician:	And would you be able to do that?
Mother:	(laughs) Yes. I really think I could. It would take her by surprise.
Pediatrician:	And you . . . would you surprise yourself by your own strength and ability?
Mother:	Probably.
Pediatrician:	What else could sabotage your new plan?
Mother:	. . . I don't know.
Pediatrician:	Think of something *you* could do to undermine it.
Mother:	(embarrassed) I guess I could decide it's not important enough after a day or so to make a hassle out of.
Pediatrician:	That's right.
Mother:	No . . . no, that won't happen. I want to change things so that they will be good for me too.
Pediatrician:	Then it will be up to you.

The mother left the session with a smile; Anna was pouting and refused to look at the pediatrician. He noted with interest that the mother and child were physically separate as they went out the door.

At a return visit in 2 weeks, Ms. Griffin reported that she had implemented her plan successfully. Anna had actually been reasonable when they were home and did not challenge the rule. The mother felt so confident about her success that she had initiated an additional rule, extending her "self-boundary." She declared the bathroom off limits to Anna when she herself was using it. Anna tested this one strenuously with banging on the door. The mother was handling this by locking the door and refusing to be intimidated. The pediatrician applauded the mother, who was providing a role of strength from which Anna could model her own behavior.

Unfortunately, a third visit was prevented by the family's semi-permanent return to Washington because of an emergency in the mother's own family. Had sessions not been interrupted, the pediatrician could have continued to amplify and support the development of appropriate boundaries between this mother and child. Their beginning moves in this direction had been encouraging. However, the degree of their mutual dependency was significant and would not disappear after only two sessions. Ongoing work would be required, and it was regrettable that the work was interrupted. Weeks later, a note that accompanied the mother's request for forwarding records reported continuing success in the areas discussed. She also asked for the name of a pediatrician "who doesn't just give shots. I want one who listens and then talks." A referral was made to one of our former trainees in the Seattle area.

This family is a fitting final case for us as pediatricians. Ms. Griffin and Anna were both demonstrating potentially handicapping difficulties around the issue of separation. Using a family view and interventions based on a family approach as proposed in this text, the clinician was able to provide an important piece of competent pediatric health care: helping a child (and family) take some necessary growth steps toward independence, individuation, and autonomy. His success illustrates our tenet one last time: effective pediatric care will often be aided by a caregiver's close attention to the family as the treatment unit.

References

1. Perrin EC. Children in diverse family constellations. Ped 1997;99:881.
2. Minuchin S, Lee W-Y, Simon G. Mastering family therapy: journeys of growth and transformation. New York: John Wiley & Sons, 1996:17.
3. Skolnick A. Embattled paradise: the American family in an age of uncertainty. New York: Basic Books, 1991.
4. Minuchin, Lee, Simon, 20.
5. Minuchin, Lee, Simon, 29.
6. Patterson CJ. Children of lesbian and gay parents. Child Development 1992;63:1025.
7. Laird J, Green RJ, eds. Lesbians and gays in couples and families: a handbook for therapists. San Francisco: Jossey-Bass, 1996.
8. Tasker FL, Golombok S. Growing up in a lesbian family. New York: Guilford Press, 1997.
9. Visher E, Visher J. Therapy with stepfamilies: basic principles into practice series. New York: Brunner/Mazel, 1996:8.
10. Visher E, Visher J. Stepfamilies: a guide to working with stepparents & stepchildren. New York: Brunner/Mazel, 1979:261–265.

Postscript

We end this volume on a cautionary note. In the first edition, the times and the field were different. We were younger, perhaps more doctrinaire, and we did not feel a postscript was necessary; however, it certainly is appropriate in this edition. Throughout this revision, our dilemma has been how to provide the hat hooks and a body of knowledge regarding strategy so that interested clinicians will consider taking up this work of family interviews. Another dilemma has been how to convey this message without leading readers to conclude that strategy is all that counts when, in fact, it is not. Technique is turning out to be somewhat less important than we once thought.

This admission is born of our growing experience with seeing what works in family interviews during the past 20 years. The topic of what makes an interview (or interviewer) effective is being increasingly studied. In one article about learning from clients, Barry Duncan, a family therapist, reports the following:

> *Senior outcome researcher Michael Lambert of Brigham Young University concluded in his 1992 review of 40 years of research that specific approaches and their techniques are responsible for no more than 15 percent of clients' improvement—roughly the same proportion ascribable to hope or to the placebo effect.*
>
> *Far more statistically significant to successful outcomes are what researchers label "extratherapeutic factors"—what clients bring into the therapy room and what influences their lives outside of it. These factors might include persistence, openness, faith, optimism, a supportive grandmother, membership in a religious community or sense of personal responsibility: all factors operative in a client's life before he or she enters therapy. They also include interactions between such inner strengths, happenstance or luck as a new job, a marriage, a change in the weather, a crisis successfully negotiated that brings a husband and wife together.*

Lambert's 1992 analysis ascribes 40 percent of improvement . . . to such client-factors. (1)

These factors have precious little to do with strategy and technique, and they are clearly outside an interviewer's sphere of influence. However, the second most significant factor—reported by this same author to be 30% responsible for client improvement—is one that the interviewer can and must shape while using technique: *the relationship between patient and interviewer.*

Outcome studies suggest that even supposedly protocol-driven behavior therapy works better in the hands of therapists who are well-liked and have good rapport with clients. A successful therapeutic alliance, defined as broad agreement on goals and approaches established early in therapy, is more predictive of success than technique or diagnosis. . . . Outcome research shows that it's what the client *thinks about the relationship that counts—not how warm, respectful or responsive the* therapist *thinks he or she is being. Orlinsky's 1986 analysis examined 40 studies . . . assessing therapist empathy. Empathy as perceived by the client significantly predicted a positive outcome in 22 out of 31 studies. Therapist empathy as perceived by the therapist predicted a successful outcome in only 2 out of 17 studies. Likewise, client's ratings of their therapists as validating, warm and accepting were far more predictive of improvement than therapists' self-ratings of these qualities. . . . This research suggests that when faced with a seeming choice between technique and relationship, a therapist is often better off focusing on relationship. (2)*

In his own family interviewing with a group of families termed "impossible cases," Duncan focuses less on techniques learned from the master teachers in family therapy. "Now we honor more simple but enduring acts: Validating our clients' resources, courting their positive experience of therapy, and honoring their (own) theory of change" (3). That chord is struck elsewhere as well: letting go of a slavish adherence to strategy and joining clients in a relationship of empathy, collaboration, and respect (4). We particularly like a slim volume by David Waters and Edith Lawrence titled *Competence, Courage, and Change* (5). These family therapists incorporate the three words of the title into an elegant, respectful approach with clients. Their work is characterized by certain assumptions:

All patients have areas of competence which need finding, strengthening, and upholding.

Individuals are defined by their competence rather than by their deficits.

Patients are often courageous in their ability to face down and deal with life's demons. They are to be commended in the struggle.

Through the therapist's respect, collaboration, and partnership, change becomes possible.

The authors speak of courage, competence, and change not only as characteristics defining clients, but as important ingredients within the therapist also. Their work articulates succinctly how pivotal the patient–interviewer relationship can be. It provides one model for exactly what comprises such a relationship that leads to family change and growth. This book is recommended for the reader wishing to go beyond an understanding of strategy in clinical encounters.

Whereas the previously mentioned authors are therapists commenting on the process of psychotherapy, some studies on *pediatric* interviews have offered parallel insights. In an article on pediatrician interview style and its impact on mothers' disclosure of psychosocial issues, Lawrence Wissow and colleagues found that certain aspects of an interviewer's style were important, particularly:

1. Asking specific questions about psychosocial issues (e.g., child development, family/parent psychosocial problems, child feelings and emotions)
2. Offering support and reassurance
3. Being a sympathetic, attentive listener. (6)

These qualities were associated with the disclosure of a larger number of patient concerns, a greater parent satisfaction with pediatric visits, reduction in parental concern, increased compliance with pediatrician recommendations, and eliciting more illness-specific information.

In another work, Strauss and colleagues reported on physicians' informing parents of their child's cleft lip, palate, or both (7). In these encounters, what parents wanted and what they experienced with the physician were often different. Parents in this study wanted more opportunity to talk and show their feelings than the physician allowed; they wanted the physician to try harder to make them feel better. These parents also would have liked the physician to show, in the authors' words, more caring and confidence. To us this sounds like a request for empathy and respect, ingredients of the "highly facilitative" (and successful) therapist we mentioned in chapter 6 during our discussion of confrontation by interviewers. And it mirrors the observation of authors cited in this chapter that such features in an interviewer are what patients want. It is the *quality of relationship* between patient and interviewer that often determines satisfactory interview outcome.

Our text has highlighted and emphasized the concepts, techniques, and strategies that prepare a clinician for a family interview. These tools must be learned, but they are not enough alone. Family therapist Frank Pittman remarked, "techniques are for occasional use" (8). We would amend that to, *once learned,* techniques are for occasional use. The beginning interviewer must have a foundation upon which to stand and work. With that foundation firmly in place, a family interviewer must also use a blend of creativity, intuition, courage, and artistry in order to build the therapeutic relationship upon which change depends. Those personal features, along with an understanding and use of the concepts in this book, and above all a healthy respect for bumbling (one's own and that of one's patients) may make all the difference in future encounters with children and their families.

References

1. Duncan BL. Stepping off the throne. The family therapy networker 1997;21:27.
2. Duncan, 28.
3. Duncan, 28.
4. LeShan L. Beyond technique: psychotherapy for the 21st century. Northvale, NJ: Jason Aronson, 1996.
5. Waters DB, Lawrence EC. Competence, courage, and change: an approach to family therapy. New York: WW Norton, 1993.
6. Wissow L, Roter D, Wilson M. Pediatrician interview style and mothers' disclosure of psychosocial issues. Pediatrics 1994;93:289.
7. Strauss R, Sharp M, Lorch S, et al. Physicians and the communication of "bad news": parent experiences of being informed of their child's cleft lip and palate. Pediatrics 1995;96:82.
8. Pittman FS III. Turning points: treating families in transition and crisis. New York: WW Norton, 1987.

Index

Page numbers in *italics* denote figures; those followed by a *t* denote tables.

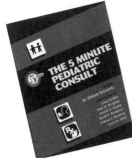
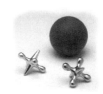

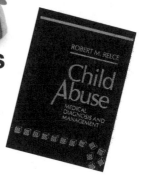
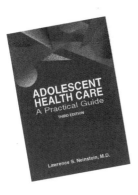
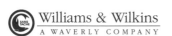